ʿAṣfūriyyeh

Culture and Psychiatry

Edited by Neil Aggarwal

ʿAṣfūriyyeh: A History of Madness, Modernity, and War in the Middle East by Joelle M. Abi-Rached

ʿAṣfūriyyeh

A History of Madness, Modernity, and War in the Middle East

Joelle M. Abi-Rached

The MIT Press
Cambridge, Massachusetts
London, England

This book was set in Stone Serif and Stone Sans by Westchester Publishing Services. Printed and bound in the United States of America.

Library of Congress Cataloging-in-Publication Data

Names: Abi-Rached, Joelle M., 1979– author.
Title: ʿAṣfūriyyeh : a history of madness, modernity, and war in the Middle East / Joelle M. Abi-Rached.
Description: Cambridge, Massachusetts : The MIT Press, 2020. | Series: Culture and psychiatry | Includes bibliographical references and index.
Identifiers: LCCN 2020004713 | ISBN 9780262044745 (hardcover)
Subjects: LCSH: Psychiatric hospitals--Lebanon--History. | Mental illness--Treatment--Lebanon--History. | Mental illness--Lebanon--History. | Psychiatry--Lebanon--History. | Mental illness--Treatment--Middle East--History. | Mental illness--Middle East--History. | Psychiatry--Middle East--History.
Classification: LCC RC451.L42 A25 2020 | DDC 362.2/1095692--dc23
LC record available at https://lccn.loc.gov/2020004713

10 9 8 7 6 5 4 3 2 1

In memory of my father, Dr. Maroun El-Khoury Youssef Abi-Rached
(1935–2014)

Contents

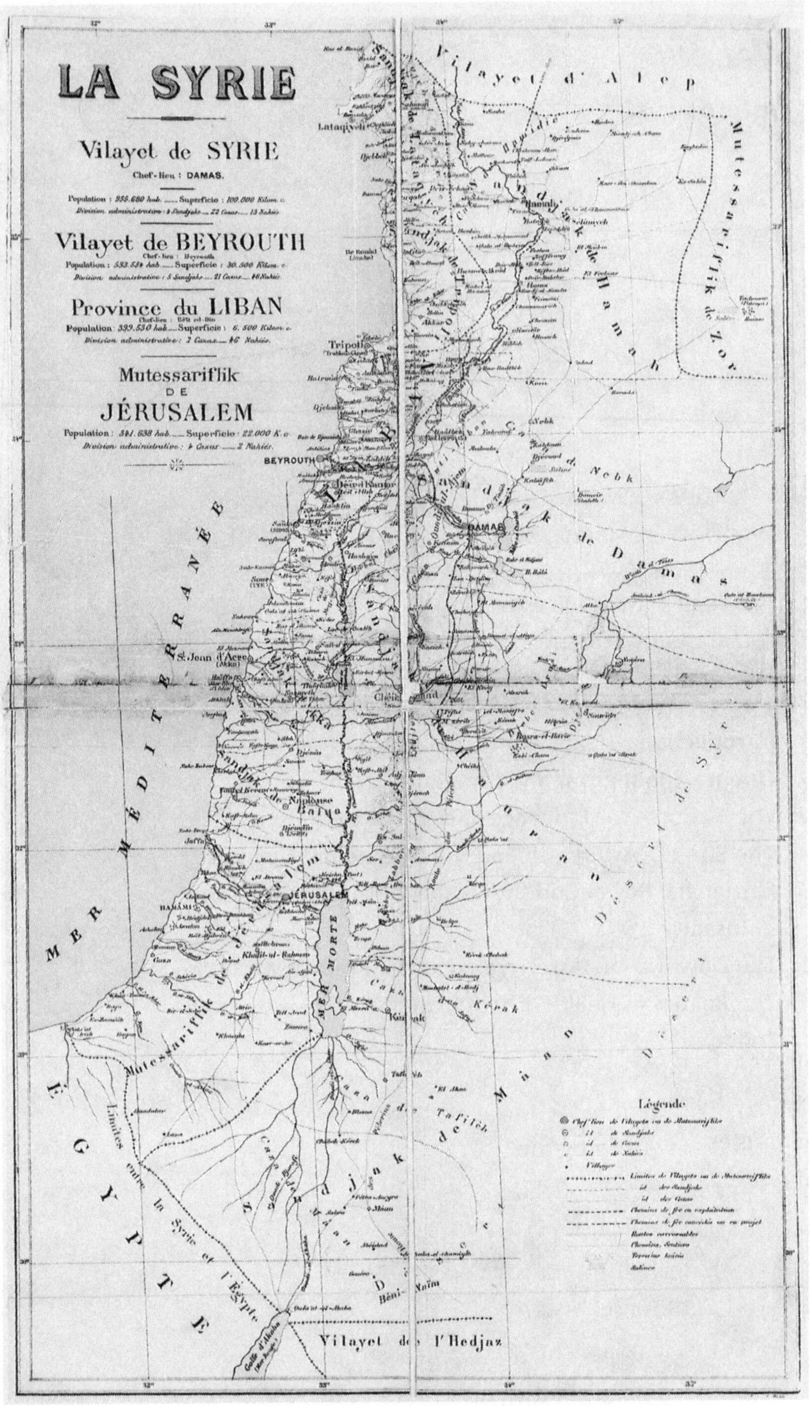

Administrative divisions of the Ottoman Near East until 1918.
Source: Fascicle no. 4, Vital Cuinet, *Syrie, Liban et Palestine: Géographie administrative, statistique, descriptive et raisonnée* (Paris: E. Leroux, 1896–1901), BnF.

List of Figures

List of Tables

Abbreviations

AA	AUB Archives
ACF	Archives des Capucins de France, Paris
ADF	Arab Dissuasion (or Deterrent) Force
ADP	Affaires diverses politiques
AR	Annual Report
a.s.* or *a/s	*au sujet* (in re)
AUB	American University of Beirut
AUB-JL	American University of Beirut, Jafet Library, Archives and Special Collections
AUB-SML	American University of Beirut, Saab Medical Library, Archives and Special Collections
BEC	Beirut Executive Committee
BnF	Bibliothèque nationale de France, Paris
CBMS	Conference of British Missionary Societies
CO	Colonial Office, Great Britain
CPCOM	Correspondance politique et commerciale
DPM	Diploma in Psychological Medicine
DSM	*Diagnostic and Statistical Manual of Mental Disorders* of the American Psychiatric Association
FFM	French Faculty of Medicine, Beirut
FO	Foreign Office, Great Britain
ISIS	Islamic State of Iraq and Syria
LBP	Lebanese pound
LGC	London General Committee
LH	Lebanon Hospital
LHMND	Lebanon Hospital for Mental and Nervous Disorders

MAE	Ministère des affaires étrangères, Archives diplomatiques, Paris
NEST	Near East School of Theology, Archives and Special Collections, Beirut
OD or /ODM	Ministry of Overseas Development, Great Britain
PLO	Palestinian Liberation Organization
PTSD	Post-Traumatic Stress Disorder
RET	The Retreat Archive, Borthwick Institute for Archives, University of York
SHD	Service historique de la défense, Ministère de la défense, Archives, Paris
SOAS	School of Oriental and African Studies, Archives and Special Collections, University of London
SPC	Syrian Protestant College
TLRSF	The Library of the Religious Society of Friends, London
TNA	The National Archives, London (previously the Public Records Office)
UNRWA	United Nations Relief and Works Agency for Palestine Refugees in the Near East
USJ	Université Saint-Joseph
UY-BIA	University of York, Borthwick Institute for Archives, York
WHO	World Health Organization
WO	War Office, Great Britain

Chronology of Major Events

1516 Ottoman conquest of *bilād al-shām*

1523 The Emirate of Mount Lebanon under the rule of the Maʿn dynasty

1540 Ignatius of Layola founds the Society of Jesus in Rome with the approval of Pope Paul III (the society's members are called Jesuits)

1697 The Emirate of Mount Lebanon under the rule of the Shihab dynasty

1805 Muhammad Ali Pasha becomes viceroy of Egypt (until 1848)

1808 Mahmud II becomes the Ottoman sultan

1810 The American Board of Commissioners for Foreign Missions is founded in Boston

1814 Pope Pius VII restores the Jesuits in the Levant

1838 Druze revolt against Bashir Shihab II and Ibrahim Pasha

1839 Ottoman Tanzimat reforms (until 1876)
Abdülmecid I becomes the Ottoman sultan

1841 Civil strife in Mount Lebanon and Damascus

1842 The end of the Emirate of Mount Lebanon

1843 Double *qāimaqāmiyya*: Mount Lebanon is divided into Druze and Christian districts

1845 Renewed civil strife in Mount Lebanon

1853 Crimean War (until 1856)

1860 Sectarian massacres in Mount Lebanon and Damascus

1861 *Mutaṣarrifiyya* of Mount Lebanon (until 1915)
Davud Pasha becomes governor
Abdülaziz I becomes the Ottoman sultan

1866 The Syrian Protestant College (SPC) is founded (renamed the American University of Beirut in 1920)

1867 SPC establishes a Faculty of Medicine

1868 Franko Pasha becomes governor of Mount Lebanon

1873 Rüstem Pasha becomes governor of Mount Lebanon

1875 The Université Saint-Joseph (USJ) is founded

1876 Ottoman Sanitation Act (*Iradé Sanié*)
Murad V is the Ottoman sultan followed by Sultan Abdülhamid II

1883 USJ establishes a School of Medicine
Vasa Pasha becomes governor of Mount Lebanon

1888 Vilayet of Beirut stretches from Latakia to Jaffa (until 1917)

1896 ʿAṣfūriyyeh is founded, a committee is formed, and a president is appointed

1900 ʿAṣfūriyyeh officially opens its doors

1914 First World War

1915 Death of Theophilus Waldmeier, ʿAṣfūriyyeh's founder

1920 In April, the San Remo Conference grants France its mandate over Syria and Lebanon and Britain its mandate over Palestine and Iraq; Greater Lebanon (Grand Liban) and the State of Syria (État de Syrie) are created

1926 Charles Debbas becomes the first president of Greater Lebanon

1939 Second World War

1941 June–July, British troops invade Vichy French Syria and Lebanon (the Syria-Lebanon campaign)

1943 The Lebanese Republic is declared independent, and Bechara el-Khoury becomes its first elected president
A "National Pact" is formed

1946 The Syrian Republic is declared independent
The Hashemite Kingdom of Transjordan is created

1948 *Nakba* (catastrophe): Palestinian exodus following the creation of the State of Israel

1958 Civil strife in Lebanon
Fouad Chehab becomes president of Lebanon

1964 Charles Helou becomes president of Lebanon

1967 June: Arab-Israeli war

1968 Palestinian *fedayeen* operate from Lebanese territory, followed by an Israeli raid on Lebanon

1970 Suleiman Frangieh becomes president of Lebanon

1975 Lebanese civil war (until 1990)

1976 Elias Sarkis becomes president of Lebanon

1977 March 16, assassination of Kamal Jumblatt, Druze leader

1982 April 10, ʿAṣfūriyyeh stops operating in ʿAramūn

June 6, Israel invades Beirut and occupies the premises of ʿAṣfūriyyeh

December 31, ʿAṣfūriyyeh offically closes its doors

1989 October 22, Ta'if Accords to end the civil war signed by fifty-eight Lebanese members of Parliament in Saudi Arabia

1990 October 13, the Syrian air force bombards the Lebanese Presidential Palace at Baabda, and General Michel Aoun, the interim prime minister, flees to the French embassy, formally ending the civil war

Transliteration, Translation, Terminology, and Monetary Values

The Arabic and Ottoman Turkish words have been transliterated according to the system used by the *International Journal of Middle East Studies*. I have retained the diacritics for many words where the pronunciation and spelling vary (for example, ʿAṣfūriyyeh instead of Asfuriyeh or Asfourieh, and ʿAramūn instead of Aramoun or Aramun). The names of prominent people and places appear in their most conventional forms (Fouad Chehab instead of Fuād Shehāb). Where the same term is transliterated differently in Arabic and Turkish, the Arabic term has been retained (*waqf* instead of *vakf*). But *millet* has been retained instead of *milla*, and *vilayet* instead of *wilāya*. I have generally limited the use of italics to non-English terms upon first use. Hebrew words have been transliterated according to the system used by the United States Library of Congress.

The psychiatric jargon used in this book is historically situated. The terms "insanity" and "insane" were routinely used in the minutes, correspondence, and annual reports of the hospital from the late nineteenth century until the early twentieth century. (Curiously, the diagnostic category "not insane" remained in the statistical tables of the Hospital until the late 1970s.) The changes in the name of the Hospital also give us an indication of when the terms "mental diseases" and "mental disorders" started to supplant "insanity" as an analytical descriptor: the Lebanon Hospital for the Insane was renamed the Lebanon Hospital for Mental Diseases in 1915 and the Lebanon Hospital for Mental and Nervous Disorders in 1950. Legally, however, it was only in 1982—the year ʿAṣfūriyyeh officially closed—that the term "mental diseases" (*amrāḍ ʿaqliyya*) supplanted the terms "insanity" or "madness" (*junūn*).[1] It is also important to note that while "substance abuse" is a clinical diagnosis (in both the *Diagnostic and Statistical Manual of Mental Disorders*, fourth edition (*DSM-IV*) and the *International Statistical Classification of Diseases and Related Health Problems*, tenth revision (*ICD-10*), it has become a loaded and normative term with negative and stigmatizing associations—which prompted its removal from the fifth edition of *DSM*.[2] Mindful of the loaded terminology of drug addiction, I use terms such as "substance abuse" and "drug addict" in a historically situated way, when what was considered "abuse" (i.e., use to the point of intoxication and incapacity) or a "drug addict" was the focus of policy, the law, and psychiatric intervention.

The term "Bible Lands," which recurs frequently in the missionary writings of the period, refers to historical Palestine and geographical Syria. The Arabic term is not Syria but *bilād al-shām* or *barr al-shām*. According to the nineteenth-century encyclopedist Butrus al-Bustani, *shām* is an Aramaic term, and thus *bilād al-shām* is a pre-Islamic term referring to the country of Sem (in reference to Noah's son) and not to "the land of the north" or "to the land on the right" (in reference to the Hijaz), as it is often misdefined.[3]

The term "Levant" is used in this book to denote a geographical area (roughly from Smyrna, Turkey, to Alexandria, Egypt) as well as cosmopolitanism. I agree with the historian Leila Fawaz that the advantages of using the term far exceed its pejorative use by the Mandate order—which, after all, was in effect for only two decades.[4]

The concept of the Middle East is perhaps more problematic, since it is the product of an imperial perspective of the world. Indeed, "Near East," "Middle East," and "Far East" are terms that can be traced back to the nineteenth century and to the various geopolitical reconceptualizations of the world at a time when French and especially American military strategists considered the Ottoman, Persian, and Chinese empires as the focal points of three influential geopolitical areas.[5] Nevertheless, I use "Middle East" in a pragmatic sense to denote the geographical area that includes the Eastern Mediterranean or Levant, Iraq, and Iran. I use "Arab world" to refer to the countries that are part of the Arab League, which was founded in 1945.

Before the Lebanese civil war, $1.00 was worth 3.00 Lebanese pounds (LBP), and LBP 1.00 was equivalent to 100 *qurush* (piastres). The Lebanese pound had been stable for decades, but by January 1985 it reached LBP 10.00 per dollar and had doubled by January 1986. The devaluation of the Lebanese pound continued until 1995, when the reconstruction of war-torn Beirut was inaugurated. In 1995, one US dollar was worth roughly LBP 1,500, and the exchange rate has remained stable until October 17, 2020, the beginning of an unprecedented economic crisis.[6] One British pound in 1897 is equivalent to 132 US dollars in 2018, and one US dollar in 1957 is equivalent to 9.14 US dollars today.[7]

Unless otherwise stated, all translations to English are my own.

Preface

> If conditions are to improve in this land some thoughts and considerations will be given to the proper care of the insane.
>
> —Annual Report, 1914–1915

According to the French alienist Alexandre Brièrre de Boismont, history can be written through the kinds of mental disorders that manifest themselves in a particular society.[1] This could not be any truer than in the case of the modern Middle East and, particularly, Lebanon. The history of madness is inescapably connected to the history of continuous sociopolitical upheavals, immigration, exile, socioeconomic struggles, war, and violence that traumatized generations of Lebanese, including me.

For my family and friends, it seemed that we lived in a huge madhouse where everyone had lost their mind, politics was an irrational discourse, and the loss of reason or sheer madness—far from being valued as the French philosopher Michel Foucault did in his influential *Histoire de la folie à l'âge classique* (first published in 1961)—was deplored and seen as the source of the many ills that had plagued the country and the entire Middle East.[2] Viewed from that part of the world, it was Friedrich Nietzsche, Foucault's *maître-penseur*, who seemed more correct in his characterization of human folly. For "too long, the earth has been a madhouse," he wrote.[3]

Yet in my first encounters with patients as a medical student, war was not the main issue. The patients at Dayr al-Ṣalīb (literally, the Monastery of the Cross, this was also known as the *Hôpital Psychiatrique de la Croix*)—whose story is covered in this book as the long-standing rival of ʿAṣfūriyyeh—were a hodgepodge of individuals: some were deeply dysfunctional; others had been abandoned as bearers of congenital malformations and, exactly like the "monsters" of a previous era, were the source of wonder and fear;[4] some were simply problematic individuals; others had been sent there ironically to escape prison; and some were not supposed to have been hospitalized in the first place.

Omar (not his real name) seemed to me to be a sane and healthy young adult. He was eighteen years old, and the reason for his admission was his homosexuality. It struck me while talking to Omar that his parents had decided to bring him to Dayr al-Ṣalīb because given the criminalization of homosexuality at the time, he could have been sent to prison instead. Omar's parents presumably preferred to say that he was suffering from some mental or behavioral illness than to allow the authorities to imprison him. Astonishingly, in her 2008 novel *Only in London*, Hanan Al-Shaykh's portrait of Samir, a middle-aged flamboyant Lebanese homosexual, who is eventually sent to ʿAṣfūriyyeh (which in Arabic means "place of the birds") to "clip his wings" of queer desire could be said to be inspired by Omar's life story.[5]

Leyla (not her real name) had been brought to Dayr al-Ṣalīb because she had directly and intentionally caused the death of her unborn child. She was in her thirties and nine months pregnant. Regardless of the reasons why she committed such an act, it was clear that the psychiatric hospital was once again a way out of prison. Instead of spending her life in the notoriously tough Lebanese prison system, Leyla's family had decided that it would be preferable for her to seek help in a psychiatric hospital.

In contrast to Omar and Leyla, George (not his real name) believed that his parents were poisoning him. He was in his forties and unemployed, and he had been a regular patient since his delusions had started a decade or so earlier.

My first encounters with psychiatric patients were hence revealing of the elusiveness of mental illness and its troubling social, personal, political, and economic implications. Mental illness was both real and a cultural and sociopolitical construct. It was real enough in the pain it inflicted on the patients and their relatives. It was real in its manifestation, logic, symptoms, and underlying biology. It was a reflection of both a broken mind and a broken society. But though real, its causes, meanings, and even phenomenology were constantly shifting. Its diagnostic grids, rationales, and underlying assumptions were also radically changing over time. It is with this "frame" of what mental illness is—a complex product that is both biological and epiphenomenal, both social and neural, both personal and political, both societal and institutional, both constructed and experienced, and both lived and performed—that I started my journey of trying to explore the history of psychiatry and its shifting mutations.[6]

As I expanded my readings and discussions about the nature of mental illness, it became clear that it may be more useful to think of mental illness as a spectrum of "forms of life" (ways of thinking about certain behaviors) and "life forms" (ways of inhabiting these states of mind, behaviors and ways of being),[7] ranging from the very biological (for example, the general paresis of the insane, or "syphilitic insanity") to the very political (for example, "protest psychosis," a form of schizophrenia invented by American psychiatrists in the 1960s to describe and medicalize the ways in which black Americans behaved during the civil rights protests),[8] with a gray zone in between containing neuro-socio-politico-psychiatric conditions such as major depression, bipolar disorder, and autism spectrum disorder.

The archives of ʿAṣfūriyyeh had been abandoned and left to the passing of time and dust. It is thanks to the personal initiative of Hilda Nassar—director of the Saab Medical Library at the American University of Beirut (AUB) until 2013—and the painstaking efforts of the archivist Linda Sadaka that the material began to be ordered, sorted, and classified. Most of the annual reports (ARs) of the Hospital (as I will sometimes refer to ʿAṣfūriyyeh) were even digitized and put online to draw the attention of researchers. Many boxes remained unopened when I commenced work on the collection. The records of the Lebanon Hospital for Mental and Nervous Disorders (LHMND) ultimately changed hands and were transferred to the AUB Jafet Library, where they are still being sorted as of this writing.

The other half of the collection is held in the Archives and Special Collections of the School of Oriental and African Studies at the University of London (SOAS). This is no coincidence, since the two committees that managed ʿAṣfūriyyeh were based in Beirut and London. At SOAS, the archives related to ʿAṣfūriyyeh have been organized into seventeen boxes. One, which will remain sealed until 2045, contains allegedly sensitive personal data. I also found relevant materials related to ʿAṣfūriyyeh at the University of York's Borthwick Institute for Archives; the United Kingdom's National Archives (previously known as the Public Records Office); and its counterpart in Paris, the Archives Diplomatiques.

Although it was impossible for me to access the archives of Dayr al-Ṣalīb (my request to do so was declined with no explanation from the mother superior, Arze Gemayel, who managed the hospital), I did find a trove of relevant material at the Archives des Capucins de France in Paris. In stark contrast to their Franciscan sisters, the French Franciscan brothers were both generous and receptive to scrutiny. I thank them for their hospitality and openness.

It is worth mentioning that the Reverend Father Jean Ducruet (chancellor of the Université Saint-Joseph from 1975 to 1995) is perhaps the only nonphysician to have had access to the medical archives at Dayr al-Ṣalīb (and all the archives related to Abūna Yaʿqūb, the founder of Dayr al-Ṣalīb, who will be discussed below). As one physician at Dayr al-Ṣalīb complained, even medical doctors struggle to get access to the archives. The alleged reason is the sensitivity of the material. The real issue, however, has to do with a deep suspicion about local researchers. After all, to borrow Jacques Derrida's terminology, at Dayr al-Ṣalīb it is the mother superior who is the "archon"—that is, both the "guardian" and the "commander" of the archives.[9] The same can be said of the Egyptian national archives, where the archon nowadays is the security apparatus.

I also relied on many primary sources in Arabic, English, and French—particularly articles from newspapers and major medical journals, as well as published monographs and travelogues from the period. Furthermore, I conducted a statistical analysis of data relevant to the patient population that spans six decades (see "Notes"), often complementing the missing data with archival material—patient records and statistical tables published in the committee minutes, rather than the official annual reports—to gain a better sense of the mutations that have taken place in terms of demographics, patterns of mental diseases, geographical behaviors, and the impact of managerial decisions. Of course, these statistics are impressionistic, but they give us a better sense of the empirical reality, based on which we could draw tangible conclusions rather than mere speculations. Finally, I conducted an online survey to which 209 people responded, and I benefited from several conversations with key actors, including a former inmate of ʿAṣfūriyyeh's forensic unit (who asked to remain anonymous). I thank him for reaching out to me and sharing his memories of his hospitalization—or, rather, his time there (he did not consider himself a patient for reasons explored in chapter 4).

This book heavily draws on my doctoral dissertation, which I completed at Harvard University in May 2017—thanks to the continuous support of my advisers, whom I was very fortunate to have on my side during this intellectual journey. For being extraordinary mentors and for their insights, inspiration, and intellectual and emotional generosity and support, I am grateful to Anne Harrington, Allan Brandt, Roger Owen, Charles Rosenberg, and Melani Cammett. Alas, Roger passed away in December 2018. His towering presence in Middle East studies and his singular mentorship, affection, and friendship are greatly missed. I am also indebted to the assistance of many patient librarians, including those at Harvard University's Widener Library—where I consulted all the volumes of *al-Muqtaṭaf* (1876–1956), some volumes of *at-Ṭabīb* (1884–1904), other periodicals and works of reference, as well as numerous primary and secondary sources. I thank Iman Abu-Nader, Kawkab Chebaro, Aida Farha, Samar Makdisi, Hilda Nassar, and Linda Sadaka from AUB's Jafet and Saab Medical Libraries. I also thank Christine Lindner at the Near East School of Theology, Monika Bem and Anne Le Bastard at the Archives de la Fraternité des Capucins de France in Paris, and Sally-Anne Shearn at the Borthwick Institute for Archives at the University of York. And I thank the librarians at SOAS and the National Archives (both in London) and the Archives Diplomatiques in Paris.

I have incurred a debt of gratitude to Adnan Mroueh (elected *mutawallī* or trustee of ʿAṣfūriyyeh in 1991) and George Sabra (a committee member of ʿAṣfūriyyeh since the 1990s), both of whom have patiently and diligently answered my numerous queries and questions over the years. I thank the psychiatrists Herant Katchadourian and John Racy for sharing their memories of ʿAṣfūriyyeh with me. I am also grateful to Dory Hachem and George Haddad, two psychiatrists from Dayr al-Ṣalīb, for their advice and encouragement. I thank Joe Bahout and Abdel-Karim Rafeq for their support early in this project. I am grateful to Chibli Mallat and Samar Howayek for their assistance on the legal aspects of mental illness in the Lebanese penal code. I also thank my cousin, Delphine Abi-Rached Darmency, a talented journalist and documentarist, for allowing me to use the wonderful picture she managed to take of the current state of ʿAṣfūriyyeh. Nadim Cortas, dean of the Faculty of Medicine at AUB until 2009, may not remember this, but it was an impromptu trip with him to the notorious caves of the eleventh-century Monastery of Qoshaiyya (mentioned in chapter 1) that convinced me to pursue this project. I thank him for inviting me to join him on the trip!

This work benefited financially from the generous support of several institutions. From Harvard University, I was awarded the following research and travel grants: the Graduate School of Arts and Sciences' Dissertation Completion Fellowship; the Weatherhead Center for International Affairs' pre-dissertation grant, the Hiebert Graduate Research Travel Award, and the exchange fellowship between Sciences Po and Harvard. From the French government, I received the Chateaubriand Fellowship in the Humanities and Social Sciences that was essential for conducting research in the French archives. At Harvard's Edmond J. Safra Center for Ethics I found the perfect setting to start putting into writing some of my thoughts in the company of a group of talented and inspiring scholars led by Eric Beerbohm. The Society of Fellows in the Humanities at Columbia University—as well as more recently the École normale supérieure and the Centre Alexandre Koyré at the École des hautes études en sciences sociales in Paris—provided a perfect setting for the completion of this book. I am also grateful to the American Association for the History of Medicine for recognizing the significance of this work with the 2019 Jack D. Pressman–Burroughs Wellcome Fund Career Development Award.

Earlier drafts of this book were presented throughout the years at different venues— notably at the annual conferences of the Middle East Studies Association, as well as at Harvard University, Columbia University, the University of California, Los Angeles, and more recently the Centre Alexandre Koyré in Paris. I have benefited from insightful conversations with too many interlocutors from these various institutions to be able to name them here.

Two early supporters of my intellectual aspirations while I was still studying medicine at the American University of Medicine were Ramzi Sabra and Malek Tabbal. It is thanks to their continuous encouragement that I was able to pursue my intellectual adventure after medical school. Meeting Nikolas Rose at the London School of Economics in 2006 was a turning point in my intellectual life for which I am forever grateful. This project would have not been possible without the many inspiring discussions with, the encouragement from, the support of, and above all the precious time I spent with family members, friends, and mentors: Alexandra Bacopoulos-Viau, Ofer Dynes, Joelle El-Amm, Ofer Engel, Mark Hanin, Michel Kabalan, Sreemati Mitter, Kathryn Schwartz, Elias Taweel, the late historian Kamal Salibi, Leila Fawaz, Mahmoud Chreih, Salim Tamari, Michael Walton and Isabel Guerrero, Allan Brandt and Shelly Greenfield, Nayla and Chibli Mallat, Hashim Sarkis and Diala Ezzeddine, Nadim and Claude Shehadi, Kavita Sivaramakrishnan, and last but not least my uncle Polo (Paul Gemayel), a surgeon who has devoted his life to caring for the sick and destitute poor. I also thank the team at MIT Press for their wonderful support for this book and meticulous editorial work. Last but not least, I thank my mother, May; my sister, Cynthia; and my husband, Ishac Diwan, for their patience and love. It is my husband Ishac, an "agnostic economist," who convinced me of the power of numbers and reawakened in me a Comtian positivist inclination. The result was the interdisciplinary approach that characterizes this book, which combines the rigor of the historical method with the quantitative and "socio-scientific" spirit of the Annales School.

The idea for this book started as a discussion with my late father on the multifaceted and fraught relationships between medicine and power. I was particularly struck by how the sectarian nature of the Lebanese civil war affected his clinical practice. He was a popular physician who on several occasions refused to bow to political pressure (including threats) from right-wing Christian parties to stop treating both Muslim and Syrian patients (when Lebanon was under Syrian occupation in the period 1976–2005). For him, medicine was above all a calling, and the Hippocratic oath to do no harm was the only injunction he could submit to. My father was a much beloved and respected physician, and it is to him that I dedicate this book.

At SOAS, I came across a letter written on April 20, 1983 by Laurence Naish, a member of the London committee of ʿAṣfūriyyeh. The letter was written a year after the Hospital officially closed its doors, and Naish suggested to a previous chairman of the London committee, Christopher M. Dalley, that "perhaps we should consider inviting someone to write a proper history of the hospital over the past 80 years."[10] Although I am not sure if the members of the committees of either Beirut or London would have approved of this present history, the purpose of the book is not to write a "proper," official, or even definitive history of ʿAṣfūriyyeh. Instead, my goal is to save this influential institution from oblivion by putting it on a par with other institutions that are worthy of exploration as windows into the histories and memories of cities, nations, and entire regions that are embedded in global dynamics of perpetual change.

Introduction

Almost a decade after the official opening of the Lebanon Hospital for the Insane in 1900, the *British Medical Journal*, one of the leading medical journals in the nineteenth century, described it as follows: "The only institution of its kind in the Turkish Empire between Cairo and Constantinople, it spreads the ameliorating influences of modern medical science and humanitarian zeal, not only among those dwelling in its neighborhood, but to far-distant countries, by travelers along the trade routes to Damascus and Baghdad, and even along the Hajj road from Damascus to Mecca."[1]

At the time of its creation and for a long time afterward, ʿAṣfūriyyeh (as the Lebanon Hospital for the Insane was known colloquially) was an international hospital—indeed, a "cosmopolitan" one, to quote the British psychiatrist Maurice Aubrey Partridge, who likely visited the Hospital in the 1940s.[2] Patients came from all over the Middle East, including Latakia, Mosul, Alexandria, Haifa, and Tehran. Foreign troops from the British Commonwealth and Africa were also treated there, especially around the times of the two world wars, when the British and French troops occupied the premises of the Hospital. Over time, however, this cosmopolitan population gradually withered, with the birth of new nations and the creation of new borders following the dissolution of the Ottoman Empire in the aftermath of the First World War.

Theophilus Waldmeier, the Swiss Quaker missionary who founded the Hospital in 1896, had chosen Mount Lebanon for several reasons. First, it was conveniently located on a hill in the vicinity of the Beirut-Damascus carriage road that connected the shores of the Mediterranean Sea to the Syrian hinterland and even to Baghdad, as the *British Medical Journal* noted. Moreover, the Hospital was only a few kilometers from Beirut, which by the late nineteenth century had become a vital port and a major source of concern for public hygienists.[3] Being on a hill protected the Hospital from possible epidemics—like cholera, typhoid, or the plague—that were ravaging cities across the trade routes of the Mediterranean.[4] Finally, the Hospital was on the margins of the city, which missionaries generally considered to be a source of sin and disease.

But geopolitics was perhaps Waldmeier's most important concern. Western missionaries remembered vividly the outbursts of civil unrest in the 1840s and the 1860s in the Ottoman provinces, especially in Mount Lebanon and Damascus.[5] Waldmeier wrote at the time, "This establishment should be erected in a healthy locality of Mt. Lebanon, where we enjoy a Christian government, good laws, great liberty, and many other privileges."[6] Thus, Waldmeier chose ʿAṣfūriyyeh—the area in Mount Lebanon that gave the Hospital its name (and not the other way around, as it is often assumed)[7]—not only for its therapeutic potential but also for the political survival of the Hospital in what was generally perceived to be a threatening and hostile milieu.

At the beginning of the 1960s—a period that witnessed mounting public criticism of mental hospitals, especially in Europe and North America—ʿAṣfūriyyeh had become so reputable that Lord Feversham (who chaired the British National Association for Mental Health and played a key role in the United Kingdom Mental Health Act of 1959) claimed that it could serve "as a model" to many British psychiatric hospitals.[8] In the mid-1970s a civil war exploded in Lebanon and engulfed the country in an infernal cycle of violence that would last for fifteen years (officially, at least). During those difficult years, ʿAṣfūriyyeh incurred enormous debts. Ironically, Christian militias that took part in the civil war became the source of much suffering, violence, and terror for patients and staff alike (see chapter 5). In 1982, a few months before the Israeli army invaded Lebanon, ʿAṣfūriyyeh closed its doors for fear of insolvency.

This book hence focuses on the life span of ʿAṣfūriyyeh, from its founding in 1896 until its closure in 1982. Had this study been restricted to a shorter period, its conclusions would have been incomplete, if not misleading. The book draws on this *longue durée* approach to examine the institutional history of psychiatry in modern Lebanon. However, as I hope the book shows, its implications go beyond the specific context of this pluralistic, if complex, society. It uses the history of psychiatry as a "sampling device" to illuminate questions related to modernity, medicalization, and social policy.[9]

ʿAṣfūriyyeh thus becomes a window into social-policy questions relating to dependency and welfare, definitions of deviance, the relation of mission to empire, and the relation of professionalism and medical authority to religion. By being deliberately comparative, the book aims to contribute to a historiography that is concerned with broader issues related to the production of scientific knowledge in a globally connected world and in the fundamental processes of social values, assumptions, and norms as well as those of institutional practice. Specifically, the book examines state-building processes and questions related to the impact of war on health and health infrastructures—an aspect that is generally either missing or treated only perfunctorily in the institutional histories of psychiatry.[10] More generally, the book uses the "biography" of an institution to examine historical processes of continuity and discontinuity and of stability and instability, and to question the politics and ethics of memory (to which I return in the epilogue).

Moral Treatment

For early twentieth century historians, such as Gregory Zilboorg and Albert Deutsch, the birth of the modern lunatic asylum marked a progressive moment in the history of psychiatry.[11] What was considered modern and revolutionary was what alienists (as medical superintendents—the precursors of psychiatrists—were called) referred to as "moral treatment" or "moral therapy."

This novel approach in effect supplanted physical constraints, like chains and straitjackets, which fin de siècle progressive alienists generally considered barbarous, inhumane, and unscientific. Not only did moral treatment entail a more humane approach to mental affliction, but above all it displaced the body with the mind as the source of insanity and thus the site of therapeutic intervention.[12] The French alienist Philippe Pinel (appointed superintendent of the Bicêtre in Paris in 1793) and the English Quaker tea merchant and reformer William Tuke (who founded a private mental hospital known as the York Retreat in 1796) are typically recognized as the pioneers of this new approach in the West.[13]

By the nineteenth century, moral treatment had generally replaced or at least supplemented physical constraints in many European lunatic asylums. However, physical methods were still much in practice in the Ottoman Empire, particularly since the decline of the *bīmarīstān*. This latter institution—which owes its name to a Persian term meaning "house [*stān*] of the sick [*bīmar*]"—emerged in the ninth century.[14] By the tenth century, the bīmarīstān was part of the common landscape of the Middle East.[15] This followed a pattern of already existing institutions deriving from the Byzantine tradition of the *xenodocheia* (literally, "lodging for strangers," charitable infirmaries for the care of the sick and poor) that became prominent in Jundīshāpūr (in what today is southwestern Iran), Nuṣaybīn (in what today is Turkey), and other urban Syriac centers in the Sassanid Empire.[16]

Unlike the Byzantine *xenodocheia*, however, the bīmarīstān made special provision for the care of the insane, who were treated by various methods: some through confinement, chains, and iron bars; others through music therapy; and still others through Galenic prescriptions, such as rest, occupation, diet, baths, bloodletting, and purgatives.[17] By the end of the nineteenth century and the decline of the Ottoman Empire, however, the bīmarīstān, which had once stood as the symbol of Muslim munificence and grandeur, had started to decay for reasons explored in chapter 1. It is precisely the decay of the bīmarīstān—and not the leprosies, as Michel Foucault tells us[18]—that enabled the birth of the lunatic asylum of European import in the context of the Middle East.

Given this context, it becomes clear why the leading alienists of the time hailed 'Aṣfūriyyeh as the first "organized lunatic hospital" in the Ottoman Empire.[19] Between Cairo and Constantinople, 'Aṣfūriyyeh pioneered a more progressive, more rational, and more humane approach to insanity.[20] Although the phrase "moral treatment" surprisingly does not appear in the annals of 'Aṣfūriyyeh, Waldmeier recognized both Pinel and Tuke as his sources of inspiration.[21] Being a Quaker, Waldmeier saw himself as the "Tuke of the Orient," and the correspondence between the York Retreat and 'Aṣfūriyyeh further attests to this influence.[22]

But in contrast to both Pinel and Tuke, Waldmeier envisioned a therapeutic approach that would incorporate spirituality and not only Quaker principles, as Tuke had established in his Retreat.[23] Nevertheless, as chapter 4 illustrates, the medical doctors at 'Aṣfūriyyeh never had recourse to these spiritual means. Rather, they resorted to all the latest therapies in use in Europe, from occupation, work, and various somatic therapies (insulin-coma, electroconvulsive therapy, etc.) to psychotherapy. And as in other European and North American contexts, the introduction of powerful drugs (notably antipsychotics and antidepressants) was generally welcomed with enthusiasm.

Modernity

Before the founding of ʿAṣfūriyyeh in 1896, two modern lunatic asylums were recognized in the Levant: the lunatic asylum in Constantinople (Süleymaniye Bimarhanesi, founded in 1560 by Suleiman the Magnificent) and the Cairo Lunatic Asylum (ʿAbbasiyya, founded in 1880). Both were in states of decrepitude before the Italian alienist Luigi Mongeri was called upon to revamp Süleymaniye Bimarhanesi in 1856, while ʿAbbasiyya passed from khedival rule to British administration in 1884.[24]

A liberal and modernizing ethos is common to the historical narratives of Süleymaniye, ʿAbbasiyya, and ʿAṣfūriyyeh. In addition, the instigators of moral treatment were all foreigners—Mongeri was an Italian physician, Frank Sandwith was a British physician, and Waldmeier was a Swiss missionary. Yet the three institutions also had marked differences. First, their motives were different. Süleymaniye rests at the intersection of two intertwined trajectories. The first, mentioned above, is the long-standing tradition of charitable institutions, which were maintained thanks to the patronage of munificent rulers (Süleymaniye was founded, after all, by Suleiman the Magnificent.) The second trajectory is the Ottoman state's centralized effort in the nineteenth century to ensure public order, which included control of disenfranchised, unwanted, and otherwise problematic people.[25] ʿAbbasiyya was also part of the new colonial apparatus that was intended to contain and control order in Egypt, which had been ceded to the British Empire in 1882. In contrast, ʿAṣfūriyyeh was part of the revivalist and millenarian movements of the fin de siècle, which were simultaneously civilizing, evangelizing, and humanitarian. But ʿAṣfūriyyeh is also set apart by the fact that the local intellectual elite as well as urban and political notables publicly endorsed it from the outset.[26]

As chapter 1 elaborates, in the cases of the Süleymaniye and ʿAbbasiyya, the reformers targeted the ossified practices and beliefs of Islam. In the case of ʿAṣfūriyyeh, Protestant missionaries targeted above all eastern or oriental Christians whom they referred to as "nominal Christians" (i.e., Christians by name only).[27] These Christians were so called because according to Protestant missionaries they held superstitious and heretical beliefs and, like their Muslim brethren, brutally treated those who were deemed insane on the assumption that they were demonically possessed.

In addition, unlike the lunatic asylums in Cairo and Constantinople, which were state-run institutions, ʿAṣfūriyyeh was a private hospital that depended entirely on voluntary donations. As we will see in chapters 5 and 6, one of the reasons for ʿAṣfūriyyeh's demise was the Lebanese state's abrogation of its responsibility toward the mentally ill amid a decline in what could be called "the missionary economy" and the rise of a new kind of moral economy influenced by new actors from the emerging oil-rich nations, such as Saudi Arabia and Iran.

Furthermore, the patient populations of these three hospitals were markedly different. While the inmate population at ʿAbbasiyya mainly consisted of the so-called criminally insane, Süleymaniye's patients were a mixture of rich and poor lunatics, people brought in by the police, and others brought in by family members.[28] At ʿAṣfūriyyeh, in contrast, patients were mostly from the working and middle classes (see chapter 4), though the Hospital was supposed to care primarily for the "poorest of the poor."[29] The patients were also generally brought by their family members rather than by the local authorities. As for the criminally insane, they were not particularly numerous. However, as chapter 4 shows, the criminalization of substance use (heroin, cocaine, and marijuana) in the 1960s contributed to a sharp increase in the patient population of ʿAṣfūriyyeh and the creation of a "forensic unit" to house them and treat them. What is not recognized is the key role that ʿAṣfūriyyeh played in the decriminalization of substance use and the medicalization of criminal insanity. Some commentators have recently begun to denounce the lack of psychiatric facilities in Lebanese prisons (see chapter 4). Few seem to remember the role that ʿAṣfūriyyeh played in prison reform—in the Hospital's participation in legal reforms, in the various psychiatric consultations and treatments it provided pro bono at various state prisons, and in the medical care it offered within its own therapeutic facility (even if the latter seems inadequate in retrospect).

More pertinently, ʿAṣfūriyyeh differed in its ethic of care. It emphasized its nonsectarian character (which was even inscribed in its constitution) despite being of "Christian foundation."[30] ʿAbassiyya and Süleymaniye, in contrast, were Muslim institutions. This difference, as we will see below, had a significant impact on the trajectory that the field of psychiatry took in Lebanon with the demise of ʿAṣfūriyyeh.

Despite the ample evidence to situate the emergence of psychiatry in Ottoman Turkey; Egypt; and, as this book argues, modern Lebanon,[31] the

Zionist Archives triumphantly claim that modern psychiatry in the Middle East was born in Ottoman Palestine with the establishment of Ezrat Nashim (Hebrew for "Women's Aid"), originally a hospice for Jewish women.[32] However, as it will become clear by the end of the book, even though Ezrat Nashim (founded in 1895) was contemporaneous with ʿAṣfūriyyeh, its historical trajectory places it closer to another psychiatric hospital, Dayr al-Ṣalīb than to ʿAṣfūriyyeh.[33] Dayr al-Ṣalīb was founded in 1919 as a general asylum for the elderly. Like Ezrat Nashim, which originally served as a refuge for vulnerable Jewish women, Dayr al-Ṣalīb served originally as a refuge for vulnerable elderly priests. Only a few decades later—in the 1920s for Ezrat Nashim and the 1950s for Dayr al-Ṣalīb—were these two hospices transformed into proper hospitals that specialized in the care and management of mental disorders.[34]

Hence while the literature has tended to focus either on Turkey or on Egypt, this book proposes a more porous and dynamic narrative that takes into consideration developments in other relevant Ottoman provinces, like Mount Lebanon and Beirut.

Competing Interests

Because conversion was difficult to achieve, Western missionaries often resorted to charitable interventions to reach their aim. They introduced the printing press and founded many institutions such as schools, hospices, dispensaries, and hospitals to teach, train, and care for a new elite that could build on these new foundations to propagate the "true" Christian faith (Protestant or Catholic, depending on the denomination of the missionaries) through the dissemination of scientific and sacred knowledge. At the same time, medical missions promoted education, science, and social justice as means of fighting superstition, idolatry, and bigotry. They saved lives, helped the needy, cared for the sick, and laid the foundations for institution building.

The assumption that missionaries were a "soft" or "gentle" extension of the colonial powers[35] hence grossly simplifies and homogenizes the complex and multifaceted reality of these missions in the late nineteenth century. Medicine, in particular, has been as ambivalent in its aims and purposes when practiced either by the secular colonial powers or by the missionaries because of the "precarious dialectic of interest and disinterest."[36] Indeed, this reductionist characterization of missionaries belies the many tensions that existed among the missionaries, as well as those between the missionaries and the political ruling class.[37] As chapter 2 illustrates, the picture is complex. There was competition and conflict between Catholic and Protestant missionaries and even within each denomination. This "clerical competition," if we may put it this way, was part of a much broader struggle for influence among the competing great powers as well as among various local political actors.

The book thus situates the development of the field of psychiatry in the context of the Middle East in this framework of competing interests—rather than in the much narrower civilizing or proselytizing frameworks that abound in postcolonial historiographies. Chapter 2 argues that while the colonial powers used medicine and psychiatry to perpetuate the existence and legitimacy of, as well as the need for, their power (as the Martinique psychiatrist Frantz Fanon aptly observed),[38] the competition between these powers paradoxically helped lay the foundation of numerous institutions, including those related to the practice of medicine and psychiatry.

It is precisely in this context of competition, struggle for influence, and monopoly of knowledge that the energetic Lebanese and Francophile Capuchin priest Abūna Yaʿqūb (Père Jacques) founded Dayr al-Ṣalīb as a response to ʿAṣfūriyyeh, which he perceived as yet another Protestant provocation. As this book shows, it is Dayr al-Ṣalīb—ʿAṣfūriyyeh's long-standing competitor—that gained the most from ʿAṣfūriyyeh's demise. With the waning of ʿAṣfūriyyeh and its ultimate closure in 1982, Dayr al-Ṣalīb became the leading psychiatric hospital in Lebanon and one of the largest psychiatric hospitals in the Middle East.

Quite often, arguments that consider missionaries to collectively be a monolithic entity or mere expansions of colonial power also assume that the theological discourse is mummified, immutable, and timeless. However, this is far from true: not only did the motivation and theological discourse change over time, but so did the role ascribed to religion.[39] As chapters 2 and 3 will show, the missionary discourse quickly subsided with the death of the founder, supplanted by an anticlerical, secular, and modernizing form of managerial politics.[40]

Arguably, then, the missionaries were far from being mere colonial brokers or "intermediaries" between the East and the West,[41] even though they depended on foreign protection and material support.[42] I have mentioned above a few elements that complicate this simplistic characterization, but other factors were at work as well. Many missionaries did adapt to local circumstances by learning the local language, traditions, and customs, and many also chose to be buried in the foreign land where they had preached, worked, and hoped for a better world to come.[43] One could dismiss these choices as reflections of a superficial engagement with the exotic—as going native. Waldmeier and especially Cornelius Van Dyck, a prominent medical missionary involved with the creation of ʿAṣfūriyyeh and a founding member of the Syrian Protestant College (SPC) (today the American University of Beirut), nevertheless gained the respect and admiration of the locals for their substantial contributions and charitable works. Van Dyck was even popularly referred to as *al-ḥakīm*, a title in Arabic that means both "doctor" and a "wise and authoritative person."[44]

Finally, proselytism may have been the means of missionary work, but it was not an end in itself. These missionaries, be they Catholic or Protestant, were firm believers in the power of the gospel as a transformative and world-redeeming message. Besides the category of the deviant "other"—the degenerate, inferior, corrupt, and depraved Oriental sects (Muslims and eastern Christians explored in chapter 1), missionaries also recognized a more universal "other" that was faceless and more generic: a conduit to divine salvation and redemption. In a letter addressed to the Society of Friends in England, Waldmeier introduced the aims and ethos of ʿAṣfūriyyeh by quoting the way in which Van Dyck had characterized the insane in the "Bible Lands" as "the dead which cannot be buried."[45]

These outcasts are faceless and universal in their misery: a reminder of our mortality, humanity, and—for the missionaries—the remnants of our sacredness. Saint Francis of Assisi saw in the suffering of lepers a spiritual renewal and a way to experience the creation and God's worldly presence through his incarnation.[46] Waldmeier thought in similar terms about the poor insane of Syria. Unlike Saint Francis, however, he did not have a theology of reconciliation and cosmic fraternity. Rather, his theological inspiration was one of redemption for both a fallen humanity and the souls then dwelling in the Bible Lands who were in need of care and awakening from a life of sin filled with affliction and illness.

Seeking to cure ailing souls and bodies was therefore a way not merely to convert heathens but also to bring people out of darkness to life and light: a project of cosmic proportions, for it meant partaking of the eternal kingdom of God.[47] The "dead which cannot be buried" were precisely the sacred link to this eschatological project.[48] It is worth being reminded of the deep theological and humanitarian motivations of such fin de siècle endeavors—motivations that tend to be buried under presentist readings that obscure the metamorphoses that such missions undergo over time.

Biomedicine versus Superstition

More than a century after Waldmeier complained about the locals consulting sheikhs or priests to treat their insane relatives, a Palestinian health promoter with Médecins Sans Frontières complained about the same practice.[49] This raises the question: Did the mission of 'Aṣfūriyyeh fail? Some have argued that 'Aṣfūriyyeh failed to convert the locals to the biomedical model due to the persistence of "vernacular" forms of healing that mainly manifest themselves as spiritual healing (for instance, in the form of the use of amulets and visits to holy shrines as protections from the "evil eye" and jinns—the evil spirits that are allegedly the cause of mental illness).[50]

This argument has several flaws, however. While it is true that beliefs in miracle cures still exist in the region, and that mental illness is still profoundly stigmatized,[51] this situation is not peculiar to the Middle East, nor is it necessarily an indication of the failure of the biomedical model. The stigmatization of mental illness is still acknowledged as a major impediment to treatment in Europe and North America.[52] Alternative or nonchemical ways of treating mental illness are also available in these Western contexts, and miracle cures are still hailed by the Vatican.[53] Yet such resistance to the biomedical model has not impeded the "psy" sciences (psychology, psychiatry, and psychoanalysis) from becoming pervasive in the West.[54] In other words, biomedicine and alternative forms to neurochemistry can coexist. One does not necessarily cancel the other. Why should this logic be different in the context of the Middle East?

As this book shows, the evidence abounds that 'Aṣfūriyyeh was successful in changing understandings of mental illness despite the persistence of superstitious beliefs and stigmatization. To be sure, local norms are still dominant in the region. Tradition and superstition still impede the treatment of mental illness and enable stigmatization, to the extent that in 2013 (four decades after the American Psychiatric Association removed homosexuality from its *DSM*)[55] the Lebanese Psychiatric Association had to publicly denounce the popular belief that homosexuality is a mental disorder.[56]

In addition, in the Arab world, the provision of mental health care remains profoundly inadequate.[57]

Yet the successive medical directors did their utmost not to turn ʿAṣfūriyyeh into a place of last resort—though as chapter 4 will illustrate, this was often difficult to achieve. The Hospital was meant to be a place of cure and hope: a demonstration of modern medicine and science, of progress and civilization. Its patient population shifted from the poor and downtrodden to a broader group that included all the victims of modernization. Although the historian Eugene Rogan dismisses the nineteenth-century European practice of psychiatry at ʿAṣfūriyyeh as "pseudoscience" (an anachronistic judgment that is problematic), he still concludes that the introduction of psychiatry displaced various local norms.[58] In fact, not only did norms change significantly but—as this book demonstrates—the field of psychiatry also grew and flourished, and demands for its services rose over the years. Ordinary life became the purview of these new mind experts.[59]

In the West, the use of powerful drugs (especially antipsychotics) and various socioeconomic forces heralded the ultimate downfall of large psychiatric institutions in a process that came to be called deinstitutionalization or decarceration.[60] By contrast, and as I discuss in chapter 4 and in the epilogue, in the case of Lebanon and more broadly the Middle East, the same factors enabled the expansion of neurochemical cures (psychiatric drugs) to all spheres of society without bringing an end to large psychiatric hospitals. On the contrary, these institutions continued to grow over the years—even if some had to close, like ʿAṣfūriyyeh.

War

Interestingly, the historiography of lunatic asylums and other institutions for the reformation of marginal and deviant populations has tended to diagnose the proliferation and spread of these institutions as a moment of crisis in the social order, be it the French society during the revolution, the United States in the Jacksonian era, capitalism in general, or the modern family.[61] The nineteenth-century Levant is no exception to this argument. The region witnessed a period of intense reforms known as the Tanzimat (1839–1876), which entailed the promulgation of more progressive laws and the reorganization of several bureaucratic institutions, including those in the military, education, and public-health sectors.[62] This period was also punctuated by the notorious sectarian massacres in Beirut and Damascus, which were followed by a significant regional reconfiguration.[63]

The sectarian clashes of 1840–1841 caused the division of Mount Lebanon into two self-governing districts (*qāimaqāmiyya*): one under a Maronite governor (*qāimaqām*) and the other under a Druze governor.[64] Twenty years later, following the 1860–1861 massacres in Mount Lebanon, a *règlement organique* (a series of international agreements among European powers and the Ottoman Empire) merged the two *qāimaqāmiyya* into the *mutaṣarrifiyya* of Mount Lebanon. The Sublime Porte appointed an Ottoman Christian governor to rule this semiautonomous enclave, which made it an ideal site for missionary work.[65]

In his memoir *Fifty-Three Years in Syria*, Henry Harris Jessup, an American Presbyterian missionary and one of the founding fathers of the Syrian Protestant College, wrote that the civil war between Christians and Druzes in 1860 was both a moment of crisis in the history of Mount Lebanon and a watershed moment in missionary work.[66] Missionaries and other volunteers had flocked to Beirut to help in the rescue and humanitarian efforts related to the conflict, which had killed thousands of Christians and left many more in total destitution.[67] Institutions proliferated in the aftermath of the massacres, including schools, orphanages, and hospitals. The British Syrian Mission, a humanitarian initiative that brought Waldmeier to Mount Lebanon, was also founded in the aftermath of the massacres.[68] Indeed, historians now recognize the nineteenth century as a crucial period in the emergence of humanitarianism.[69]

War in particular is a constant undercurrent in the story of ʿAṣfūriyyeh. Remarkably, the Hospital managed to survive the two world wars unscathed. During the First World War, the Ottoman authorities had granted protection to ʿAṣfūriyyeh on the grounds that it was a *waqf* (a pious and/or charitable foundation) and an international hospital that cared for all patients regardless of creed or ethnicity. However, the civil war of 1975–1990 marked a stark departure from previous war episodes, as the militias that took part in the civil war used religion as a political weapon. Chapter 5 illustrates how the belligerents deliberately targeted ʿAṣfūriyyeh for the first time in its history; militias frequently kidnapped or killed, staff members, students, and patients, or perpetrated other physical violence against them; and they also used the premises for their military operations, thus exposing the remaining civilians at the hospital to more shelling, bombing, and killing from the opposing warring parties. This is not to romanticize any elements of the Ottoman past but to underline the fact that the indiscriminate and often intentional targeting of hospitals as a tool of war, a tragic characteristic of modern warfare, was not always a feature of war.

In terms of psychopathologies, war and civil unrest brought to the fore new symptoms, illnesses, and mental disorders, from "mental degeneration" caused by emigration at the beginning of the twentieth century to "toxicomania" during the civil war. The book ends in 1982 with the closure of ʿAṣfūriyyeh. Two years earlier, post-traumatic stress disorder (PTSD)—the diagnosis par excellence of trauma—was introduced in *DSM-III* after much lobbying by Vietnam War veterans.[70] Thus, this new traumatic discourse is almost absent in the period the book covers, though, as mentioned in chapter 4, psychiatrists used earlier iterations of PTSD (like "shell shock" or "war neurosis") to make sense of the new psychological and behavioral complaints that combatants as well as veterans manifested, especially on the battlefield. In contrast, publications that examined PTSD per se took hold from the 1990s onwards and in the context of the Lebanese civil war focused mainly on civilian patient populations.[71] That is why the conceptual shift that PTSD enabled must be rethought as the product of new kinds of wars where civilians rather than combatants become frequent (and often deliberate) targets rather than mere bystanders.

Sectarianism

The politics and impact of sectarianism and nonsectarianism on the ethic of care and the health infrastructure may be what make the story of ʿAṣfūriyyeh peculiar and idiosyncratic. This is also a pertinent illustration of how a specific context can affect the trajectories of health infrastructure and behavior.

From the outset, ʿAṣfūriyyeh was open to people from all religions and denominations. Jews, Muslims, and Christians from Baghdad to Alexandria and the Arabian deserts found shelter in the foothills of Mount Lebanon. Some historians have interpreted this nonsectarian appeal as a mere "public relations" effort or arrogance on the part of the missionaries to show how uncivil and uncivilized the inherent sectarianism of the East was.[72]

As this book shows, however, these claims ignore the long-term transformations this core character of ʿAṣfūriyyeh underwent over the years. While "unsectarian" and "international" remained the two constant characteristics of the Hospital, the significance of these terms changed over time: from a politics of inclusion in the wake of the sectarian massacres of the 1860s to a model of coexistence during a civil war in which the norms and rules of tolerance and solidarity had eroded on the national level.

Despite its original British superstructure, ʿAṣfūriyyeh's executive committee in Beirut was composed of prominent Lebanese members from different religious backgrounds. Gradually, the new local medical elite started to colonize the Hospital's administrative structures, culminating in the ascendency of Antranig Manugian (the first Lebanese medical director of the Hospital) in the 1950s and the Beirut committee's taking over of the affairs of the Hospital after being the target of much suspicion from the overseeing London committee. More relevantly, ʿAṣfūriyyeh was one of the very few functional institutions where people from different sectarian groups could live and work together during the height of the civil war in the 1970s. The Hospital remained faithful to its nonsectarian credo until its official closure in 1982, despite tremendous pressure during the civil war to forego this distinctive feature (see chapter 5). Arguably it was the Hospital's pluralistic character that made it the target of violence during the civil war.

As chapters 5 and 6 further demonstrate, in contrast to the case of most psychiatric hospitals in Europe and North America, the downfall of ʿAṣfūriyyeh was not due to the process of deinstitutionalization that followed the antipsychiatry movement of the 1960s.[73] Instead, ʿAṣfūriyyeh was a casualty of the civil war and a changing moral economy in the region that followed various shifts in geopolitical interests. But its closure during the civil war marked what I call the birth of the sectarianization of health care, and mental health care in particular (see chapter 6). The closure of an emphatically nonsectarian hospital allowed the flourishing of two other institutions that had been founded to cater to two different religious groups, Christian (Dayr al-Ṣalīb) and Muslim (*Dār al-ʿAjaza al-Islāmiyya*, or the Islamic Asylum for the Elderly). Moreover, the Protestant religious court's efforts following the official end of the civil war in 1990 to reclaim ʿAṣfūriyyeh as a Protestant waqf (see chapter 6)—and hence as a Protestant legacy or property—was a natural outcome of the rise of a health-and-welfare politics that had been drawn on sectarian lines amid the weakening and eventual breakdown of the state in the 1970s.

Historicizing Madness

Let me now turn to how historians have written about the history of madness and how this book departs from such histories. To quote E. H. Carr, we live in "the most historically-minded of all ages."[74] No one writing on the history of madness or any matter can any longer fail to situate his or her work in relation to the literature, especially when it comes to such a contentious topic as mental illness.

In 1949, at the fiftieth annual meeting of ʿAṣfūriyyeh in London, the celebrated Middle Eastern historian Albert Hourani, whose father Fadlo was an active member of ʿAṣfūriyyeh's London committee as will be mentioned in chapter 5, delivered a speech in which he spoke of the ways in which ʿAṣfūriyyeh's history had similarities with the evolution of Lebanon from a "primitive" country to a modern republic: "From being a place for the segregation of the mentally afflicted, and then a place for their treatment and relief, [ʿAṣfūriyyeh] had become a centre of demonstration, experiment, and training for work in mental diseases in the Middle East."[75] These triumphalist pronouncements about ʿAṣfūriyyeh were made at a time when historians such as Deutsch and Zilboorg were embracing medicine and psychiatry enthusiastically and uncritically. This prevalent Whiggish posture is understandable, since after all this period witnessed the most dramatic increase in life expectancy thanks to the marvels of the newly discovered antibiotics.[76]

By the 1960s, however, mental hospitals had become dilapidated and overcrowded—places of suffering, neglect, and desolation. This made them the target of numerous revisionist historians and the subject of journalistic exposés as part of a broader critique of the coercive measures of the state.[77] Detractors denounced the psychiatric enterprise as a tool of social control and conformity that standardized, classified, and socially coerced those deemed mentally unfit for the sake of the bourgeois values of liberal democracies.[78] Like jails, factories, sanitariums, and military encampments, lunatic asylums were increasingly seen as inhumane—"total institutions," as the sociologist Erving Goffman described them in his seminal study of asylums, published in 1961.[79] Several influential works from this new institutional history of deviance that built and expanded on the work of these early social critics were published in the 1970s and began to be more widely discussed.[80]

Notably, it was Michel Foucault's *Histoire de la folie à l'âge classique* that delivered the most crushing verdict on psychiatrists and psychiatry. And despite its problematic philosophical, historiographical, and methodological assumptions,[81] that work remains so influential that reading it is an obligatory rite of passage for anyone writing on the history of madness. Perhaps Foucault's most interesting, provocative, and counterintuitive thesis is that moral and hence psychological treatment was more insidious and perverse than the physical shackles used to restrain the insane, for it trained and turned the will against itself—to use a Nietzschean terminology. Hence, Foucault argued, the revolutionary appeal of psychiatry was mythical if not disingenuous, since it obfuscated the silenced internal mental world of perpetual self-judgment and self-scrutiny that the mad had now been confined to.[82] The silencing of the mad and the isolation of madness through psychological methods marked a radical shift, Foucault argued, from a more tolerant approach to managing insanity (in the medieval past) to a crueler model of coercion despite the humanitarian cloth of moral treatment. In the context of the Middle East, the historian Michael Dols's magisterial analysis of madness in medieval Islamic societies shares this narrative of lost innocence with Foucault (though Dols does not share Foucault's view that the function of lunatic asylums is to confine the greatest numbers possible of socially undesirable individuals).[83]

The 1980s saw a departure from this binary way of viewing psychiatry as either a tool of social control or a revolutionary moment in the progressive history of medicine. The historiographical works of that decade, which were more empirically detailed and nuanced than their predecessors, tended to emphasize the ambivalent nature of the psychiatric profession as both coercive and therapeutic, normative and liberating. Scholars argued that because of the intractable nature of mental illness and the complex and ambiguous character of both individuals and institutions, it was difficult, not to say disingenuous, to provide a definitive assessment of the nature of those institutions.[84]

This last historiographical wave, neither triumphalist nor radically revisionist, resisted a monolithic understanding of historical truth, simple dichotomies, and master narratives.[85] Although inspired by Foucault's insights from his influential history of madness, this body of literature was critical of grand theorizations and univocal critiques of psychiatry that tended to silence patients and families alike, while singularly demonizing the state and its apparatuses. This historiographical wave (which continues to attract scholars today) has managed to display through contextual specificities the multiple functions of asylums and the porousness of the institutional politics of mental illness that together involve different actors with diverse resources and interests.[86]

Postcolonial Madness

In the colonial context, many scholars have criticized asylums and hospitals, as well as public health policies in general, as fulfilling broader (if ultimately insidious and damaging) civilizing and expansionary goals.[87] Some scholars have invariably assumed (and in many cases established the truth of that assumption) psychiatric practice to be exploitative and dehumanizing.[88] Even when scholars tried to challenge Foucault's *grand renfermement* (great confinement) thesis—for example, in the African context there is no evidence of statewide confinement of problematic individuals into one large institution, as Foucault claimed was the case in the Parisian *Hôpital général* (General Hospital) during the ancien régime[89]— they still seemed to find something insidious in colonial psychiatrists and the very practice of psychiatry itself.[90]

Recently, however, scholars have tried to complicate and undermine the use of colonial psychiatry as a "tool of empire."[91] In her examination of the history of the Indian mental hospital at Ranchi (the largest mental hospital in India from the 1920s to the 1940s), Waltraud Ernst illuminated important local efforts and engagements that had a bearing on the development of psychiatry in British India.[92] In a similar vein, the historian Richard Keller has shown how the psychiatric hospital at Blida in French Algeria, where Fanon worked, was also innovative, experimental, ambitious, and progressive.[93] Can any of these insights be applied in the context of ʿAṣfūriyyeh and the *Mashreq* (the East) more generally speaking as opposed to the Maghreb, the focus of Keller's work?

Although, as mentioned above, Hourani provided an assessment of the Hospital in the late 1940s that fits Keller's thesis, there are stark differences between the Hospital's Mashreq context and the case of French North Africa. In contrast to the situation in the Maghreb—where psychiatry was used in the political and moral economy of *mise en valeur*, a nineteenth-century French colonial ideology that entailed a rational, scientific, and progressive program of economic exploitation of colonized territories that the French deemed decadent[94]—ʿAṣfūriyyeh was not part of any metropolitan moral-economic policy of improvement. Under mandatory rule (1920–1939), the French in fact tended to undermine ʿAṣfūriyyeh, because they considered it a rival institution in the hands of "Anglo-Saxons" (see chapter 2). And while there were constant exchanges in terms of know-how, expertise, money, and commodities between the metropoles of Europe and North America and the provincial peripheries of the Ottoman Empire, 'Aṣfūriyyeh was certainly not a space of innovation where new therapeutic tools of modern psychiatry were tested before being exported back to a European metropole. 'Aṣfūriyyeh was innovative, experimental, and progressive in the sense that the latest therapies were made available at the Hospital soon after their success in the West. If anything, 'Aṣfūriyyeh served as an experimental setup for the kinds of therapeutics the population that lived outside the walls of the Hospital and avoided being hospitalized for fear of being stigmatized would end up consuming.

As for Ernst's insights, two in particular are germane to the history of 'Aṣfūriyyeh and the development of psychiatry in the broader Middle East. These include the importance of local (rather than merely colonial) contributions on the development of psychiatric practices and an examination of the dynamic flow of local and global exchanges (rather than merely exported forms of knowledges) in shaping institutional practices. The difference, however, is contextual. As we will see in this book, different contexts have different implications for the various conceptual, practical, professional, and structural configurations of (mental) health behaviors and understandings. Another difference is Ernst's temporal framework of analysis, which does not account for the postcolonial or postimperial period: indeed, the process of "Indianization" of the colonial medical services that Ernst studied occurred under British rule not after independence (1947).[95]

Toward a Global History of the Middle East?

A critical, albeit thin, historiography that examines psychiatry and deviance in the context of the Middle East has emerged in recent years.[96] The few other conventional histories though informative, still operate within a teleological framework.[97] The very few works that have tackled 'Aṣfūriyyeh are still stuck in the Foucauldian and postcolonial frameworks. Rogan has argued that 'Aṣfūriyyeh was used as a tool for the control and coercion of the native population, "by which the Europeans sought to colonise the Middle East," while Rogan's student Jens Hanssen has stated that the Ottomans supported 'Aṣfūriyyeh "to cleanse Beirut's streets from unwanted and unaccountable elements of society."[98] In a recent doctoral dissertation on the history of psychiatry in Syria and Lebanon, Beverly Ann Tsacoyianis complements the narrative on the civilizing and colonizing motivations of this missionary endeavor with another emphasis on proselytism.[99]

What these three historical accounts have in common is a parochial perspective that exclusively focuses on the missionary phase of ʿAṣfūriyyeh at the expense of a much longer, more relevant, more nuanced, and richer historical trajectory. These accounts also feed on a priori denigration of missionaries, which consequently obfuscates two important aspects: first, the catalytic role these missionaries played in institution building as well as in changes in collective norms and behaviors; and second, the role and impact of local agencies (i.e., local actions and choices) in the history of the Hospital in terms of the long-term implications of the institutionalization of psychiatry.

Instead of focusing on one specific period, this book takes a longue durée perspective, bearing in mind the entire life span of ʿAṣfūriyyeh as well as the much longer history of care and charity in the region to show how the Hospital transformed and reinvented itself while the social, political, and economic climate of the region, indeed the very borders within which it was situated, changed dramatically over time.[100] It is with the notion of "global history" as a perspective that looks at the past in an unprejudiced, integrated, and connected way, looking at the dynamic exchanges between local and global influences and agencies, from our perspective, which is inevitably situated in the present, more specifically in our globalized present, that I delineate three key features of the history of psychiatry in the context of the Middle East.[101]

First is the emergence of mental illness as an object of concern or the ways in which mental illness became visible. In contrast to more romantic narratives à la Dols, this book highlights an important shift that occurred in the nineteenth century with the displacement of the bīmaristān by the modern lunatic asylum of European import. Rather than silencing madness through a more psychological approach to mental illness (which, Foucault tells us, was the key feature of the lunatic asylum—and psychiatry, by extension), in the context of the Middle East the impact of this new institution was to render visible a new kind of individual who had previously managed to live and die quietly and invisibly. One of the features of the modern lunatic asylum all over the world was its location generally at the margins of the city and sociopolitical life.[102] While this brings ʿAṣfūriyyeh closer to such institutions, it also marks a major departure from the bīmaristān, an institution that was part and parcel of the social and urban fabric of medieval Islamic and Ottoman societies.

Second is the recognition of the pivotal role of both local and global forces in institution building, particularly in a geopolitical area that is fraught with competing political actors and stakeholders such as the Middle East. Contingent factors are necessary but not sufficient to understand historical developments. What scholars in Middle East studies (and, arguably, in postcolonial studies more generally) have understated is the crucial impact that local actors had on the future of such institutions following the age of empire. As this book demonstrates, local actors directly participated in the growth and flourishing of the fields of medicine and psychiatry, not only by demanding services but also by contributing to these fields' institutionalization (chapters 1–3) as well as to both their successes and failures (chapters 4–6). In other words, the growth of the field of psychiatry (and medicine more broadly) was possible not only because of contingent factors—notably, the rivalry among competing political actors and stakeholders—but also because of popular demand by the locals who welcomed the modern ways of engaging with medicine.

Indeed, ʿAṣfūriyyeh's motives, message, and reach changed dramatically through the years because of local demands as well as expectations. Over a period of almost nine decades, the Hospital became a lesson in management and institutional governance, private and public engagements, and the training of a new professional elite that came to be dispersed all over the Middle East and beyond. The Hospital's role mutated from that of a home for the downtrodden and forgotten to that of an institution of modern psychiatric practice and of national pride and regional influence. Indeed, many psychiatrists, psychiatric nurses, social workers, and psychologists who became pioneers in Lebanon, elsewhere in the Arab world, and beyond were trained at ʿAṣfūriyyeh. And the mental health policies of many Arab countries from Syria to Saudi Arabia were shaped according to the recommendations of ʿAṣfūriyyeh's successive medical directors (chapter 3).

This is why in the end ʿAṣfūriyyeh cannot be viewed solely as a product of missionary work. Instead, it must be viewed as a hybrid institution that was the product of global as well as local efforts, interests, choices, actions, and encounters. It was the product of all these collective flows of agencies. This can become apparent only if instead of focusing on what I call the missionary phase of ʿAṣfūriyyeh, as some scholars have done, one takes a much longer and a more global approach.

Third is the complex nature of mental illness and its irreducibility to either a uniquely biological or uniquely sociological process. In general, narratives that simplify or make a caricature of missionary efforts while using them as a way to articulate broader critiques of imperialism and colonialism also romanticize and glorify traditional practices and understandings of mental illness, even if these refer to superstitious beliefs that have often perpetuated the stigmatization of mental illness and demeaned certain life-forms and choices. This book instead takes an approach that recognizes the complexity of mental illness without reducing it to an entity that is either socially constructed or purely neurobiological. As I wrote in the preface, mental illness falls on a spectrum that goes from the biological to the political and cannot be reduced to the former or the latter. Psychiatric discourse is the product of particular mind-sets, styles of thinking, cultures, and jargons that are situated in certain societies and epochs. Nevertheless, recognizing the contingency of that discourse does not necessarily mean denying its universality or reality. At the heart of this book is a clear recognition of the suffering of those who are mentally ill. Rather than objectifying them under hypnotizing prose about the coercive power of the state and the psychiatric gaze,[103] I try to attend to the various articulations and conceptualizations of mental illness as well as to the various efforts—both local and global—that enabled the "disciplinization" of psychiatry and the institutionalization of a discourse about normality and pathology.

By 1966, according to Manugian, ʿAṣfūriyyeh had become a "miniature mirror image of the social, political, and economic insecurity and unsettled state of Lebanon."[104] It is in this spirit that the book uses ʿAṣfūriyyeh as both "metonymy and metaphor"[105] of modern Lebanon and the wider Middle East. ʿAṣfūriyyeh played an important social and institutional role in shaping modern Lebanon, both through changing common perceptions of what was normal or abnormal, modern or regressive, and through the complex relations the Hospital had with the different state apparatuses of the time. But ʿAṣfūriyyeh may also be viewed as a microcosm of the wider geopolitical region. The diverse political, economic and demographic, pressures are reflected in some of the manifestations of the various mental ailments and their causes. The history of madness is situated in time and place, and ʿAṣfūriyyeh is no exception.

1 Oriental Madness and Civilization

> Leaving that place, Jesus withdrew to the region of Tyre and Sidon. A Canaanite woman from that vicinity came to Him, crying out, "Lord, Son of David, have mercy on me! My daughter is suffering terribly from demon-possession." Jesus did not answer a word. So his disciples came to Him and urged Him, "Send her away, for she keeps crying out after us." He answered, "I was only sent to the lost sheep of Israel." The woman came and knelt before Him. "Lord, help me!" she said. He replied, "It is not right to take the children's bread and toss it to their dogs." "Yes, Lord," she said, "but even the dogs eat the crumbs that fall from their master's table." Then Jesus answered, "Woman, you have great faith! Your request is granted." And her daughter was healed from that very hour.
>
> —Matthew 15:21–28

> Junūn (madness): from the Arabic root j-n-n, the dissolution of the mind or its corruption, or its possession by a jinn.
>
> —Butrus al-Bustani, *Muḥīṭ al-Muḥīṭ*

To start making sense of the birth of the modern lunatic asylum in the Levant, this chapter reconstructs the knowledge of the various understandings of madness—its nature, manifestation, and prevalence—in the few decades prior to the founding of ʿAṣfūriyyeh in 1896. The first part of this chapter examines the foreign medical and travel literature of the time. Two observations can be made. First, not only were the Western characterizations of "oriental madness" condescending and self-serving (a truism from a post-postcolonial perspective), but perhaps more pertinently, they were simplistic and generally oblivious of the long tradition of Islamic or Arab medicine (the term is contested).[1] That history includes the landmark institution of the bīmāristān—a medieval general hospital that had specialized wards devoted to the care of the mentally ill and whose vestiges were still visible at the fin de siècle.

Second, what transpires is an early ethno-psychiatric description of the oriental mind. The Orient was invariably defined in terms of deficiency and lack.[2] The oriental mind consequently was considered to be doubly pathological: it was morally deviant, due to its alleged religious inferiority and turpitude, and pathological for being incapable of folly except in its most "primitive" form—notably, religious insanity.[3] The oriental mind was conceived of as a bare life-form: incapable of insanity and of sublimation and barely affected by the ills of progress and civilization (for it was incapable of either).

The second part of the chapter examines the local medical discourse. Although madness was still popularly understood to be a form of supernatural manifestation, for the intellectual elite it was always defined in naturalistic terms. Viewing demonic possession as a cause of insanity was condemned as unscientific and irrational. More interestingly, madness was not merely conceived of as a product of modernity and civilization (as was the case in the West). In the writings of the Nahḍa intellectuals (the Nahḍa movement is discussed in detail below), pathology became a trope for social, political, and moral myopia. What was bare was the politics of life, not the "oriental mind" per se.

The striking dissonance between the Western and Eastern discourses in the late nineteenth century reflects profoundly divergent understandings of historical and epistemological processes. While for Western writers, reason and progress seemed to advance triumphantly and always linearly, for the intellectual elite of the Nahḍa, the production of knowledge was a dynamic process of cultural and intellectual exchange between East and West—even though Western ideals and values were the driving force, the inspiration, and ultimately the model to follow.

A Menagerie of Wild Beasts

Visitors to the fin de siècle Levant—from Constantinople to Cairo—seemed to have been repulsed by how people who were deemed insane were treated. They spoke of dilapidated institutions, filthy and overcrowded cells, agitated "wretched" souls chained with iron shackles, and lunatics who looked and sounded like "wild beasts" and gave the asylum the appearance of a "menagerie."[4] Asylums have long attracted curious visitors, tourists, and travelers. Lunatic asylums are mentioned in a nineteenth-century travel guide to Syria and Palestine as sites of potential interest to the curious visitor en route to Palmyra or Jerusalem.[5] Of course, this attraction is not restricted to asylums in the Orient. In the seventeenth century, for example, London's notorious Bedlam became part of the tourist trail and was one of the city's top attractions.[6]

One traveler to Constantinople wrote of his disappointment upon seeing the unexpectedly shocking state of the asylums given that it was commonly believed that the "Turks" treated their insane as spiritual creatures who had experienced prophetic inspiration.[7] Instead of a devotional care "full of respect and indulgence," travelers were shocked to find "cells with iron gratings": "The first sound we heard," recounts one traveler, "was the heavy clanking of chains. On the outside of each window was a strong staple driven into the wall, to which one end of a chain was fastened, and on following it through the bars with our eye we saw the other was attached by an iron collar round the neck or body of a naked human being, who was either crouched in some attitude, or crawling about the bars inside, like a wild beast in a menagerie."[8] In Cairo, a medical visitor reported to the *Boston Medical and Surgical Journal* a similar sight: "We at length arrived at an open court, round which the dungeons of the lunatics were situated. Some who were not violent were walking unfettered, but the poor wretches within were chained by the neck to the bars of the grated windows. The keeper went round as he would do in a menagerie of wild beasts, rattling the chain at the windows to rouse the inmates, and dragging them by it when they were tardy of approaching."[9] Even Gustave Flaubert, the acclaimed French writer, noted that the insane were "screaming in their cells" at the Cairo lunatic asylum, which he visited in 1849 during his two-year journey in the Orient.[10]

The situation seems to have been even worse in Syria.[11] Epileptics were a common sight in the streets of Beirut, according to George E. Post, a medical missionary and professor of surgery and medicine at the SPC in Beirut.[12] "Idiots and imbeciles" were also commonly found in the city, "uncared for" and begging for alms.[13] Labib Jureidini, a Syrian medical graduate of the SPC, concurred: "The demented are allowed to go at large, wandering along the streets, sometimes objects to the jeers and practical jokes of heartless fellows … often presenting sights that are shocking to all sense of decency."[14] As for the "troublesome lunatics," the dangerously violent, and the harmful "raving maniacs," they were usually confined and chained up.[15]

The insane bore the signs of cruelty and violence. John Warnock, medical director of the Egyptian government hospital for the insane at 'Abbassiyya, near Cairo, reported that "29 patients admitted in 1901 bore the marks of ropes or chains and their friends rub hot irons into their heads and backs, disfiguring them for life and causing weeks of needless torture."[16] In the first few annual reports (ARs) of 'Aṣfūriyyeh and related publicity material, one also frequently sees pictures of the chains in which the patients were brought to the hospital or of their cauterized heads.[17]

According to medical missionaries and medical travelers to the Orient, the main reason for the inhumane treatment of the insane was widespread ignorance of the medical causes of insanity and the entrenched superstitious beliefs in demonic possession. In an address to the Société impériale de médecine de Constantinople, Luigi Mongeri, the medical superintendent of the lunatic asylum in Constantinople, observed that the oriental masses were deeply convinced that insanity was of a supernatural origin rather than the result of natural causes.[18] The *Lancet*, the leading British medical journal, put it clearly and simply: "The chief form of insanity acknowledged in the East is demoniacal possession."[19]

Of course, these statements are an oversimplification and reflect ignorance of the varieties of forms of madness that may be expressed in Arabic.[20] As an Arabic proverb puts it, "madness comes in various forms (*al-junūn funūn*)." Indeed, according to 'Alī ibn Rabbān at-Ṭabarī, author of the influential ninth-century compendium of medicine *Firdaws al-Ḥikmah* (*Paradise of Wisdom*), there were at least "thirteen different kinds of mental illnesses."[21] But as mentioned below, the hospitals that initially had been founded to care for insanity among other ailments—the bīmāristāns—were in a derelict condition by the end of the nineteenth century. And that erudite Greco-Islamic past when the insane were cared for using a variety of therapeutic approaches had fallen into oblivion. Indeed, the entry on "insanity" (*junūn*) in Butrus al-Bustani's nineteenth-century encyclopedia (cited in the second epigraph to this chapter) relied primarily on the medical missionary Cornelius Van Dyck's textbook on pathology, which had been written in Arabic with only a superficial reference to this forgotten past.[22] The definition of insanity, according to al-Bustani, referred not only to a state of jinn possession (the traditional understanding of insanity) but also to the corruption or veiling of the mind—corruption in the moral as well as the biological sense.

Western medical literature abounds with violent and dramatic cases of exorcism, which vindicated the claim that the treatment of the insane was in the hands of superstitious religious men, whether they were sheikhs or priests.[23] According to Frederick Sessions, a Quaker who collected testimonies on folkloric customs and traditions in Mount Lebanon, the demons of insanity were "exorcised by priests and magicians, through chaining, beating, and starving, till the miserable victim recovers or dies—generally the latter."[24] Jinns seemed to be everywhere, including in stones and in wells. They not only protected against the evil eye (*'ayn*) but were also capable of attacking and hurting. That superstition was pervasive could be seen through the flourishing business in charms and relics worn by patients to keep them safe from falling sick.[25] According to Van Dyck, "a great majority of all classes and ages have usually some paper, or image, or relic, about the person, which confers many imaginary benefits; and during illness, various charms of this nature are employed both by patient and physician, in order to enhance the effect of the remedies used."[26]

However, Henry De Forest—the third American medical missionary to have joined the British Syrian Mission after the 1860s massacres—reported that a medical form of insanity was also recognized.[27] A doctor and a priest were commonly summoned to assess the condition of a patient. If an exorcism did not work, then the patient was dismissed on the assumption that the symptoms were a result of a medical disorder, not possession.[28] De Forest mentions the case of a woman who was struck by a hereditary form of insanity precipitated by an episode of puerperal fever. A priest was summoned, prayers were said, and blessed water was sprinkled. But when the woman still refused to obey the priest's orders, the priest beat her violently until she bled.[29] Because she remained violent and did not respond to the priest's exorcism attempts, the priest concluded that there was no evidence of possession. Instead, he only found "simple melancholy," which required medical rather than divine intervention.[30]

The most notorious sites where such exorcisms were performed in Mount Lebanon was the "holy cave" of the Maronite Monastery of Qosḥaiyya (*Dayr Mār Anṭūniūs Qosḥaiyya*), where "scores of insane of all sects of nominal Christians, of Druses, and even Moslems" were brought every year.[31] In this eleventh-century monastery (which remains a popular pilgrimage destination to this day), the Egyptian monk St. Anthony the Great (c. 251–356) is believed to have cured the insane by miraculously unchaining them at night (figure 1.1).[32] In this convent, we are told, the Maronites "maintain a very mysterious power over their fraternity, and this is even extended [to] and felt among the Musselmen."[33] The insane were dragged into the cave, where they were left, chained by the neck, until the saint appeared. If the chain were to be unfastened, then a miracle was said to have occurred.[34] Many people are believed to have died there following cruel treatment.[35] As Jureidini wryly remarked, "At any rate, they often succeed, and oftener they succeed too much. They drive not only the evil spirit but even the very life spirit out of their patients."[36] One young man who developed acute mania was taken to the holy cave, where he was left in chains for four years until he starved to death.[37] This young man was a nephew of Asʿad Khairallah,

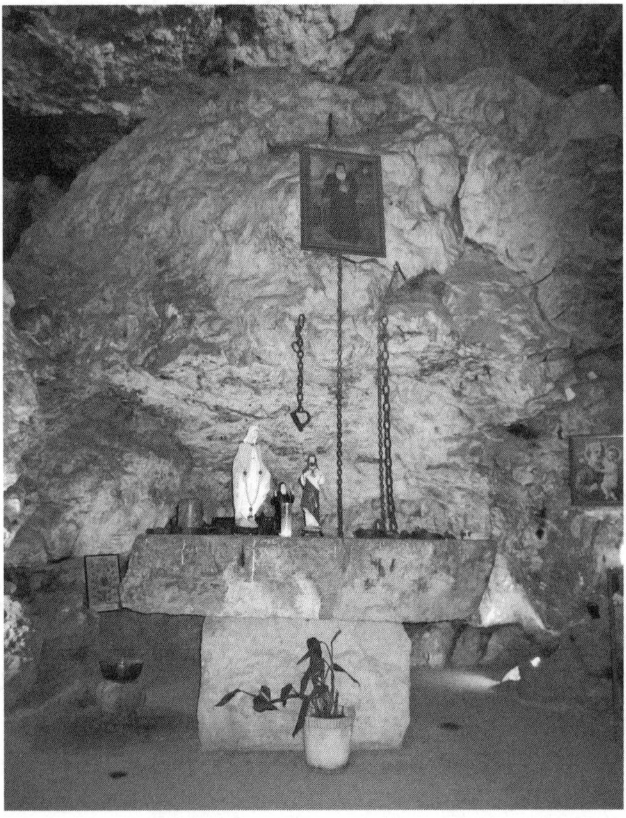

Figure 1.1
The cave where the insane were chained at the Monastery of Qosḥaiyya in Mount Lebanon, 2011.
Source: Photo by the author.

one of the members of ʿAṣfūriyyeh's founding committee.[38] Although we lack written evidence, it is easy to think that the ordeal and fate of his nephew may have motivated Khairallah to participate in a reformist institution that denounced the inhumane treatment of people deemed insane.

The holy cave of Qosḥaiyya was not the only site of the miraculous curing of insanity. Missionaries mention other caves, shrines, and mosques where exorcism was practiced, such as the site near Mount Carmel in Palestine where the prophet Elijah was believed to have healed the insane who were abandoned there.[39] And in Nablus, the Muslims had a cave named after Saint George (El-Khudr), where the saint showed his power in casting out devils from the *majanīn* (the mad).[40] The insane were chained in the holy cave, kept naked day and night, and deprived of food and light. A sheikh would bind amulets around the insane person's arms and feet as charms, bleed him in different parts of the body, read portions from the Quran, and implore the prophet Elijah "to cast the demon out from the man."[41]

For Van Dyck, however, only Muslims drew any distinctions among different forms of insanity.[42] "Acute frenzy and raving mania" were usually considered "cerebral diseases," whereas only some forms of violent insanity were viewed as the work of jinn or an "unclean spirit"—and only in such cases was the lunatic said to be "majnun [mad] and a subject for incantation and exorcism."[43] Other forms of insanity, including epilepsy, imbecility, and melancholia, were even considered sacred diseases.[44] Salvator Furnari, a distinguished Italian medical doctor who lived in exile in Paris for many years, wrote that "throughout the Orient madness is generally regarded as a sacred disease, sent to men by a deity or some good or evil spirits."[45] Generally the insane were tolerated, and sometimes they were venerated. Only rarely did madness assume a "furious character."[46] A physician who had traveled to Damascus made similar observations. Besides being rare, this physician noted, madness was often mild—to the extent that many of the dervishes who were insane "are allowed to go wherever their inclination prompts them, and they rarely do much mischief except to throw stones at Christian boys along the streets, and to curse Franks [French or European people] who may happen to pass near them."[47] Those who developed a more serious form of insanity were either kept at home or sent to the bīmāristān, where they were abandoned in chains and left to starve to death.[48]

Nevertheless, according to Jacques-Joseph Moreau (de Tours), an alienist at the Bicêtre, Muslims venerated all those afflicted with forms of insanity as "chosen by Allah": namely, "the idiots, the imbeciles and the demented."[49] Many travelers confirmed Moreau's claims, frequently mentioning this worshipping of the insane among their observations of the mores and traditions of the inhabitants of Syria. For instance, Baron Isidore Justin Séverin Taylor mentioned the special treatment the insane received in Damascus, precisely because such people were "considered to be inspired and chosen by God."[50] In her description of Syria, Lady Isabel Burton also confirmed that the insane were "much respected, as their souls are supposed to be already with God."[51]

Yet according to Van Dyck, who had spent more than five decades as a practicing physician in Syria, there was no "actual worship of the insane."[52] Rather, he saw a respect for some forms of insanity as "a sort of inspiration or veiling of the mind, caused by contemplation of the Deity, and such are said be 'veiled,' or 'concealed by a curtain,' or 'drawn out of themselves.'"[53]

The belief in demonic possession was not restricted to the Muslim and Christian sects (or to the African tribes commonly invoked in the medical literature of the time). Based on a variety of anthropological, historical, and religious sources, Henry Wetherill, a physician at the Philadelphia General Hospital and the Pennsylvania Hospital, showed how widespread, long-standing, and deeply entrenched the belief in demonology was among the Jews of Palestine and neighboring lands, and how all forms of insanity—from epilepsy to catalepsy—were often understood to be the work of evil spirits.[54]

Moral Deviance

Intolerance toward Muslims and the stereotyping of their beliefs as a source of disease and corruption were common in the medical and travel literature of the nineteenth century. In an 1851 letter to the editor on the state of general health in Palestine published in the *Boston Medical and Surgical Journal* (today the *New England Journal of Medicine*), the author blamed Islam for being a source of decadence, corruption, and depravity.[55] The therapeutic solution, the author suggested, was not proselytism but rather the eradication of the inhabitants of the land, since they appeared to be irremediable. In his address to the graduating class of the Marion Sims College of Medicine (today the Saint Louis University School of Medicine), Jureidini does not hesitate to identify the characteristics that make Islam an "unhealthy religion" whose only advantage seems to be "total abstinence from all intoxicating drinks."[56] Although Jureidini cites superstition, fatalism, the belief in the "evil eye," and polygamy, he singles out the lack of hygiene—"very common among the poorer classes, especially among the Mohammedans"—as "one of the most productive causes of disease."[57]

For the medical missionaries who had been working and living in Syria since the early nineteenth century, it was the "nominal Christians" rather than the Muslims who were to blame for spreading "mental and physical" diseases.[58] These nominal Christians were criticized for their propensity for moral laxity, indulgence, and liberal mores. In contrast, Muslims were considered immune from such forms of mental and physical decadence, since they abstained from alcohol and had a more regulated and constrained form of sexuality. According to Post, nominal Christians' laxity in morals was due to human imperfections and not to the eastern Christian doctrine, even though he described it as decayed and corrupt. Instead, the "Mohammedan system" simply legalized depravity, as he put it. His consolation was that the Oriental churches at least maintained "the Christian idea of monogamy, and family and personal virtue."[59] In contrast, for people like Jureidini, polygamy was a source of unhealthy influence over both physical and moral constitutions.[60]

Of course, the logic and practice of stigmatizing, marginalizing, or eliminating those who are deemed unfit and racially inferior—and thus sources of corruption and pollution—were not uncommon in the nineteenth century. Eugenics was an influential ideology, and "ethnic psychology" or "ethno-psychology" (*der Völkerpsychologie*, as it was originally dubbed by Moritz Lazarus in 1851)[61] was emerging as a discipline in its own right. This was the age of evolutionary theories that were marked by widespread beliefs in the superiority of the civilized European or Western race and a growing recognition of the detrimental impact of progress on health and fitness.[62] I return to these new relations between madness and civilization below. Suffice it to say here that these explanations of sources of pathology were generally predicated on assumptions of religious, moral, and racial superiority.

Madness and Civilization

Interestingly, all the historical sources concur that mental diseases were far less common in the Orient than in the so-called civilized world. De Forest reassures us that "the disease is far less frequent than in our own [American] land."[63] Benoît Boyer, a professor of therapeutics and hygiene at the French

Faculty of Medicine (FFM) in Beirut, noted that "the diseases of the nervous system in general are extremely rare in Syria." However, he did see sporadic cases of epilepsy, neurasthenia, hemiplegia, and general paresis.[64] Hysteria, rampant in Europe at the time, was also infrequently observed, though the laxity of morals, women's material preoccupations, and increased celibacy were all causes of concern for Boyer.[65] Mania and melancholia were generally thought to be totally unheard of in the "savage nations" (*nations sauvages*) and only rarely found among those considered to be barely civilized peoples such as "Arab Bedouins."[66] Criminal insanity was similarly thought to be less prevalent than it was in Europe, for it was generally assumed that the most violent cases were usually confined and only the harmless left to wander freely.[67] According to Van Dyck, cases of suicides in Syria were allegedly rare, and "religious fanaticism" was not a cause but rather a consequence of insanity.[68] In others words, some missionaries did not believe that fanaticism was "inherent" in the minds of the locals but symptomatic of a pathological behavior.[69]

Similar observations about the low prevalence of insanity were made about the wider Orient. Moreau (de Tours), a physician at Bicêtre, who had been traveling in Egypt for several years, noted that at the Cairo lunatic asylum "affections of the head (congestion and apoplexy) are exceedingly rare."[70] He also reported that he had not seen a single case of insanity—"not even one idiot"—in all of Nubia, and as for Sanaa (in Yemen), Kurdufan (in Sudan), and Abyssinia, "only a few imbeciles" could be found there. Moreau quoted a Polish doctor who, during his seven years of practice in the Egyptian army of Muhammad Ali Pasha, claimed to have seen only two Syrians afflicted with nostalgia.[71] In fact, in 1843 Moreau had published a monograph on oriental madness based on his observations during his visits to the lunatic asylums in Malta, Smyrna, Constantinople, and Cairo.[72] He hesitantly concluded that their numbers were much lower than in Europe.[73] But he also made the sweeping conclusion that it is the total moral and physical apathy of Orientals that make them immune to insanity—a claim similar to those made by medical missionaries and other commentators mentioned above.[74]

Thus, in contrast to the more romantic and orientalist depictions in which the Orient tended to be viewed as an exotic place of insanity—an "empire of unreason" and permissible unreasonableness—it is apparent that it was not a "space of insanity."[75] The "oriental brain," to borrow Burton's words, was believed to be immature, both emotionally and intellectually, to the extent that its cerebral matters remained unaffected by insanity.[76] This assumption, as chapter 4 shows, dramatically changed in the twentieth century, though remnants of such cultural prejudices still remain embedded in the psychiatric jargon—especially in the discursive practices of ethno-psychiatry.[77]

It was commonly believed in the nineteenth century that modernity and civilization were predisposing factors for developing insanity.[78] François-Emmanuel Fodéré, a professor of medicine at Strasbourg, put it in a typical pronouncement of the time, "civilization has induced a change in our human nature which, though advantageous to society, has also made us subject to many diseases."[79] This is why, according to the influential French medical doctor Adolphe Kocher, it was only when the "Arabs" started to appropriate the vices of European civilization—especially alcohol consumption—that criminal insanity started to become more frequent and more visible.[80] Similarly, for Van Dyck, it was only when nominal Christians started to adopt Western manners, such as intemperance, that cases of insanity increased among them.[81]

European and American alienists were convinced that insanity was less prevalent among the people of less civilized and uncivilized nations, because their immaturely developed emotional and intellectual faculties had been spared the intoxicating and enervating way of life of civilized nations.[82] What preserved their sanity was thus a less sophisticated and exciting life, less exposure to the "abuses of civilization," abstinence, and a "more natural mode of life, very early marriages and less sentimentality."[83]

For the French alienist Étienne (Jean-Étienne-Dominique) Esquirol, it was not civilization per se that caused insanity but the excesses that civilization enabled.[84] Alexandre Brière de Boismont, another famous French alienist went even further. In his 1839 *Mémoire lu à l'Académie des sciences*, he very forcefully inscribed the history of madness and sanity within a linear, continuous, and progressive temporal history of humankind.[85] Drawing on the works, observations, practices, and classifications of the moral causes of insanity by French and English alienists, Boismont showed how the impact of political events was at the root of insanity, especially among the civilized nations.[86] As he put it, "the expression of madness follows the national character of a people," for madness reveals "the character or the prejudices of a nation."[87] The manifestation of madness mirrored the characteristics of a nation and vice versa: the latter determined the indigenous types of madness, with the individual and the nation forming one organic whole. Boismont wrote that in France and other civilized nations, madness was caused by "vanity, arrogance, ambition, ebullient passions, skepticism and love," which he contrasted with what he referred to as despotic countries—such as Turkey or Egypt—where madness was rare precisely because people's passions were stifled by the local mores, education, and religion.[88]

During his time in Turkey and Egypt, Boismont noted, he failed to encounter a single case of suicide.[89] Presumably, these souls were so oppressed that they had become impervious even to despair.[90] The way in which Boismont described the inhabitants of Turkey places them at the lower end of the *scala natura*: humans who barely exist, living in the present with some kind of animal instinct for survival; passive and fatalistic recipients of life who are incapable of anticipating (let alone grappling with) future worries and incapable of engaging with (or even imagining) the existential and metaphysical aspects of life.[91] In both their sane and insane states, these people had what amounted to the most primitive definition of life: living without even being aware of doing so.

A common problem in the thesis of the impact of civilization on insanity was the puzzlingly large number of paupers found in European lunatic asylums. For some, this was an indication that the civilized world did harbor within its confines some barbaric people: paupers, for instance. But John Bucknill and Daniel Tuke (authors of *A Manual of Psychological Medicine*, which later became a classic)[92] thought otherwise. Insanity "is not, as some assume, a condition of barbarism," they reasoned, "but one of the complex unfavourable elements of a civilized nation."[93] The evidence, they argued, was the higher percentages of literacy among the insane pauper populations of civilized nations, compared to those of their uncivilized pauper counterparts.[94]

Another complication was the positive correlation between insanity and the extensive use of intoxicants in the Ottoman Empire. Consumption of intoxicants was becoming such a major public health issue that in 1857 all the coffeehouses in Constantinople were ordered to close following an epidemic of *folie furieuse* (frenzy) caused by the consumption of narcotic electuaries.[95] Again, the way to reconcile the thesis that madness was a by-product of civilization with the observation that intemperance was a major cause of physical insanity in less civilized nations was to show how benign the kind of insanity that did manifest itself was. "Thus we shall see," Bucknill and Tuke assure us, "that in China, and among the Mussulmans in Egypt, by whom opium is so much used, there is comparatively little evidence of mental disease; and that travellers attribute the immunity enjoyed by the former to the … limited use of alcoholic drinks."[96]

And despite the often-acknowledged methodological shortcomings, most alienists would have concurred with Tuke "that insanity attains its maximum development among civilized nations, remaining at a minimum among barbarous nations, as well as among children, and animals below man."[97] As with most medical treatises of the time, Tuke's review of the prevalence of insanity in the less civilized nations consists of anecdotal evidence. Although these observations should be examined with much caution, Tuke alerts his readers, they should not be dismissed "but be accepted as the nearest approach we can make to the statistics of insanity in uncivilized countries."[98]

The Decay of the Bīmarīstān

As we have seen, reports of cruelty and inhumanity in the treatment of the insane paint a picture of a premodern, dark, uncivilized, and savage world that contrasted with the moral and enlightened Western world. This is a picture of the Bicêtre before Philippe Pinel, a picture of medieval and unenlightened Europe.[99] The almost ritualistic emphasis on holy caves, shrines, and superstitious practices conveniently depicted an Orient plunged into utter ruin, both physically and morally. The Orient had descended into deep torpor and was in desperate need of awakening.

The sense of the linear progress of the civilized nations, in contrast to the immutability and stagnation of the Orient, was pervasive in the literature of the period. In one typical pronouncement, the French journalist Gabriel Charmes captured how the oriental sense of time, and hence epistemic and existential possibilities, were perceived. "The most fertile countries on the Mediterranean," he wrote, "are condemned to remain unfathomable and sterile."[100] For some Western observers, the Orient was preserved in its pristine state and therefore was an excellent laboratory for self-discovery, self-identity, and self-assertion to those who dared to venture there.[101] For a very few others, it was a pitiful sight to witness.[102]

Some, of course, did not shy away from reminding their audiences of how lunatics were mistreated in Western asylums and that in the not-so-distant past superstition had been similarly rampant in Europe. For instance, Boismont mentioned how beliefs in magic and witchcraft had led to a dismaying number of executions in Europe, even during the so-called Age of Enlightenment.[103] However, for him this tragic state of affairs was symptomatic of poor judgment (*erreurs de la raison*), because for him—and others who shared his teleological view of history—reason was resolutely marching toward a more enlightened future.[104] In contrast, Mongeri of the lunatic asylum in Constantinople used this chapter in the history of Europe precisely to put in perspective some of the denigrating descriptions of oriental mentality. While he attributed the lack of progress in the care of the insane in the Orient to the prevalence of superstitious beliefs in the region, he also noted that such beliefs were still held even in enlightened French circles.[105]

With a few exceptions, most medical doctors and travelers failed to acknowledge the long history of charitable and institutional care of the insane in the Orient, the vestiges of which were still visible in fin de siècle Levantine cities such as Aleppo or Damascus.[106] If they did, it was still part of a triumphalist view of progress, but one that had a twisted trajectory: a cyclical notion of history with its ebbs and flows, in which the West was now advancing ahead of the rest. Such is the way Western alienists made sense of the disappearance of lunatic asylums in North Africa. Although the Moroccan city of Fez had had a hospital in the seventh century with a ward specifically devoted to the insane, Boismont tells us that such hospitals had disappeared precisely because madness had become rare in Africa.[107] Less elaborately, the *Boston Medical and Surgical Journal* mentions the twelfth-century Damascene bīmāristān Nūr al-Dīn, a public institution "founded by some benevolent Muslim in the time of the later Caliphates—a stately building, but now as destitute of every comfort as any prison in this barbarous land."[108] Van Dyck also mentioned the continuous, if decaying, functionality of the Damascene bīmāristān, where the lunatics were confined in cells and received little if any treatment.[109]

Henri Gûys—the French consul to Aleppo from 1838 to 1847—mentions Aleppo's major but desolate lunatic asylum. Unlike the majority of Western medical doctors, who generally denied or undermined the long history of charitable care, Gûys seemed to have been aware of that heritage. He saw in the facades of the hospital a testimony to what had once stood as Muslim charity.[110] Although he does not name it, he was most likely referring to the bīmarīstān Arghūn al-Kāmilī (founded in 1354 by the Mamluk Sultan Arghūn al-Kāmilī),[111] which was renovated in the late nineteenth century.

(Its structures remained intact until it was damaged by the ongoing civil war in Syria which began in 2011.)[112]

Unusually, too, for the French consul, what caused the degradation of care was not an inherent decadent race but cupidity and negligence—as well as political and institutional corruption: a claim that members of the rising Arabic-speaking intelligentsia also made, as we will see below.[113] Gûys also underlined similarities in the attitudes toward the insane in the East and the West. "Madness is no more a disease in the Orient than in the Occident," he noted. "Here the insane are given the same kind of attention as they get back home."[114] What explained the low prevalence of insanity in the Orient, he believed, was not some inherent cerebral numbness but a more family-oriented care for the insane. Families took it upon themselves to care for their insane relatives instead of abandoning them in institutions or on the street. But his pronouncement was a rare departure from the consensus about the prevalence and causes of oriental insanity.

By the end of the nineteenth century, the Ottoman Empire had fallen into a "state of decrepitude" (to borrow the words of Tsar Nicholas I).[115] Along with the empire went the institution that had once stood as a symbol of Muslim munificence and grandeur—namely, the bīmarīstān. Evidence points to a substantial usurpation of charitable endowments and the corruption of political power as being at the root of the decline of the bīmarīstān.[116] The intellectuals of the Nahḍa movement spoke of a general state of degeneration or decadence (*inḥiṭāṭ*), especially moral and political, in the Ottoman provinces on the eastern Mediterranean. But the decline of the bīmarīstān may have been linked to a shift in the Ottoman priorities in the mid-nineteenth century to meet the needs of the new army during the Tanzimat era (1839–1876)—a shift that led to the establishment of several military institutions, including a military medical school and modern military hospitals (mentioned in chapter 2).

Some observers saw other causes for the decay of the bīmarīstān. Van Dyck lamented the lack of philanthropic impulses in the rising Beirut bourgeoisie. As he informed the Pennsylvania Board of Public Charities, "A good hospital for the insane is one of the greatest needs in all the Orient, and I have been trying for years to induce the wealthy residents of Beirut to establish one; but scarcely hope to see it accomplished."[117] Theophilus Waldmeier, ʿAṣfūriyyeh's founder, concurred, noting that "the Oriental and his wife are proud of a great number of children and relations; but it seems to me that, opposed to this natural feeling, there is another almost its contrary—namely, the little care felt for others, and for the general public welfare."[118] As we will see shortly, however, for the Nahḍa intellectuals it was a broader and more insidious pathological state of decay—moral, political, and social—that was the source of the inadequate management of madness. Indeed, it was the source of madness.

It is telling that the term *māristān*—the corrupted form of the term "bīmarīstān"—came to mean lunatic asylum at some point at the end of the fifteenth century or early in the sixteenth (when exactly this shift happened is disputed),[119] just when these institutions started to decay and become inhabited solely by the majanīn. This would remain the case until the birth of the modern lunatic asylum at the fin de siècle, when the lunatic asylum's status as a recognized site within the urban landscape would change dramatically, and the meaning of those who inhabited these asylums would acquire new dimensions. The insane—once an invisible, if pedestrian, sight among the urban landscape, including people treated in the bīmarīstān—would soon be treated in special hospitals found on the margins of society and its urban centers. Their marginalization made them more visible: they became the object of study of a new science and a new politics of life. This is the "epistemological rupture" (to use a Bachelardian term)[120] that occured with the birth of the lunatic asylum of European import. By the end of the nineteenth century, the term "bīmarīstān" and its arabized version *dār al-marḍa* (house of the sick) had been displaced by a new word, *mustashfa* (house of healing), that came to refer to a hospital not as the house of the sick but in more positive terms as the house of cure or healing.[121]

The New Sciences of the Mind

From the 1870s until the beginning of the twentieth century, the Levant witnessed an intense intellectual, cultural, and scientific revival known as the Nahḍa—usually translated as "Renaissance" or "Reawakening."[122] Although many members of the Nahḍa movement had been trained at the SPC, which was founded in 1866 by American Protestant missionaries (see chapter 2), they were not passive recipients of their Protestant-inspired education. Many resisted the missionary discourse, while the missionaries themselves were not always in agreement about the pedagogic nature of their missions (see chapter 3). It is with this notion of the Nahḍa as a dynamic, progressive, and above all critically self-reflexive movement that I now turn to the movement members' understandings and views of mental pathology.

The Nahḍa was marked by a proliferation of scientific and medical periodicals. Besides *al-Jinān* (The gardens; 1870–1886), which was chiefly a political and literary journal with sporadic (yet sophisticated) articles on science, medicine, and technology (including several early articles on the clinical typology of insanity),[123] *al-Muqtaṭaf* (The digest; 1876–1952) may be considered the first popular scientific digest. First published in Beirut in 1876, *al-Muqtaṭaf* was jointly edited by Ya'qub Sarruf, Fares Nimr, and Shahin Makarius. Most of the founders of these new periodicals (including *al-Jinān*, which was published by the encyclopedist, teacher, translator, and public intellectual Butrus al-Bustani) were associated in one way or another with the SPC. Sarruf and Nimr were early graduates of the college and were recruited to teach there, while Makarius was involved in the printing of *al-Muqtaṭaf*.[124] The three were Van Dyck's protégés and worked under his mentorship, while al-Bustani, an early Protestant convert, was his close friend.[125] Indeed, it was Van Dyck who encouraged the three to found *al-Muqtaṭaf* and use the college's facilities, and he even suggested the name of the journal.[126] They all shared the faith and belief that moral, social, and political progress could be achieved only by embracing democratic and liberal values, such as women's emancipation and intellectual enlightenment.[127] Sarruf, Nimr, and Makarius ultimately moved to Egypt in 1884 for various reasons—including their persecution by the Maronite patriarch, who declared anathema against the Protestant missionaries, and Ottoman authorities, who accused them of belonging to a secret society of agitators aiming to foment rebellion against the Turks. But their dismissal from the SPC following their support of Edwin Lewis—a Protestant missionary and professor who became persona non grata at the college (see chapter 2) after declaring his Darwinian proclivity—had more weight in their decision to relocate in Cairo.[128]

In that same vein, *al-Muqtaṭaf* showcased the pervasive interest in the latest developments in the brain sciences as tools of social progress and reform. It included articles on the latest theories of the brain, on the nature of the mind and the nervous system, and on mind-body and mind-brain interactions. Several articles also discussed the social, personal, and economic benefits of mental hygiene and the detrimental consequences of civilization (*tamaddun*) on the mind. The work of contemporaneous eminent scientists, like the French neurologists Jean-Martin Charcot and Charles-Édouard

Brown-Séquard, was often mentioned and discussed.[129] Furthermore, the nature of intelligence, dreams (which had been a topic of interest long before the 1900 publication of Sigmund Freud's *The Interpretation of Dreams*),[130] free will, morals (*akhlāq*), mental fatigue, the brains and minds of criminals, and the new techniques of studying the mind (such as phrenology, animal magnetism, hypnotism [*al-naum al-maghnaṭīsī*] and psychology) were also frequently debated. The sciences of the soul (*an-nafs*) and reason (*al-ʿaql*) were old epistemological concepts that Avicenna (Ibn Sina, d. 1037)—the preeminent philosopher and physician of the Islamic world—had explored in his prolific writings on the rational principles and nature of the soul.[131] But *al-ʿulūm al-ʿaqliyya* (generally used in the plural to refer to the "sciences of the mind" or "rational sciences," the meaning in Avicenna's time) were given a new scientific foundation in *al-Muqtaṭaf* through a neologism, which the editors of the journal used to distinguish the old science of the soul from the new science of the mind—the latter being steeped in the contemporaneous discoveries and techniques discussed in the journal. They used the term *bsīkhūlūjīā* (the Arabized version of the English term "psychology") for the first time in an 1887 article (a few years after it was used in Ottoman Turkish) to refer to the "science that investigates the nature of the mind, its structure, and the drives that control it."[132]

Articles on madness per se appeared sporadically, however, and were much fewer in number compared to articles about the various other medical, scientific, and technological concerns and topics covered in the journal—which was only to be expected in an age that was more concerned with the ravages of epidemics.[133] Nevertheless, these articles always reflected the sociopolitical agenda of the Nahḍa. The general lack of reliable statistical data—which, as we saw above, was underlined repeatedly in the medical and travel literature of the time—was also acknowledged in *al-Muqtaṭaf*. For example, the author of an article on the incidence of madness in Russia speculated that if the causes of insanity were alcoholism and poor living conditions, then insanity should be more prevalent in bilād al-shām (i.e., Palestine and geographical Syria).[134] But the author was quick to add that this was mere speculation, since there were no statistical data (*iḥṣāʾ*) to rely on. Rather than stopping there, the author used the opportunity to articulate a subtle social and political critique of both the people and the government of the region. The lack of reliable statistics, the author argued, reflected a general lack of national concern or interest in gathering such data, and hence a lack of willingness either to understand the deep-seated causes of social malaise or to improve the social and economic conditions of the local population.

This ties in well with *al-Muqtaṭaf*'s social and political critique: the journal felt that the ills of the East lay in the people's failure to embrace a modern and positivist epistemology. In the journal's view, such an epistemology was the key to progress and prosperity, both individually and collectively.[135] Rather than explaining the alleged low incidence of insanity as an indication of a lack of civilization—that is, as an inherent character flaw of the oriental mind—*al-Muqtaṭaf* instead highlighted a more pertinent aspect of the subject: namely, the lack of a positive science of the state, which is the very definition of statistics.[136]

When insanity was discussed in *al-Muqtaṭaf*, it was always in accord with the progressive and liberal undertones of the journal. An ongoing theme was the benefits of knowledge, literacy, and education as the antidotes par excellence for charlatanism and superstitious, uncritical, and unscientific beliefs—all of which, the editors believed, were at the root of the decline of the Orient. They promulgated education and knowledge as antidotes to mental and societal afflictions. If madness is prevalent, the reader is told, it is because of poverty, illiteracy, and ignorance.[137] Knowledge and education were thought to immunize the self against what the editors referred to as the "germ of insanity" (*jurthūmat al-junūn*),[138] while socioeconomic stability and moderation were allegedly bulwarks against suicide and certain other forms of madness.[139] (Just a few years before the French sociologist Émile Durkheim published his seminal *Suicide*, the editors of *al-Muqtaṭaf* seemed to have identified something like anomie—a state of normative breakdown due to lawlessness—as a potential cause of madness.[140])

Following the prevailing views on the relationship between madness and civilization, the editors argued that it was the excesses of civilization that brought mental ills: those excesses caused geniuses to lose their mental faculties and industrialized nations to suffer from suicide epidemics. *Al-Muqtaṭaf* published several articles in an attempt to raise awareness "of this ill before it propagates among us."[141] The editors argued that rigorous education, mental pressures, and other burdens of civilization (not education per se) were the causes of brain damage and a predisposition to disease.[142] Interestingly, this perspective humanizes the oriental mind, since it allows it to have the potential—indeed, the luxury—to become insane (which, as we have seen, was perceived as a sign of civilization).

The editors of and various contributors to *al-Muqtaṭaf* invariably gave mental afflictions a naturalistic explanation. They defined madness as a disease of the brain and the nervous system (*maraḍ al-dimāgh wal-jihāz al-'aṣabī*),[143] even though they provided other reasons for madness—such as heredity, intense intellectual activity, or other "organic" causes.[144] When one reader of the journal asked the editors to define madness, the answer was "a deficiency in the brain, for the brain is the instrument of the power of the mind."[145] When another reader asked whether a distinction existed between the soul (*an-nafs*), the mind (*al-'aql*), and the spirit (*al-rūḥ*), the answer was categorically in the negative.[146] Several years later, when another reader asked the same question, the answer—though slightly more nuanced (perhaps in a nod to the contested nature of the debate), essentially remained unchanged.[147] For the intellectual elite of the time, madness was perceived as a disease of the body (*da' min adawā' al-jism*), just like tuberculosis or smallpox, which were common medical ills.[148]

The authors invoked demonization only to highlight how medieval concepts of madness had been supplanted in the Age of Enlightenment by a more naturalistic definition (*waṣfan ṭabī'iyyan*).[149] They noted how France, to reinforce that new belief, had found it necessary to pass a law in 1838 in which madness was redefined as a disease of the brain.[150] Incidentally, this same law formed the basis of the 1876 Ottoman Regulation for Lunatic Asylums (*Bimarhaneler Nizamnamesi*), and it was Mongeri who influenced the Sublime Porte to adopt it.[151] (More on this subject is presented in chapters 3 and 4.)

The positivistic and naturalistic descriptions of madness and mental afflictions were not only part of *al-Muqtaṭaf*'s Victorian faith in science and medicine. These descriptions were also indicative of the journal's more comprehensive view of human nature and human possibility.[152] The editors and contributors seem to have been quite sensitive to the complex nature of the mutual influences between East and West in the production of knowledge, which was also a major theme of the journal. In the first part of a series of articles titled "Jihād al-'Ulamā'" (Striving of the scientists), they showed how exorcism and demonization had been dispelled as medieval practices in the West only at the beginning of the nineteenth century, though they acknowledged that these practices were still prevalent in certain parts of the world—including the Orient.[153] In another article, the editors bemoaned the inhumane and archaic treatment of the insane in bilād al-shām. They contrasted these old-fashioned and prejudiced practices with the more rational

European approach to managing madness, which was reflected in Europe's grand, clean, and orderly hospitals that specialized in the alleviation of humanity's mental afflictions.[154] The editors showed how supernatural beliefs had been supplanted by a new understanding of madness as a natural disease (*maraḍ ṭabīʿī*) and a new therapeutic approach that relied on kindness, humanity, and moderation (they were referring to "moral treatment" without naming it). Interestingly, they insisted on reminding their readers of how Avicenna had indicated that this is the proper way to treat the insane, and how his naturalistic description of madness as a brain disease was now being vindicated in the West.[155] These sporadic pronouncements are not trivial. They should be viewed as an attempt to redeem the glorious past of Islamic and Arabic medicine, since the editors frequently attempted to redeem the lost and glorious past of Islamic civilization.[156]

Criminal insanity was another recurrent topic in the journal. Phrenology had become an influential school of thought in the nineteenth century, especially in terms of understanding the behavior of people who were known as degenerates, including the criminally insane.[157] In line with the journal's aim of disseminating the latest scientific theories, discoveries, and findings, *al-Muqtaṭaf* published a series of articles on madness and crime, both of which were major preoccupations in the nineteenth century.[158] The articles covered the nature of criminal behavior; whether such behavior was innate or developed; whether certain traits, characters (*ṭawābiʿ*), or morphological features in the brain could be identified; and whether such erratic behaviors could be reformed. These inquiries were conducted allegedly in the service of enlightening the people of the region.[159]

The journal published many articles on the health and fitness of the people of the East, as well as ways to improve people's behavior. This was in line with the preventative, reformist, utilitarian, and evolutionary mode of thought of fin de siècle Europe, which was concerned with degeneration and was therefore preoccupied with finding ways to improve the efficiency, fitness, and productivity of the general population. However, the editors of *al-Muqtaṭaf* were critical readers of Western literature. They were aware of problems with the validity of the methodology and the underlying assumptions and implications of the various philosophies and ideologies they scrutinized. One example will suffice. An article titled "Fasād al-Frenūlūjiā" (The corruption of phrenology) systematically and critically enumerated the many flaws in the scientific pretensions of phrenology.[160] Yet on the whole, this exchange of ideas and interpretations between East and West was a dialogue of the deaf, with the West rarely acknowledging the novel and critical ways in which the intellectual Levantine elite was engaging with (and contributing to) global knowledge.[161]

Doctoring the Nation

Two other journals were dedicated to medicine at the time. One was *at-Ṭabīb* (The doctor), which was initially published as *Akhbār Ṭibbiyya* (Medical news). First published in 1874, this was the first medical journal in Arabic. The second was *ash-Shifā'* (Healing), which began publication in 1886. Both shared the ethos and aims of *al-Muqtaṭaf*: to popularize the latest discoveries in medicine and technology, and advocate for more progressive attitudes to improve the health and wealth of bilād al-shām. Both journals were also widely read and distributed. Like *al-Muqtaṭaf*, local authors who had strong associations with the SPC contributed to these new medical journals. Shibli Shumayyil, the founder of *ash-Shifā'* and a prominent intellectual in the Nahḍa movement, was among the first medical graduates of the SPC (class of 1871).[162] And although two SPC professors and medical missionaries—namely, Post and Van Dyck—had founded *at-Ṭabīb*, the journal became a professional forum for the rising medical elite and a focus of national pride. The editors of *al-Jinān* welcomed the new journal, which was edited by the man they referred to as the "illustrious" George Post. They saw the journal as contributing not only to medical knowledge in general but also to the Arabic language, which itself was undergoing radical transformations during the Nahḍa.[163] *Al-Muqtaṭaf* also hailed the new journal as a great contribution to the "nation": when the publication of *at-Ṭabīb* was suspended between 1877 and 1880, the editors of *al-Muqtaṭaf* considered supporting the journal to be a national duty (*wājiban waṭanyyan*), since its impact was far-reaching.[164]

Unlike *al-Muqtaṭaf*, however, these two journals were dedicated to medicine and its allied sciences, with the aims of influencing public health policy; informing the rising medical and professional elite of the latest findings, technologies, and theories; and helping different health professionals exchange expert opinions.[165] Ultimately, the two journals aimed to provide their readers with a critical lens into the emerging medical and scientific literature, disseminate the ethics of clinical practice, raise awareness of the history of various aspects of the profession, and inform about other institutional developments in the East in the hope of serving both the nation and the broader *umma* (the supranational community).

Thus, both journals included sophisticated articles on madness, simply because they were targeted towards medical professionals. The journals adopted a naturalistic approach to mental illness and insanity while also recognizing the difficulty of distinguishing reason from unreason.[166] Epilepsy and other forms of madness—previously thought to be incurable were now described as medical conditions that were amenable to treatment by various medical interventions.[167] Authors frequently provided classifications of mental diseases, such as neurological disorders (*amrāḍ al-ʿaql*) versus other forms of madness (melancholia, mania, delusions, and so on).[168] Others discussed pharmacological treatments and expanded on specialized topics related to specific mental and nervous disorders.[169] And whereas *al-Muqtaṭaf* primarily relied on reviews of the pertinent medical and scientific literature, both *al-Muqtaṭaf* and *at-Ṭabīb* adopted case-based reasoning, complementing this new approach with expert opinion and hospital statistics—a style of thinking that was becoming increasingly popular in nineteenth-century European and American medical journals.[170]

Yet all three journals, like most of the periodicals of the Nahḍa, shared a moralistic and normative discourse. Their editors firmly believed in the enlightening nature of popularized science, instilling in their readers a critical way of thinking, and opening their minds to the benefits of civilized life. However, civilization entailed something more than simply embracing liberal values and ideals: it meant above all a duty to serve one's nation. (The terms *waṭan, bilād,* and *umma* were used interchangeably to refer to the latter.) This required contributing to the intellectual elevation (*irtiqā'*) of the nation and improving its social conditions by spreading knowledge as a means of achieving justice and progress.[171]

The motivation was an acute awareness of the decay and degeneration of the East (*al-sharq*), which had become a recurrent leitmotif in these periodicals in the mid- to late nineteenth century.[172] The journals sought to "enlighten the minds of ordinary people"[173] through a rapprochement between the private and public domains (*al-khāṣa wul-ʿāmma)* in a process that might anachronistically be called public engagement.[174] In an advertisement for *at-Ṭabīb* published in *al-Muqtaṭaf,* the editors of the former noted that their medical journal had decided to broaden its topics to reach a more general audience. Punning on the name of the journal (The doctor), the article concluded that the journal had become a "doctor for both the family and the nation."[175]

The basis of true and sustainable progress, the editors of *at-Ṭabīb* believed, was above all moral, and not merely material. They argued that real progress occurs through an altruistic ethos of care and the sense of a duty to help others (*khedmat al-ghayr*).[176] Therefore, the Victorian values of self-governance and thriftiness that influenced some of the founders of *al-Muqtaṭaf*[177] were not enough. The values had to be deployed in the service of the nation. And while *al-Muqtaṭaf* secularized this transcendental (almost "categorical," in Kantian terms) duty to help both the individual and the nation, *at-Ṭabīb* reminded its readership of its more sacramental nature: "Medical doctors should follow the steps of the Christ and visit the poor and love his neighbor ... but also visit the poor and rescue him and attend to the need of the rich ... also speak frankly with the mad and children and should not lie about false hopes of recovery and should not profit from them."[178] The last statement clearly reflects the still obvious, if dwindling, missionary tone of the journal.

The intellectual elite of the Nahḍa was also avant-garde in its critique of the West. At least six decades before the widespread indictment of colonialism and imperialism, the editors of *al-Muqtaṭaf* unwaveringly denounced the Western powers' exploitive imperialistic goals as well as their condescension toward the rest of humanity. In perhaps the most caustic critique of the West, Shumayyil denounced the dehumanizing nature of the East's sycophantic dependence on the West. In an article titled "The Mental and Moral Decline of the Orient," he noted that "due to the struggle for survival, Orientals are exposed to humiliation and misery, working for their masters, the Westerners, who are manipulating them ... because the law of struggle for existence in nature is merciless, the weak are inevitably doomed either to annihilation or assimilation."[179] But ultimately he blamed the Orient for its own downfall and for its corruption of morals, its despotic regimes, and its ossified religious practices that stifled the mind. "No wonder if we see the West dominating the Orient and yearning to occupy it," he concluded.[180] Yet this was a constructive critique, since most of the Nahḍa adherents seem to have internalized parts, if not all, of the Western discourse.[181] Statements like these were also a reflection of a crisis of modernity that the new elite was going through, as well as its need to legitimize itself in its revolutionary claims: that of being part of an awakening amid a decadent and degenerating present.

The intellectual elite was aware that the Mashreq's developmental lag had social, economic, cultural, and intellectual causes. However, in contrast to the views of many Western commentators (or Orientalists, in the pejorative Saidian sense), their views were not fatalistic, and their notions of time and epistemic possibility were not condemned to sterility and immutability. The prolific publication and dissemination of works and ideas in philosophy, literature, theology, medicine, and science were an indication that the current situation was not an inevitable state of affairs. The intellectual elite was consciously aware of being in the midst of a scientific renaissance (*nahḍa ʿilmiyya*)[182]—one that was to last only until the First World War.

Conclusion

By the nineteenth century, traces of the glorious past of medical munificence in the Islamic world were all but gone. Bīmāristāns (the hospitals that had been the pride of the Islamic rulers) had degenerated into māristāns, which were now in ruins: places of desolation where the insane were abandoned, chained up, and uncared for. These places had become synonymous with madhouses and were part of the new landscape of the dying Ottoman empire.

Instead of blaming Orientals for their primitive minds, inclined only to superstition and irrational beliefs, the local intellectual elite used insanity and the deterioration of the māristāns to mount a sociopolitical critique of both the state and the people. The Nahḍa intelligentsia took upon itself the responsibility for convincing the oriental mentality to change the sociopolitical foundational structures upon which nations are built and that they believed correlated with the "health of nations" (*ṣiḥḥat al-ummam*).[183] While they acknowledged the mistreatment and neglect of the insane in the Mashreq and denounced the prevalent irrational and superstitious belief in evil spirits as a causative explanation for insanity, they also bemoaned the loss of the glorious history of charitable and rational care. They looked to the past for both inspiration and legitimacy, much as those involved in the Italian Renaissance had sought inspiration from the Greco-Roman classical traditions that had come before them. But in contrast to the Western view of the Orient as immutable, sterile, and only potentially salvageable, the Nahḍa views were more malleable—opening the possibility of change for both individuals and societies.

When the founding of ʿAsfūriyyeh was announced in 1896, *at-Ṭabīb* endorsed the project as a much-needed initiative that would significantly benefit the nation. The journal referred to ʿAsfūriyyeh as "the Lebanese bīmāristān" (*al-bīmāristān al-lubnānī*).[184] This is significant because starting in 1884, the journal was edited not by foreign medical missionaries but by well-known intellectual figures of the Nahḍa—namely, Ibrāhīm Yāzijī, Bishārah Zalzal, and Khalīl Anṭūn Saʿādah (the last two were also physicians who had studied medicine at the SPC in Beirut).[185] Rather than dismissing the effort to create ʿAsfūriyyeh as an attempt to proselytize or civilize the natives, the editors of *at-Ṭabīb* decided to underline the birth of the new Hospital as part of a moment in the history of the modernization of the region. As the primary critics of Western imperialistic ambitions, they could easily have dismissed this initiative as yet another instrument of colonial rule, yet they decided to endorse it wholeheartedly and unapologetically.

2 The Struggle for Influence and the Birth of Psychiatry

> For there will never cease to be poor in the land. Therefore I command you, "You shall open wide your hand to your brother, to the needy and to the poor, in your land."
>
> —Deuteronomy 15:11

"I am going to open two schools—one which I shall establish, and one which the Jesuits will found to oppose it."[1] This is what the medical missionary Cornelius Van Dyck is quoted as having said upon opening a school in ʿAbay, a village in Mount Lebanon. A few decades later, the competition and rivalry continued unabated. In 1956, Louis Roché, the French ambassador to Lebanon, lamented in his correspondence with the French minister of foreign affairs that as soon as he had reached Beirut, he had been "plunged into the atmosphere of the long Franco-British rivalry around this curious political and religious chessboard that is Lebanon, where one feels so many foreign hands ready to cheat, every movement is watched."[2]

Roché was right, the French and British had a long history of rivalry that predated the collapse of the Ottoman Empire.[3] But, the French had more to lose and therefore more reason to be suspicious. Their privileged position as the protectors of Catholics in the Levant was threatened by an increasingly ambitious and powerful Great Britain and an ever more visible American presence.[4] This gave the French more reason to view any "Anglo-Saxon" activity in the Orient with deep suspicion. However, as we will see in this chapter, these profound and existential suspicions maintained a productive competition that, ironically, benefited the region through the flourishing intellectual and educational atmosphere it created. The historian Jean-Pierre Filiu has called the paradoxical combination of colonial exploitation and cultural proliferation *"évènement-Janus."*[5] I argue in this chapter that the birth of psychiatry in the Levant, and in the broader Middle East, may be considered such a "Janus event."

This chapter situates the birth of psychiatry in the Levant within the power struggles of the late nineteenth century between diverse local and global actors. Knowledge in that century became intensely politicized. "Zones of influence" (*zones d'influence*)—a term French diplomats frequently, if casually, used to refer to universities and, as we will see below, medical schools—were created, developed, and sustained from the humanitarian interventions of 1860s to the Cold War a century later in the aim of using knowledge to coopt the rising elite. Medicine in particular played a prominent role in this long competition over epistemic influence in the region. In contrast to the modernization of medical practice that was motivated by a will to reform the army, be it in Egypt or Constantinople, the founding of medical schools and hospitals in the Levant was an opportunity for diverse political actors to expand their influence and interests and perpetuate their presence in the Middle East.

The chapter retraces how the psychiatric profession flourished from the age of empire to the end of the French Mandate. Rather than positioning the history of ʿAṣfūriyyeh within the proselytizing crusades of the fin de siècle, as scholars have done so far, I argue that its history should instead be analyzed within a broader framework of a struggle for power and monopoly. The chapter begins by sketching the medical landscape that began to emerge in the mid-nineteenth-century—an important infrastructure in the production of the medical elite in the region. It then explores how the idea of a "home for the insane" was first conceived of, and how different actors and factors helped materialize this endeavor. The chapter underlines the role that local elites—professionals and notables from across religious denominations—played throughout the history of the Hospital as well as the ongoing struggle for power, influence, and a monopoly on knowledge. Another important observation that emerges in this chapter and the next is the withering of the missionary ethos that had driven the proliferation of many institutions dealing with education and health care in the Levant.

A New Medical Elite

Beginning in the nineteenth century, a new class of physicians who were trained in the increasingly influential modern and scientific medical practice started to supplant traditional healers. The latter included barbers, oculists, midwives, bonesetters, lice removers, and bleeders as well as the itinerant herbalists (or *moghrabis*—so named because they were thought to come from the Maghreb), who concocted herbal treatments, ointments, infusions, cure-alls, and other therapeutic oddities.[6] The rational and experimental method in science—with its new theories of the body based on advances and discoveries in physiology, experimental pathology, germ theory, and an emphasis on anatomo-clinical observation—was slowly displacing the humoral- and manuscript-based medical thinking that had lasted for centuries.[7]

At that time two medical schools started to attract students from the Levant. The first was Qasr al-ʿAini Medical School, founded in 1827 by the French physician Antoine Barthélémy Clot Bey at the instigation of the Egyptian viceroy, Muhammad Ali Pasha, who ruled Egypt from 1805 to 1848. Initially built near the Abu-Zaʿbel military camp to serve the army, it was founded as an effort to modernize and reform the country.[8] It was relocated to Qasr al-ʿAini (near Cairo) in 1837 to serve a much wider patient population.[9] Although European teachers staffed the medical school, its language of instruction was initially Arabic (the language changed to English following the British occupation of Egypt in 1882).[10] When Clot Bey visited Mount Lebanon in 1837 to recruit students for his new medical school, Emir Bashir II entrusted him with four students: Ibrahim Najjar, Yusuf al-Jalekh, Yussuf Merhej, and Ghaleb Khoury.[11]

Less than a month after Muhammad Ali Pasha opened his own school, Sultan Mahmud II established the Imperial School of Medicine *(Tiphane-i Amire)* in Constantinople primarily to support the new Ottoman army.[12] Its language of instruction was French. As Sultan Mahmud II advised medical students, "my purpose in having you taught French is not to educate you in the French language; it is to teach you scientific medicine and little by little to take it into our language ... work to acquire a knowledge of medicine from your teachers, and strive gradually to take it into Turkish and give it currency in our language."[13] After 1870, however, the curriculum shifted to Turkish in an attempt to prioritize the majority of Muslim students, who were falling behind their Christian and Jewish peers.[14] Although this move helped introduce a new medical terminology into Turkish, it somewhat homogenized medical practice due to the loss of minority physicians (Greeks, Armenians, and Jews)[15]—some of whom ended up continuing their medical studies in Beirut, as discussed below.

Medicine became an important tool of foreign penetration in the Levant in the nineteenth century. In a revealing letter to the French minister of foreign affairs, the procurator-general of the French Congregation of the Mission (of Lazarists—members of the Congregation of the Mission, a Catholic organization founded in Paris in 1625 by St. Vincent de Paul) noted that every foreign power had its own hospital in the major Levantine cities.[16] However, France lacked a proper hospital that could compete with the Protestants and serve as a bastion of French influence. Indeed, the only major civilian hospital in Beirut was the Prussian hospital (also known as the Johanniter hospital), which the Knights of St. John in Berlin had established first in Sidon and then in Beirut, following the notorious massacres in Mount Lebanon in 1860.[17] The other civilian hospital in Beirut was the *Hôpital français* (French hospital), which the French Sisters of Charity *(Filles de la charité de Saint Vincent de Paul)* had established in the mid-1840s.[18] But the main hospital in the city was the Ottoman military hospital, which was built in the 1840s, 1850s or 1870s (the exact date is not clear).[19]

Six years after the sectarian clashes in Mount Lebanon, the American Presbyterian missionaries (who had been in the Levant since the early nineteenth century) founded the SPC in Beirut, and a year later they founded a school of medicine.[20] The Prussian hospital became their teaching hospital; the professors of medicine—most of them American missionary doctors—became the hospital's attending physicians, and nine deaconesses from Kaiserswerth (in the Prussian Empire) served as nurses.[21] Over the years, the Prussian hospital became so reputable that Emperor William II of Prussia visited it during his grand tour of the Near East, which was part of the new *Weltpolitik* of securing for the Prussian Empire a "*Platz an der Sonne*" (a place in the sun) in an age of new imperialism.[22] On that memorable visit the emperor bestowed a decoration on George Post, the American medical missionary and professor of surgery at the SPC who helped establish the first medical journal in Arabic (see chapter 1).

The Lazarist procurator-general concluded his report to the French minister of foreign affairs by complaining that the French hospital was much smaller (thirty-six beds) and less well funded than the Prussian hospital.[23] He also complained about the lack of help from the French government, which he believed was under Jesuit influence (a suspicion that turned out to be well founded).[24]

When the Protestant missionaries changed the language of instruction of the SPC in 1880 from Arabic to English to "keep pace with the rapid developments that were then taking place in the West,"[25] the Jesuits perceived the move as a threat to Catholic and French interests in the Levant.[26] Three years later, with the support of the French government, the Jesuits opened their own faculty of medicine in Beirut (the French Faculty of Medicine, or FFM) to counter what they perceived as an increasing threat posed by the Protestant influence.[27]

To avoid any further clashes with the Lazarists, whom the Jesuits accused of trespassing on their territory,[28] the Jesuits struck a deal with the Sisters of Charity: the sisters would assume administrative and nursing responsibilities at the French hospital (which was now affiliated with the FFM, just as the Prussian hospital was affiliated with the SPC), while the doctors and medical students of the FFM would be responsible for medical care.[29]

The Jesuits, who had founded the Université Saint-Joseph (USJ) in Beirut in 1875 precisely to counter the growing Anglo-Saxon influence, could not have founded a school of medicine without the support of the French government—which, though anticlerical, was nevertheless opportunistic.[30] Léon Gambetta, the anticlerical French statesman, had famously declared in the French parliament that although clericalism is the enemy "it is not an article to be exported," thus justifying paradoxically the support of religious missionaries in the Orient as a way to propagate and extend French interests.[31]

According to the chancellor of the FFM, the Jesuit Lucien Cattin, there were two reasons for having a French school of medicine in Beirut: "to expand and deepen the traditional influence of France in the Orient" and "to resist the American and German influence" (the latter was usually combined with everything English and referred to as Anglo-Saxon).[32] While much has been written about the former, an examination of the latter can help us better understand the different developmental paths the region has taken as well as the complex political entanglements there.[33] Medical and educational institutions were widely regarded as centers of influence and propaganda. The elites who were in the process of forming were the future allies that the foreign powers would need to maintain their presence and power in the region. This alliance was doubly advantageous, since these elites, experts, and skilled technicians also formed the human capital necessary for Western economic expansion.

Nevertheless, when Jules Ferry, the French minister of public instruction, granted the Jesuits 15,000 francs to build a medical school to fight Anglo-American propaganda, he did not give them full control of the school.[34] The French government decided that it would have "direct and permanent control" over the medical curriculum, the distribution of diplomas, and the appointment of professors.[35] Every year the government sent to Beirut a French professor of medicine to sit on the jury that examined medical students. The professor was expected to produce a report for the government on the state of the university and medical education in the region, more broadly. The aim was clear and simple (if a bit deceitful): use the Catholic missionaries to destroy Protestant and Anglo-Saxon influence.[36] The French government's subsidies consequently allocated an annual budget to the FFM, the status of which was now generally considered a barometer of French influence in the Orient.[37]

The aim was to surpass the Americans and ultimately oust them from what the French saw as their natural territory, the so-called French Levant. Reports were produced to monitor the quality of teaching at the FFM, for the students needed to be irreproachable and superior to their American-educated counterparts.[38] In the first report commissioned by the Quai d'Orsay (headquarters of the French ministry of foreign affairs), a Dr. Villejean, a French professor at the University of Paris, suggested somewhat portentously that these aspiring doctors should remain in the Levant "if we want to disseminate French ideas and influence in those lands that will have to return to France during the liquidation of the Turkish Empire."[39] He wrote this in 1887, almost three decades before the dissolution of the Ottoman Empire. As the French newspaper *Le Journal* confirmed a few decades later, "spread today throughout the Orient, in Syria, Palestine, Egypt, and Turkey, all these doctors, who owe their pursuit of science to the French, have remained friends of our country and our culture, and everywhere they spread our influence and make us loved."[40] These were the agents through whom France would expand its influence.

One way to compete with the American medical school was to make the Jesuits' medical diploma more valuable. To be able to practice medicine in the Ottoman Empire, students had to pass an exam in Constantinople called the colloquium (introduced in 1888) in either Turkish or French.[41] This was also the case for graduates of the FFM until 1894, when the French government decided to grant them the right to practice in France, thus bypassing the need to pass the colloquium. But the Sublime Porte refused to acknowledge these state diplomas (*diplômes d'État*). A compromise was eventually reached: a jury of French and Ottoman examiners would judge the competence of medical graduates at the Jesuit campus in Beirut, without the need for a colloquium.[42] Every year at the Jesuit campus, a pompous ceremony was held in honor of the jury—whose members, including the Ottoman professors, received several *Légion d'honneur* awards for services rendered to France.[43]

The SPC in turn started to pressure the American minister-resident in Constantinople to intervene on its behalf after the college failed to attain recognition of its diplomas from the Porte.[44] However, the American minister-resident failed to persuade the Ottomans, who instead agreed to examine SPC students in Beirut through an imperial commission assisted by the American faculty to confer on these students the imperial medical diploma.[45] In 1909, the Porte designated Colonel Yusuf Rami Effendi and adjutant-majors Mechet Osman and Midhat Effendis (professors at the imperial faculty of medicine) as members of a mixed jury for the examinations of SPC medical graduates in Beirut.[46]

The Ottomans had agreed to collaborate with the French, a major imperial power, as a way to counter Russian expansion, since there were rumors that Russia was now envisaging the creation of a university in Damascus.[47] Indeed, the Russians had been enhancing their influence and expansion in the Orient ever since the Treaty of Küçük Kaynarca of 1774, mainly through financially supporting the Orthodox Church and any initiative that concerned the Orthodox community.[48] As the historian Abdul Latif Tibawi has argued, this was partly due to "Protestant and Catholic inroads on the Orthodox in Syria-Palestine."[49] Henry Harris Jessup, one of the founders of the SPC and general secretary of the American Presbyterian Mission in Syria, had documented that the Russians were "intensely active in resisting the aggressions of the Papists and Protestants on the Greek Church constituency" by opening schools and hospitals, exactly as their competitors were doing.[50] In 1878, local philanthropists from the increasingly wealthy and influential Greek Orthodox community established the Greek Orthodox hospital (known as the Saint George Hospital). However, donations also came from the Russian Orthodox Church, to the extent that the institution became known as "the Russian hospital."[51] Russian support continued over the years. As late as the 1960s, Russia was making financial donations, sending equipment, and supplying technical assistance to the Greek Orthodox hospital in Beirut.[52]

The other elephant in the room that is usually ignored is the Sublime Porte. It is not incidental that the medical school in Damascus, founded by Sultan Abdülhamid II in 1901, became a weapon for the Turks to counter French and Anglo-American presence and influence. Of course, there may have been other reasons why the sultan thought it vital to build yet another medical school in the Arab provinces (such as rallying Muslim public opinion behind him to support his pan-Islamism).[53] The irony is that later, during the Mandate of Syria and Lebanon, the French used the same medical school in Damascus as a French center of influence among the Muslims.[54] In any case, the sultan's intentions were clear to the French: his move was a way to counter their influence. In a report to the French government, Allyre-Julien Chassevant, a professor of medicine, was very explicit: "In 1901, the Turkish Government created a Turkish School of Medicine in Damascus organized on the model of German universities to counter the influence of medical doctors who graduate from the French Faculty of Medicine in Beirut."[55]

For the Turks likewise this competition for influence was a direct threat to their own propaganda. As a journalist for the Turkish newspaper *Stamboul* wrote at the time:

> It would be naive to think that the French investment in science is completely disinterested. One only has to hear what the French themselves say about their aim, which consists of the expansion of their influence in Syria.... Should we remain indifferent spectators while both the French and the Americans themselves are investing so much in this influence? ... We, too, should work on expanding our influence, or rather prove that we are the worthy masters of this country.... We, too, have a technical way to compete with the foreign medical schools in Beirut ... and this is through the medical school in Damascus.[56]

The Birth of Psychiatry

For the Protestant missionaries, the mind and human rationality were the royal road to defeating Catholicism and Islam. According to Jessup, Protestants "fear nothing in the region of logic, nothing from the light of truth," while Jesuits preferred indoctrination out of their fear of cultivating the powers of reasoning.[57] This was because the Protestant missionaries believed that logic and reason would naturally lead to the true (i.e., Protestant) faith. Science was one way to expose both Muslims and nominal Christians to their religions' respective inconsistencies.[58] As Daniel Bliss (the first president of the SPC, who held that position from 1866 until 1902) wrote regarding the importance of teaching mental philosophy, "Mental and moral science are so intimately connected with man's spiritual nature that opportunities are continually occurring in the classroom to enforce the great fact upon the mind of the student that a pure morality and a rational religious faith are in accordance with the constitution of the human mind, and a necessity to its highest well-being."[59]

One of the first members of the original faculty of the SPC, the Rev. Dr. Harvey Porter became an instructor in mental sciences and history in 1871 and a professor of psychology and logic in 1885.[60] A little more than a decade later, psychology replaced the mental sciences at the college. This heralded the shift from "metaphysical psychology" to a more positivistic science, or what John Dewey called the "new psychology."[61]

Psychology, which was taught to senior undergraduates, was described in the SPC catalogue for the year 1897–1898 as "a study of the mental powers as revealed in [the] consciousness, with due reference to their physical basis as determined by physiological investigations, and to the distinction between the physical and psychical elements of mental processes."[62] The American psychologist James Baldwin's influential *Elements of Psychology*, published in 1893, replaced the previous standard textbook of instruction, *Mental Science* (an 1882 revision of the 1854 *Empirical Psychology*), by the theologian, metaphysician, and psychologist Laurence Perseus Hickok (and edited by Julius H. Seelye), which Porter had used as a textbook for ten years.[63] This was an interesting choice, because although Baldwin's psychology combined Darwinian and Lamarckian elements, it was a functionalist and intuitionist form of psychology that rejected "crass materialism" and positivism.[64] It is thus no surprise that Porter's commencement address in 1883, in which he argued against an animalistic or instinctual origin of the human intellect, was received enthusiastically. It was widely considered a healthy antidote to Professor Edwin Lewis's controversial commencement address from the previous year, which the board of trustees condemned for endorsing Darwinism.[65]

The board had forced Lewis to resign, which had caused an uproar on campus. The student protests were so disruptive that they had to be contained by the police. More strikingly, a few professors—most notably Cornelius Van Dyck and his physician son William (both of whom shared Lewis's natural theology and disapproved of the board's decision)—in turn resigned in the wake of the "Lewis affair."[66] After leaving the college, the Van Dycks joined the newly founded hospital for the poor, the Saint George Greek Orthodox Hospital.[67] The Jesuits followed the incident closely and saw in it signs of the inevitable downfall of their rival institution. In a note to the French minister of foreign affairs, Pierre Mazoyer—a Jesuit and procurator of the Missions of the Society of Jesus in Syria, Egypt, and Armenia—predicted the ultimate downfall of this "major American achievement."[68] Of course, this turned out to be merely wishful thinking.

The Missionary Phase of ʿAṣfūriyyeh

On April 17, 1896, Jessup invited a number of residents of Beirut to his house to hear from Theophilus Waldmeier, a Swiss Quaker missionary, about his plan to found a "home for the insane in Bible Lands."[69] Waldmeier had started to develop an interest and sympathy in "the cause of the poor insane" two years earlier.[70] He was now sixty-four years old, having spent the previous twenty-five years building a school and a hospital in Brummana, a town in Mount Lebanon, and a decade before that doing similar work in Abyssinia (Ethiopia).

Born a Roman Catholic in a Swiss canton not far from Basel, Waldmeier graduated from St. Chrischona Mission College, a Protestant missionary school in Basel, in 1858.[71] Shortly after that, he was taken under the wing of the Swiss Lutheran Samuel Gobat who was bishop of Jerusalem from 1848 until his death.[72] With Gobat, Waldmeier traveled to France, Egypt, and Palestine before finally reaching Abyssinia where he spent ten years before he was forced to leave, following the British expedition in 1868 that put an end to the Ethiopian emperor's irascible behavior and secured British interests in the region.[73] Waldmeier moved with his wife and daughter to Beirut in 1869, where he joined the British Syrian Mission as an inspector of the mission's schools in Beirut, Damascus, and Mount Lebanon.[74] It was in connection with his work in Mount Lebanon that Waldmeier became a Quaker, after meeting two influential American Quaker missionaries (Eli and Sibyl Jones) in Beirut in 1869. A Protestant convert himself, Waldmeier decided to embrace the Quaker principles as "the right basis for a true spiritual Church."[75] It was thanks to the financial support of the Joneses that many of Waldmeier's undertakings were possible, including ʿAṣfūriyyeh—a project he embarked on at the age of sixty-four with the support of his second wife, a Lebanese woman called Fareedy Saleem who is buried today alongside her husband in the Quaker cemetery in Brummana.[76]

Ten of those present at the meeting at Jessup's house consented to act as an executive committee—what would become known as the Beirut Executive Committee (BEC). The Rev. Dr. John Wortabet (a highly respected local doctor and distinguished professor of anatomy at the SPC's faculty of medicine since the academic year 1866–1867)[77] was elected president, Jessup was secretary, an English banker named Charles Smith was treasurer, and Waldmeier was recognized as the founder and named "business superintendent." The other members included two locals: Esbir Shukayr (a dragoman at the British general consulate in Beirut) and As'ad Khairallah (a Protestant convert and clerk at the American Mission Press, whose nephew, mentioned in chapter 1, perished in one of the notorious holy caves where the insane were brought in the hope of a miraculous cure).[78] Two English physicians named Brigstocke (who had a private practice in Beirut and had served as first chair of the obstetrics and gynecology department at the SPC from 1875 to 1884) and Graham (a physician at the Prussian hospital and professor at the SPC faculty of medicine) also joined the BEC; as did the American physician William T. Van Dyck and a German pastor named Otto Fritze (see figure 2.1).[79] Also present that day was Thomas Smith Clouston, the director of the Edinburgh Royal Asylum at Morningside and acclaimed doyen of British alienists.[80] He had returned to Beirut that day after a journey in the Holy Land and was very supportive of the idea of a lunatic asylum in the Levant—an idea he had discussed at Wortabet's house in Beirut a few weeks earlier in the presence of another prominent English alienist, David Yellowlees.[81] He then pledged to help raise funds in Edinburgh and donated ten British pounds to the cause.

Both Clouston and Yellowlees were advocates of a medical approach to mental diseases based on a proper training in what was then called mental science.[82] In 1879 Clouston became the first lecturer on mental diseases at the University of Edinburgh, and Yellowlees had trained with him at the Royal Edinburgh Asylum, where both had been residents. Yellowlees went on to become physician-superintendent at the Royal Glasgow Asylum, and Clouston became superintendent at the Royal Edinburgh Asylum.[83] Physical restraint, they believed, was not curative and only to be used when appropriate, instead exercise and occupation needed to be encouraged—especially in the early stages of insanity.[84] Both were also advocates of separating chronic and acute cases, an idea that marked the managerial strategy of ʿAṣfūriyyeh (see chapter 4).[85]

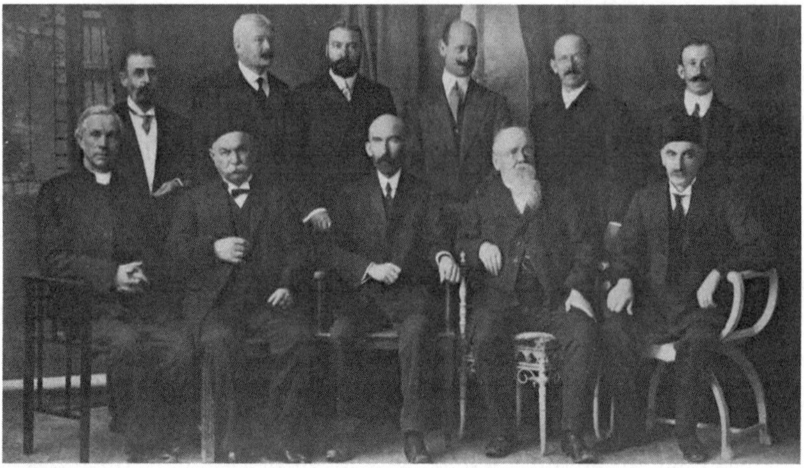

Figure 2.1
The Beirut Executive Committee, 1911. Standing: Mr. Glockler, Dr. Adams, Dr. Moore, Dr. Graham, Dr. Hoskins, Dr. W. Smith. Seated: Dr. Mackie, Mr. Shoucair, Dr. Webster, Mr. Sigrist, Mr. Khairallah. (The founder was ill and unable to be present when this picture was taken.)
Source: AR, 1953–1954, n.p., LHMND, AUB-SML.

In his suggestions for the reform of the British Lunacy Act of 1845, Clouston had proposed a provision that would allow "the removal from asylums and for suitable guardianship elsewhere of patients who have so changed in mental condition, without having recovered since their admission, that they no longer need asylum care."[86] A lunatic asylum, in his view, was supposed to be a place of cure, not a dumping place for people who had become a burden to their families and society. This, too, had clear resonance in the way in which ʿAṣfūriyyeh's medical directors later came to manage the Hospital (see chapter 4).

Perhaps the most prominent endorser of Waldmeier's hospital for the insane was Percy Smith, who by then had become superintendent of the Bethlem Royal Hospital. Smith had joined Bethlem as a resident physician at a time when the chief physician was the famed George Savage—who for a while had attended to Virginia Woolf's mental turmoil.[87] Like his mentor, who was recognized for having transformed Bethlem into a "place of clinical instruction," Smith was eager to transform the profession into a prestigious specialty that was scientific and modern.[88] Following in Savage's footsteps, Smith (who became president of the Royal Medico-Psychological Association in 1904) urged the Royal College of Physicians to institute a diploma in psychiatry.[89] This is how the certificate in psychological medicine instituted in 1885 came to be known as the Diploma in Psychological Medicine (DPM) in 1910.[90]

Other supporters provided political legitimacy. From the beginning, both the Ottoman governor of Mount Lebanon and the British consul general were very supportive of Waldmeier's initiative.[91] Their interventions turned out to be crucial at different stages of the Hospital's existence. When the old Damascus road threatened to bisect the premises of the Hospital, the Ottoman governor of Mount Lebanon, Nahum Pasha, ordered the closure of the old road, thus preserving the integrity of the estate.[92] And, as we will see below in this chapter, during the First World War, Governor Djemal Pasha allowed ʿAṣfūriyyeh's British medical director to remain on the Hospital grounds, when he could have been arrested as a prisoner of war.

British support for the Hospital throughout its history was equally vital, financially, technically, and even politically. Although the Hospital was above all an international hospital, it had often been perceived as a British institution of a sort since the beginning. This was because of the Quaker connection and also because the Hospital recognized the British consul general, Drummond Hay, as "the protector of ʿAṣfūriyyeh."[93] Indeed, the subsequent British ambassadors became ex officio presidents of the BEC, which was responsible for the day-to-day affairs of the Hospital while the London General Committee (LGC) had full authority.[94] In addition, the members of the Hospital's senior medical staff (including the matron) were generally British, while the attending medical doctors—who had generally studied at AUB (and in some cases at the French Jesuit faculty of medicine), had to acquire their DPMs from the Maudsley Hospital in London before they could pursue a career at ʿAṣfūriyyeh. (The Hospital was given the right to grant the DPM in 1956.[95]) The rest of the staff members, who were drawn from the local population, were frequently trained by the British personnel or sent for further training in Great Britain, where the Ministry of Overseas Development (ODM) financed their stay. This "technical assistance," as the ODM called it, would last into the 1970s.

After the meeting at Jessup's house, Waldmeier set off with his new wife to Europe and beyond aboard a French steamer headed for Marseilles.[96] During their two-year tour, Waldmeier raised funds in Switzerland, Germany,

Great Britain, Ireland, Canada, and the United States. Waldmeier and his wife familiarized themselves with the administration and treatment of patients while residing at the Frankford Asylum for the Insane in Philadelphia, which had been founded by the Society of Friends in 1813.[97] Over the years, the Society of Friends in Philadelphia turned out to be the most generous of the Societies of Friends around the world, financing the erection of four buildings at ʿAṣfūriyyeh.[98]

The tour also gave Waldmeier and his wife the opportunity to acquire firsthand knowledge of lunatic asylums with eminent alienists and superintendents. In Britain, Waldmeier visited the York Retreat, where he said he "learned a great deal" about the architectural and managerial requirements of an asylum.[99] He met with the greatest authorities on mental diseases in Switzerland, Germany, and Great Britain to learn more about the best therapeutic approaches. He organized auxiliary committees and appointed local treasurers in numerous European cities and towns for future fund-raising activities.[100]

Finally, he wrote public appeals to Christian philanthropists in Europe and the United States in which he pleaded the cause of the insane. A general committee of the Lebanon Asylum for the Insane (which was soon renamed the LGC) first met at Bethlem in London on March 11, 1897 under the chairmanship of Percy Smith.[101] (The name of the Hospital was changed to the Lebanon Hospital for the Insane a few months later.[102]) Waldmeier and his wife then returned to Beirut, having successfully raised a few thousand pounds in donations.[103]

Waldmeier bought two plots of lands in 1897 from Hussein Hikmat Jumblatt, and the Waldmeiers settled a few months later in an existing house on the premises of what would become the Hospital.[104] When the Hospital officially opened in 1900, there were two buildings for patient admissions: one for male patients (the "Swiss House," which the Swiss auxiliary committee had funded) and another for female patients (the "American House," funded by the American auxiliary committee).[105] Additional plots were purchased in 1902 and 1905. And several houses were built in the vicinity of the Beirut-Damascus carriage road, which over the years became a vital highway connecting the Mediterranean with the Syrian hinterland.[106] By 1912 the property contained thirty-six acres, with twelve houses on its premises in addition to a reception hall, an engine house for light and heat, domiciles for the farmers who cultivated the land, and several water reservoirs, one filled through a windmill.[107]

Conveniently located in the foothills of Mount Lebanon and only a few kilometers from Beirut, ʿAṣfūriyyeh benefited from salubrious weather and rich, cultivable land that the Hospital used for work therapy through the encouragement of gardening and other manual labor (figure 2.2).[108] It was in fact three doctors—Bedford Pierce, Yellowlees, and Clouston—who recommended that ʿAṣfūriyyeh be built on the so-called cottage system.[109] This celebrated architectural type had been popularized in the Belgian city of Gheel, whose lunatic asylum was organized into small houses or villas surrounded by arable land, giving patients a homey setting.[110] The organization and management of lunatics into therapeutic communities was at the heart of the cottage system, which came to define ʿAṣfūriyyeh's therapeutic philosophy.

The editors of the medical journal *at-Ṭabīb* (mentioned in chapter 1) welcomed the new initiative at Jessup's place as one that was possible thanks to concerned "patriots and foreigners" (*waṭaniyyīn wa-ajānib*), underlining its

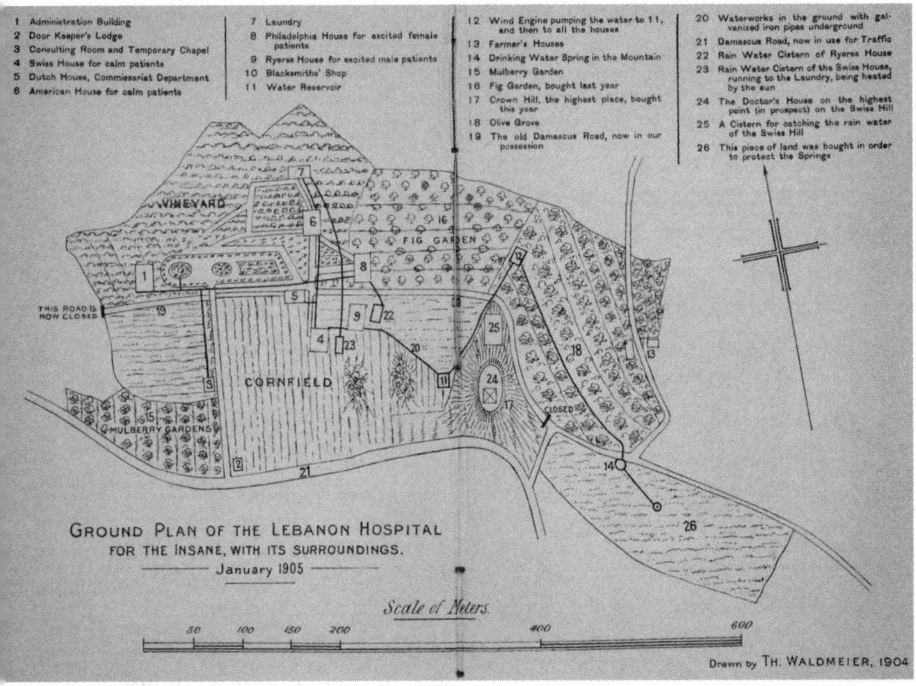

Figure 2.2
Plan of ʿAṣfūriyyeh.
Source: LH/12/01, box 16, LH, SOAS.

international cachet.[111] They emphasized the nonsectarian character of the Hospital: it would be open to everyone, regardless of religion or nationality. Local Muslim, Druze, and Christian notables were on the general committee based in Beirut along with thirteen Europeans (ironically including one Jesuit).[112] And although these local members were only honorary, they played an active part in the success, survival, and flourishing of ʿAṣfūriyyeh throughout its long history.

A constitution was drafted as early as 1896.[113] The Hospital's properties were turned into *waqf* (pious or charitable endowment) to guarantee that the Hospital would pursue its aims in perpetuity. Calls for donations from various Quaker-related committees established throughout Europe and the United States were constantly made and invariably met. This was an age when interest in proselytizing and civilizing missions was still present in the collective conscience, meaning that largesse for such purposes was easily procurable.[114] However, this phase was also marked by continuous friction between the founder and the successive medical doctors, all of whom became increasingly annoyed by his interfering in the affairs of the Hospital.

Because it was becoming customary in Europe and North America to recruit medical doctors with some experience in lunatic asylums, the Hospital administrators decided that its head should not merely be an administrator or a general physician but one who was acquainted with the new "alienistic science."[115] Article 11 of the 1896 constitution made this position clear: "The medical officer of the Asylum shall be not only a thoroughly qualified physician but a specialist in Mental Diseases, who shall have had experience as House Physician in an Insane Asylum for at least eighteen months, and who shall be specially recommended by competent authorities, both for professional qualifications, personal character and administrative ability."[116] Emil Sioli, a noted German alienist and director of the Frankfurt Asylum, was appointed president of ʿAṣfūriyyeh for 1896–1898. However, nothing came out of his tenure, and it is not even clear if he ever made it to Beirut. Waldmeier simply wrote that the committee "fell into a sleepy condition."[117] A Dr. Maag—a graduate of the University of Zurich, in Switzerland, who had some experience in mental diseases and who had offered his services for free—was appointed in 1898, and the committee asked him to get to Mount Lebanon as soon as possible so that he could become acquainted with the customs of the people and above all learn Arabic.[118] He never made it, however (for unknown reasons), and the committee decided to appoint another doctor in his place.

The committee then chose Otto Wolff, a specialist in mental diseases from the well-known Münsterlingen Asylum in Switzerland.[119] Wolff traveled to Constantinople to get his diploma legalized from the Imperial School of Medicine so that he could practice in the Ottoman Empire.[120] But because of an outbreak of the plague in Beirut at the time, he had to be quarantined when he arrived in the city, which delayed the opening of the Hospital until August 1900.

Wolff did not renew his three-year contract due to escalating conflicts with the committees in London and Beirut, both of which became increasingly wary of his intentions when he started a private medical practice on the premises of the Hospital.[121] The committees were not a priori against his having a practice outside the Hospital, but they believed it was inappropriate of him to open a general medical clinic on the Hospital premises. Above all, Wolff's desire to open another practice in Beirut directly interfered with the interests of the Hospital and was therefore deemed questionable.[122]

Wolff's reasons for doing so were both professional and financial. He was, after all, meagerly paid. He also complained that a medical superintendent who was not involved in scientific research or general medical practice was doomed to become alienated from the medical community and lose legitimacy.[123] There was more to this situation, however. Waldmeier saw his own power challenged by a man whom he accused of acting as a dictator: "an unlimited ruler" who wanted everyone to bow to him and who had a preference for acute cases. (Waldmeier's aim, in contrast, was to fill the Hospital to capacity to show how popular it had become.)[124] Waldmeier also accused Wolff of being incapable of learning the language and customs of the Orient. "Notwithstanding his great knowledge of psychical and mental diseases," Waldmeier complained in confidence to the LGC, "as an expert he could not get on here without us [the Waldmeiers] and it will be so for the next three years until he knows the language."[125]

Even Waldmeier's wife, Fareedy, complained about Wolff. In a private letter to Francis Brading (secretary of the LGC), she accused Wolff of being a materialistic, individualistic, and rude alcoholic.[126] She also took the opportunity to criticize the matron, who she said had a bad influence on the patients due to her habit of not attending Sunday prayer services. Clearly, the Waldmeiers were becoming uneasy about the growing medical influence. Fareedy concluded, "These people are only working for money and it can't be expected otherwise from people who are atheists, without any humble principles they seek their own interests."[127] This had nothing to do with Wolff's idiosyncratic behavior. Until the founder's death in 1915, the Waldmeiers constantly clashed with all medical doctors for the same reason: a rising secular medical authority.

Harry Thwaites, another specialist in mental diseases, replaced Wolff in November 1904. Thwaites had trained at Claybury Hospital in Essex and had held various appointments at major hospitals in London.[128] The committees soon criticized Thwaites for struggling to learn Arabic and for failing to acquaint himself with "the customs and habits of the people": two required skills they found necessary for the successful treatment of patients. Most importantly, Thwaites was found to lack a "missionary spirit."[129] Once again, Theophilus Waldmeier was complaining—this time about Thwaites's incompetence in spiritual and linguistic matters. As Waldmeier wrote to the LGC, Thwaites failed to show "Christian love, sympathy, and interest."[130] Waldmeier asked the LGC to make it clear to Thwaites that his job depended on his taking "a special interest in the spiritual welfare of the natives in attending the Arabic services held at Asfuriyeh on Sundays and other times."[131] On May 13, 1908, Thwaites announced his resignation.

Waldmeier took the opportunity to remind the committees that not only does an alienist need asylum experience and a "true linguistic gift of learning the Arabic language ... and much patience and love with the Syrians in order to win their hearts," but the alienist should also "be a total abstainer from alcoholic drink, he needs to be a protestant Christian with a missionary spirit because he has in the future to conduct divine service on Sunday."[132] Nevertheless, Waldmeier's vision of the missionary mental specialist would never materialize on the premises of ʿAṣfūriyyeh.

A new medical superintendent was appointed in October 1908: Henry Watson Smith, who had studied medicine at the University of Aberdeen in Scotland before becoming interested in mental diseases under the influence of his uncle, who ran a private lunatic asylum in Norwich, East Anglia. After graduating in 1901, Watson Smith had held appointments at Aberdeen, became house surgeon at the West Suffolk General Hospital, in Bury St. Edmunds, and then gone on to Peckham House in London before taking up a position as second assistant medical officer at the Durham County Mental

Hospital (in northeast England). It was on the strong recommendation of this last institution that the LGC chose Watson Smith as the next head of ʿAṣfūriyyeh, which now had seventy-five beds. He took up his official duties in February 1909 after obtaining the requisite Turkish medical degree at Constantinople—as all his predecessors had done.[133]

The friction between the Waldmeiers and Watson Smith was the subject of most of the correspondence between Theophilus Waldmeier and the LGC before Waldmeier's death in 1915. Waldmeier often clashed with successive medical doctors because he had no faith in their medicine. In 1913, two years before he passed away, he wrote that time and experience had taught him that "even a medical specialist can do very little for the recovery or cure of an insane patient by medicine."[134] He also believed that medical doctors were needed in asylums not for their curative prowess but for their ability to maintain sanity in places of insanity.

This time, however, the Hospital committee saw in Waldmeier's continuous meddling in the management of ʿAṣfūriyyeh and patient care an obstacle to the progress that the Hospital had made. The LGC complained about the Waldmeiers' interfering in the administration of the Hospital (especially with the admission of patients) and their lack of consultation with the local committee on important issues.[135] In addition, the committee accused the Waldmeiers of feeding misinformation about Watson Smith to the press.[136]

The Hospital could not afford to lose Watson Smith, who within a few years had gained a working knowledge of Arabic and proven to be an excellent administrator and physician. He had become a respected authority in the country and according to the LGC, he had "the fullest confidence of the public."[137] These factors all brought legitimacy, success, and prestige to ʿAṣfūriyyeh. An anonymous member of the local executive committee suggested that the time had come to marginalize the Waldmeiers. "The fact is," he said, "we will never have peace at Asfuriyeh until the Waldmeiers are outside of the grounds of Asfuriyeh entirely."[138] His was not a lone voice. Another member reiterated the determination of the Beirut committee "to take away from him [Waldmeier] all share in the active management of business."[139]

It was soon decided that the Waldmeiers would be asked to retire from the management of the Hospital, which they did in 1910 on their own initiative—although they requested to remain on the premises of the Hospital. This request was granted, and the Waldmeiers were given an annual honorarium of £200.[140] Nevertheless, the Waldmeiers continued to cause trouble.[141] The BEC finally decided to house them outside ʿAṣfūriyyeh—a decision that did not go unnoticed by the Waldmeiers' patrons. The Swiss threatened to withdraw all financial contributions.[142] Even after the death of Theophilus Waldmeier in 1915, his daughter Lily asked for the dismissal of Watson Smith in an angry letter to the chairman of the LGC.[143]

Despite the successive resignations and short tenures of the first three medical superintendents, the founding or "missionary" phase of ʿAṣfūriyyeh brought more publicity to the Hospital and saw the erection of new houses and other buildings as well as a flow of donations, technical expertise, and various commodities (such as linen, medical instruments, and water pumps, all of which were shipped from all over Europe). In the years before Waldmeier's death, at least ten houses and other buildings had been built.[144] However, the death of ʿAṣfūriyyeh's founder in 1915 heralded a new era under the uncontested leadership of Watson Smith.

Consolidation of ʿAṣfūriyyeh

Through his long tenure (1909–1934), Watson Smith witnessed many of the major political transformations of Mount Lebanon, from the Ottoman regime of the mutaṣarrifiyya (1861–1915) and its dissolution following the First World War to the French Mandate order (1920–1939).

During the First World War, Watson Smith remained on the premises and kept the Hospital functional while battling the disastrous famine that eventually claimed a third of the population of Lebanon.[145] Although the subjects of belligerent nations were supposed to be sent to Damascus as prisoners of war, Watson Smith was allowed to remain on the premises of the Hospital thanks to the intervention of Ohannes Pasha Kouyoumdjian, governor of Mount Lebanon.[146] Despite the abolition of capitulations (special privileges issued to Europeans by Ottoman sultans) at the beginning of the war, the Ottomans recognized that ʿAṣfūriyyeh was a charitable institution with an international character and thus did not close it—making it one of the few institutions under European management in the Ottoman Empire that managed to continue functioning during the war.[147]

Not only did the Ottomans not shut the Hospital down, but they also seem to have assisted it by helping supply vital commodities. Azmi Bey, governor general of Beirut, allowed the Hospital to be supplied with petroleum from the municipality of Beirut.[148] The Ottoman military authorities also sent regular supplies of flour and wheat.[149]

The American government may have also played a part in keeping the Hospital open and functioning. Before British troops entered Syria and Palestine, following the fall of the Ottoman Empire, the British had asked the United States government (which had remained neutral for the first three years of the war) to provide protection and financial aid to the Hospital if the need arose.[150] In a consular dispatch to Washington, the United States embassy in Constantinople reported that ʿAṣfūriyyeh was running normally and that Watson Smith and the British matron, a Mrs. Gibb, had been allowed to remain at the request of the American consul general at Beirut. The report added sardonically, "Whatever the Turks may do they may be trusted not to molest the insane whom they regard as under the special protection of Allah."[151]

Despite the generosity of Ahmed Djemal Pasha—the military governor of Syria, who sent a gift of one hundred sacks of wheat to the Hospital—inflation and the scarcity of food and other vital commodities hampered the treatment and care of the patients.[152] The years 1915–1916 were a time of "the greatest pecuniary difficulties," as one annual report of the Hospital put it.[153] Indeed, 1916 marked the climax of famine and starvation in Mount Lebanon. The wheat supply was so disrupted that the Hospital administrators even envisaged closing ʿAṣfūriyyeh. However, this was avoided by the political intervention of Ismail Hakki Bey (the last governor in Mount Lebanon) and Lady Halide Edib, a renowned Turkish novelist and feminist who took interest in the Hospital.[154]

Help for the Hospital continued to arrive from different relief organizations. In 1915, the Hospital was temporarily put under the protection of the American Red Cross.[155] Together with the American Committee for Relief in the Near East, they sent clothes, sheets, blankets, and gowns for patients as well as other vital supplies,[156] while the department of public assistance of the city of Beirut supplied the Hospital with flour, rice, sugar, and coffee.[157] All the local committees scattered around Europe mobilized to send donations.

In 1917, in the aftermath of the collapse of the Ottoman Empire, British troops occupied the premises of ʿAṣfūriyyeh (which had been renamed the Lebanon Hospital for Mental Diseases in 1915). During an influenza epidemic, Watson Smith had treated over four hundred men under the command of British General Edmund Henry Hynman Allenby, for which he later received the Order of the British Empire.[158] Members of the Beirut committee welcomed the occupation of the Hospital by these troops as liberation from Turkish oppression.

When French troops entered Beirut in 1918, negotiations for a peace treaty between the great powers had already begun. In anticipation of the Treaty of Sèvres (signed on August 10, 1920) that dismantled the Ottoman Empire, the French government decided in 1919 to turn the medical diploma into a *diplôme d'État,* which would grant medical students of the FFM the right to practice medicine not only in France but also in other places where France was to become the occupying power.[159] This strategic measure put the Americans in an inferior position, since the United States was the only foreign power that did not gain any territory from the treaty. Thus, medical students who graduated from the SPC were left without any official jurisdiction.[160] Remarkably, Article 146 of the treaty obliged the Turkish government "to recognize the validity of diplomas granted by recognized foreign universities and schools, and to admit the holders thereof to the free exercise of the professions and industries for which such diplomas qualify."[161] The article also applied to nationals of the Allies who resided in Turkey—the so-called Levantines, who constituted an important portion of the FFM's student body.[162]

The conference in San Remo, Italy, on April 26, 1920, granted France its mandate over Syria and Lebanon and Britain its mandate over Palestine and Iraq.[163] This is how the French-mandated territories came to be—including Greater Lebanon (Grand Liban), the State of Syria (État de Syrie), the State of the Alawites (État des Alaouites), the Jabal al-Druze (Djebel Duruz), and the Sanjak of Alexandretta (Sandjak d'Alexandrette).

To show that the French were now in charge, the Mandate authorities replaced the Ottoman professors who had previously sat on the colloquium examinations of SPC medical graduates with a jury made up of French military medical doctors and two professors from the Jesuit FFM. (In 1920, the SPC was renamed the American University of Beirut, or AUB.) But the AUB diploma was purposefully a much less valuable diploma than the FFM diploma, since the former allowed its holders to practice only in the mandated territories and not in all of the French colonies.[164]

Now that the mandates had been established in Syria and Lebanon, the French started to organize their territories and impose their rule. In 1921, a short note to the ministry of foreign affairs warned the ministry that it would be wise to "keep an eye on the American College in Beirut, which is anti-French at all levels," and in particular had a "bad influence on the Arabs."[165] The French authorities did keep a close eye on AUB, which they continued to characterize as a center of Protestant propaganda.[166] They also favored graduates of the Jesuit university for governmental posts.[167]

The Mandate authorities reiterated that the USJ should continue playing its role as one of the Mandate's main tools of influence in Syria and Lebanon, and it did all it could to make this possible. It was during the Mandate that the French General Maxime Weygand inaugurated the new teaching hospital of the FFM, the Hôtel-Dieu de France.[168] The explicit purpose of building this new hospital following the clash between the professors at the FFM and the Sisters of Charity over the latter's "authoritarian behavior"[169] was to maintain French superiority over what the Jesuits saw as their ever-growing wealthy competitor, AUB and its hospital.[170] It was also during the Mandate that new laboratories were built and new academic chairs created at USJ.[171] This was all done to expand French influence—and above all to counter the continuous progress of AUB, which was described as being considerably wealthier, more hurried, and more audacious than the FFM and therefore in an advantageous position.[172] Indeed, in 1929 and 1930, the Rockefeller Foundation helped finance major developments on the American campus in Beirut: new medical and science laboratories, various clinics, a medical library, and dormitories for medical students.[173] The foundation's financial support of AUB's medical school continued until at least the 1960s.[174] And this was most likely part of the foundation's wider mission in building a progressive and rationalized scientific medical practice in line with corporate capitalism in the United States.[175]

At the same time, however, the French Mandate's welfare policy indirectly helped ʿAṣfūriyyeh initiate a new phase of financial growth and possibility, marked by a shift in the paying population from private to government-supported patients. The first decree of the French High Commissioner, General Henri Gouraud, on December 10, 1919, concerned the creation of a welfare system—the *Service de santé, d'hygiène et d'assistance publique*—allegedly out of benevolent concern for the poor.[176] But in a confidential document, the delegate to the high commissioner in Damascus, Georges Catroux, urged the French government to invest in projects that would bring "moral profits" (*profits moraux*) and a sense of security and prosperity to the locals, thus making the Mandate more acceptable.[177] The assistance publique—modeled on the French rationale of the *état providence* (providential state)[178]—was perceived as the embryonic beginning of a public health service at the state level, the first in the region.[179]

In the French context, the assistance publique turned out to be an important tool in the anticlerical politics of the French republic.[180] One can similarly argue that in the new Mandate order, this embryonic form of welfarism was equally vital for the persistence of French influence. Indeed, the French authorities considered the program to be a continuation of their politics of assistance to their *oeuvres* (benevolent endeavors mostly initiated and managed by French Catholic missionaries, whom the authorities recognized as being vital in the dissemination of French influence).[181] The French authorities were well aware of the daunting task they might have faced had these charitable and religious organizations not existed. The existence of this network of private initiatives (both secular and religious)—which was more developed in Greater Lebanon than in the rest of the mandated territories (and perhaps the other French colonies)—was possible as a result of the ongoing competition between the various groups of missionaries and the rival imperial powers that sought power and influence.[182]

The French Mandate ironically turned out to be a boon for the flourishing of psychiatry in the region. During the First World War, the Ottomans had imposed a five-year educational program to conform to the curriculum at the Imperial Medical School. After the war, however, the SPC decided to revert to its four-year curriculum, and it was the FFM chancellor who alerted the mandatory authorities of the change.[183] The French high commissioner, finally in a position of power, demanded that AUB change its curriculum to a five-year program, threatening that otherwise AUB's students would be refused the right to practice medicine (the Jesuit chancellor was convinced that students were attracted to AUB's curriculum because it was one year shorter than that of the FFM).[184] Ironically, it was out of the need to fulfill the wishes of the Mandate authorities that AUB introduced clinical psychiatry (including visits to ʿAṣfūriyyeh) in its new curriculum in order to fill part of its new five-year curriculum.[185]

Although Watson Smith had envisaged a course in psychiatry as early as 1918, he was appointed the first lecturer in psychiatry at AUB in 1921.[186] In 1922, AUB became formally affiliated with ʿAṣfūriyyeh, and the training of students started four years after that, when a deal was finally reached with the Rockefeller Foundation—which granted the Hospital a large sum

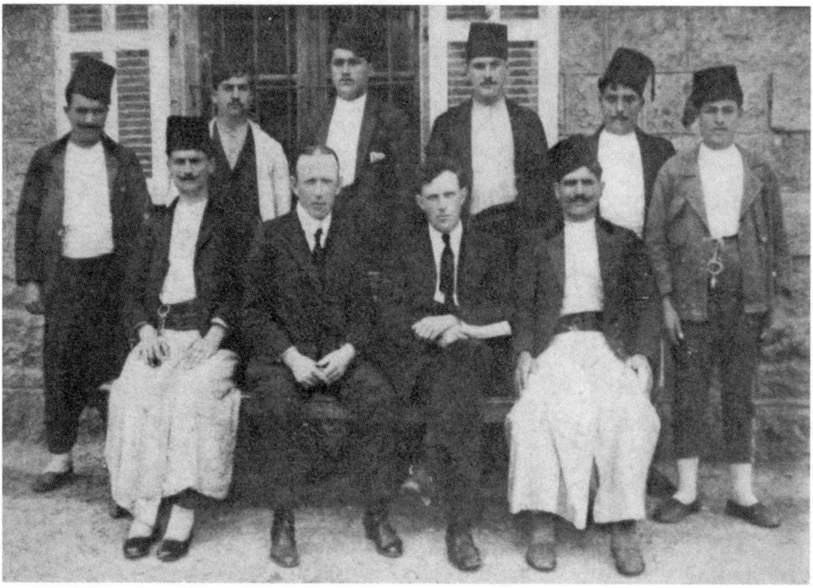

Figure 2.3
Henry Watson Smith (seated, second from left) with the head attendant and the male nurses at ʿAṣfūriyyeh.
Source: The Lebanon Hospital for Mental Diseases, c. 1920, n.p., box 125, CBMS, SOAS.

of money for the support of a graduate medical student at ʿAṣfūriyyeh.[187] In 1924, Watson Smith became lecturer in nervous diseases in addition to continuing his clinical work in psychiatry.[188] His title was changed the following year to clinical professor of neurology and psychiatry, a post he held from the academic year 1925–1926 until his unexpected death in 1934 (figure 2.3).[189]

It was under Watson Smith's leadership that ʿAṣfūriyyeh became an academic center for teaching and training in psychiatry. An oral exam in neurology and psychiatry was introduced in 1921,[190] and two hours per week of psychiatry and neurology were introduced the following year.[191] In 1926, when a clinical internship at ʿAṣfūriyyeh was initiated, psychology (a prerequisite to psychiatry) became part of the premedical courses.[192] Indeed, in addition to the fifth-year medical students—who now resided for two months on the premises of ʿAṣfūriyyeh—psychology and sociology students started to visit the hospital to get familiarized with psychopathology.[193]

Watson Smith was also an entrepreneur à la Thomas Kirkbride, the renowned superintendent of the Pennsylvania Hospital, who designed and built the hospital he managed.[194] With only meager funds, Watson Smith restored and reequipped the Hospital buildings.[195] New pavilions were built under his personal supervision, with neither architect nor contractor. He put in place an economic plan to make the Hospital self-sufficient in terms of water, olives, and soap supplies, and he also managed to build a new house for women entirely from local funds: a first in the history of the Hospital. Watson Smith was also an advocate of mental health and social responsibility. His reputation kept soaring, and patients kept flocking to the Hospital.[196]

When ʿAṣfūriyyeh officially opened its doors in 1900, the French totally ignored the initiative in contrast to the praise and publicity the Hospital received in many English and American missionary and medical journals. During the French Mandate, however, the secretary general of the LGC approached French Protestants living in Great Britain "to enlist the support, both moral and financial, of the French people" to "widen and strengthen the international basis of the hospital"[197] (this latter aspect is further explored in chapter 6). Both the French consul in Paris and the high commissioner in Syria and Lebanon believed this to be a good opportunity to extend French influence in an institution that was now under French Mandate jurisdiction.[198]

But the French mandatory authorities decided to forgo the opportunity to get involved in ʿAṣfūriyyeh for several reasons. First, they were already invested in another hospital that now served the state of Syria: the Ibn Sina Mental Hospital (*Asile d'Avicenne de Damas*) outside Damascus, which opened on May 12, 1923, primarily to serve French military personnel.[199] Before the French established this new asylum in Damascus, however (and even long after its establishment), they continued to send their sick soldiers to ʿAṣfūriyyeh. In 1921, three *aliénés* (insane people) were sent to ʿAṣfūriyyeh for treatment, and sixty-two soldiers from the Légion syrienne and the French Foreign Legion were admitted for physical and nervous exhaustion in 1920–1921.[200] High Commissioner General Henri Gouraud even sent an official letter thanking the medical director for the care the French soldiers had received at ʿAṣfūriyyeh.[201]

Second, the French were hoping that the Association of French Protestants in Lebanon and Syria (*Oeuvres protestantes françaises du Levant*), which had been created in 1925 to take over German properties (including the Prussian hospital) after the war,[202] would contribute financially to ʿAṣfūriyyeh on behalf of the French state: something that did not happen.[203] There was also no benefit from an official investment in ʿAṣfūriyyeh unless, as the high commissioner suggested, a French House could be erected (to accompany the English and American Houses on the premises of ʿAṣfūriyyeh).[204]

Because the priority was to fund and support French oeuvres—and since ʿAṣfūriyyeh was considered a British institution (and sometimes even a German institution due to its Swiss founder, who had strong links to German and Swiss Protestants)—the high commissioner did not see any reason for investing in ʿAṣfūriyyeh. However, there was more to the story than that. When the procurator of the Capuchin order requested financial help from the French government in the early 1950s, listing all the works his order had accomplished (most notably the establishment of a psychiatric hospital that had become the rival par excellence of ʿAṣfūriyyeh) and describing the Capuchins as "true artisans of French prestige overseas," the government did not dismiss his request so lightly.[205]

In 1933, during the opening ceremony of the new pavilion for women at ʿAṣfūriyyeh, in the presence of many notables and consuls, the president of the state of Greater Lebanon, Charles Debbas, bestowed on Watson Smith the Lebanese Medal of Merit for his twenty-five years of public service.[206] Watson Smith was honored as one of the country's "most distinguished, valuable, and honored citizens."[207] He unexpectedly died a few months later of heart failure at the age of fifty-five, while on furlough in England, and a pavilion in his memory was erected the following year. It is perhaps ironic that the inauguration of the Waldmeier House took place on the same day as that of the Watson Smith House given the friction between the two men. The ceremony was attended by a large and influential gathering, including the representative of the president of the state of Greater Lebanon as well as the American, French, and British consuls general. Ironically, music was provided by a forty-member French military band loaned by General Charles Huntziger, commander in chief of the French troops in the Levant and probably himself a descendant of Huguenots.[208]

In 1943, during the Second World War, Lebanon was declared independent—bringing an end to the French Mandate.[209] During a visit to ʿAṣfūriyyeh that year, Jeanne Wallon Helleu—wife of the French high commissioner, who it should be remembered had refused to financially support the Hospital—made a personal donation of 300 Lebanese pounds. "Not that this sum will go very far," she said, "but it is given with all my heart."[210]

While ʿAṣfūriyyeh was at the apex of its success, creating new conceptual and institutional frameworks for the management of mental illness in the region, the USJ appointed its first professor of neuropsychiatry, the French psychiatrist Maurice Potet, only in 1942.[211] In 1945, Potet brought several senior medical students to study psychiatric cases at ʿAṣfūriyyeh.[212] Two years later, Potet, who also had visited ʿAṣfūriyyeh several times, was succeeded by another French psychiatrist, Albert Brousseau—who held his position until 1949 and was known for his strong stance on neurobiological psychiatry.[213] This late institutionalization of psychiatry at the FFM is intrinsically linked to the history of ʿAṣfūriyyeh's foremost competing institution (Dayr al-Ṣalīb), which is discussed more thoroughly in chapter 3.

Conclusion

This chapter has situated the development of psychiatry and the growth of psychiatric hospitals not in the usual framework of modernization or proselytism but as part of a continuous struggle over influence and power, which is an analytical framework more pertinent to the Levant.

As this chapter has demonstrated, the "psy" sciences (notably psychiatry and psychology, but also the philosophy of mind and logic) continued to expand over the years for a number of reasons, some of which were paradoxical. First, many Protestants believed that a knowledge of the workings of the mind and a sound mental philosophy were the best weapons to use in proselytizing Muslims and the nominal Christians as well as in combating their sworn enemies, the Jesuits. Second, what allowed ʿAṣfūriyyeh to grow as a new site of expertise about normality and abnormality was its growing partnership with AUB. This situation was indirectly made possible as a result of the new five-year curriculum imposed by the Mandate authorities to lessen and control the competition between its own faculty of medicine and that of AUB. This fortuitous action enabled the introduction of new courses in neurology and psychiatry, caused new links to be forged between theory and practice, and led to the birth of a new generation of psychiatrists.

As we will see in chapter 3, it was only when Dayr al-Ṣalīb became a proper psychiatric hospital that the Catholics (the Jesuits and the new order of Franciscan sisters) seized the opportunity to expand their influence over yet another scientific territory of tremendous political, social, and (increasingly) economic leverage.

3 The Rise of ʿAṣfūriyyeh and the Decline of Missions

> Woe unto them that call evil good, and good evil; that change darkness into light, and light into darkness; that change bitter into sweet, and sweet into bitter!
> —Isaiah 5:20

The development of ʿAṣfūriyyeh unfolded in several stages. Chapter 2 examined the first two phases. The missionary phase (1896–1915) focused on the original objectives of the Hospital: pioneering a more humane approach to treating and managing the insane, making the approach more palatable to the locals, and finding ways to sustain this new charitable endeavor. The second phase, which followed Theophilus Waldmeier's death in 1915 and continued under the leadership of Henry Watson Smith until the latter's unexpected death in 1934, was one of consolidation and growth—specifically, with the birth of psychiatry as a new academic and scientific discipline.

This chapter continues the exploration of the Hospital's shifting mission by examining three additional phases. The third phase (1934–1949) was one of continued growth and consolidation as well as of institutionalization under the leadership of R. Stewart Miller, who forged new and long-lasting relations with the nascent Lebanese republic that was declared independent in 1943. The fourth phase (1950–1973) was marked by the transformation of the Hospital from a national institution to one with influence throughout the Middle East. The fifth and final phase, which started with the sale of the original estate of ʿAṣfūriyyeh in 1973 and is ongoing, was aborted by the civil war that erupted in 1975. This last phase was supposed to see the metamorphosis of the hospital into a modern psychiatric institute, an idea first proposed by Antranig Manugian (ʿAṣfūriyyeh's first Lebanese medical director) in 1957 but adopted only in 1976 when it was already too late.

Chapter 2 showed how ʻAṣfūriyyeh and the birth of psychiatry were the products of a competition for influence between rival actors, local and global, secular and religious. While this chapter continues to explore this dynamic—especially vis-à-vis the rise of ʻAṣfūriyyeh's competing institution, Dayr al-Ṣalīb—it will illustrate how the Hospital was also the product of its successive leaders as well as various contingent factors. Each medical director, with his own managerial style and ideals, shaped the institution and contributed to its transformation over the years. This chapter, like the previous one, will also document the withering of the missionary zeal that marked the earlier periods of the Hospital's history. Religion as an ethos of care became a footnote in the history of the Hospital.

The Monastery of the Cross

Abūna Yaʻqūb—or Père Jacques (Father Jacob), as he was known locally (his real name was Khalil Haddad)—was a Lebanese Capuchin priest born in 1875 in Ghazir, Mount Lebanon, to a Maronite family. He was beatified in a grand mass in Beirut in 2008 and is remembered today for his prolific charitable contributions, for which in 1938 he received the Golden Medal of Lebanese Merit (incidentally, only a few years after Henry Watson Smith received the same honor).[1] Abūna Yaʻqūb founded the Franciscan Sisters of the Holy Cross; more than 160 schools; and numerous hospitals, hospices, orphanages, and churches—the most famous being Christ-Roi.[2]

It was the misery of the First World War, which he witnessed firsthand, that pushed him to undertake a monumental project. In 1919 he bought land in Jal al-Dib on a hill facing the Mediterranean 15 km north of Beirut that already housed a chapel built by a monk in 1867. In 1925 he erected a sanctuary known as Our Lady by the Sea (Notre-Dame de la Mer) with a ten-meter-long cross. In 1926, on the occasion of the seven hundredth anniversary of St. Francis of Assisi's death, Abūna Yaʻqūb turned the convent into an asylum for elderly priests who suffered from dementia and other mental illnesses. Over the years, the asylum also came to care for orphans and the disabled.

We learn from Abūna Yaʻqūb's private correspondence with his superior in Lyon that he had both an impressive entrepreneurial spirit and an aversion to the growing Protestant influence in the region. At the root of the success of what came to be known as Dayr al-Ṣalīb (the Monastery of the Cross) was not, as claimed by Abūna Yaʻqūb's biographer (the Capuchin priest Théophane de Deir el-Kamar) simply serendipity or the good will of the government in encouraging philanthropic institutions.[3] Instead, two main reasons explained this success: competition with ʿAṣfūriyyeh, which Abūna Yaʿqūb referred to as the "Protestant hospital," and the latter's ultimate closure.

As early as 1906, in a few articles written and published in *Le petit messager de Saint François* (the official magazine of the French Capuchins), Abūna Yaʿqūb wrote about the two evils that needed to be fought: emigration to the Americas and what he called "the Protestant invasion."[4] He denigrated emigration to the Americas for its material pursuits. He also criticized the Protestants' heretical teachings and indifference toward France (the mother country of the persecuted Christians of the East). Revealingly, Théophane de Deir el-Kamar omitted from his biography any of Abūna Yaʿqūb's writings that mention how he had "snatched" patients from the "Protestant asylum at ʿAṣfūriyyeh" (*l'asile protestant de Asfourieh*) and how the ministry of health had sided with him against ʿAṣfūriyyeh's director, who allegedly accused him of stealing the hospital's clients.[5]

According to the biographer, it was a French officer named Captain Théomy who informed the ministry of health of the existence of a new asylum for the chronically and mentally ill.[6] Théomy sought help at Abūna Yaʿqūb's new asylum, for a friend whom, he claimed, every other hospital had rejected. It was thanks to Théomy's connection with the French Mandate's Service d'hygiène et d'assistance publique that a contract was signed in 1937 with the Lebanese government to send poor patients with all kinds of disabilities to the new asylum be treated at very low cost. But the story is more convoluted and less triumphalist than the official religious sources would have us believe.

To be able to snatch those patients, Abūna Yaʿqūb had had to negotiate the hospitalization fee, asking for half the regular fee (in 1937, this was twenty *qurush* [piastres] per day instead of forty-five).[7] In 1939, he signed another contract—this time with the municipalities of Beirut and Tripoli, which sent 130 and 30 patients, respectively.[8] The ministry of health, which had financial difficulties during the Second World War, decided to send patients en masse—especially those who were considered incurable—to Dayr al-Ṣalīb.[9] The situation was repeated in the late 1940s.[10] Of course, this did not go unnoticed—either by the committee of ʿAṣfūriyyeh, which faced increasing pressure to gain the patients back, or the press, which lambasted the transfer of these vulnerable patients as "scandalous" and accused the government of negligence.[11]

An article in the Beirut-based newspaper *L'Orient* reported that the decision was purely based on financial reasons, with no regard to the quality of care for the mentally ill.[12] The journalist added that Dayr al-Ṣalīb was inadequately equipped to cope with mental illness and that the families of the patients were outraged by the decision to transfer them to a medically deficient facility. Was this mere propaganda against Dayr al-Ṣalīb, or was there genuine concern on the part of the families and the general public? And could this be an indication that people seemed to accept—indeed, now demanded—a more scientific approach to mental illness? In any case, what is revealing about the history of Dayr al-Ṣalīb is how it situated itself within its own crusade against Protestantism. Remarkably, in a summary of Abūna Yaʿqūb's achievements (in support of his beatification), one reads that his merit was in establishing a Catholic psychiatric hospital that countered the only mental hospital in the country, which was managed by American Protestants.[13]

ʿAṣfūriyyeh coped with this new competition with diplomacy and caution. Its strategy was to emphasize the scientific nature of its philosophy of care as opposed to the mere nursing care provided at what the staff and trustees of the Hospital referred to as a monastery-cum-asylum, a mere nursing home with occasional medical supervision.[14] This description, of course, contrasted with that of ʿAṣfūriyyeh, which the committee members depicted as a hospital dedicated to the treatment and cure of mental and nervous pathologies based on modern and rational principles and the latest technological and therapeutic approaches. Indeed, committee members hailed visits by politicians such as Prime Minister Saeb Salam, the minister of health, and the head of the municipality of Beirut as crucial to convincing government officials of the vital role that ʿAṣfūriyyeh played as a center for treatment and cure.[15] It is within this dynamic of continuous competition that Dayr al-Ṣalīb continued to expand. In 1944 the number of patients treated at Dayr al-Ṣalīb had reached 348, and the hill that once had been known as the hill of jinns (*tallat al-jinn*) was now known as the hill of the cross (*tallat al-ṣalīb*).[16]

Institutionalization Phase

Many of the conditions that made the steady growth of the Hospital possible in the 1950s and 1960s—indicated by the increasing numbers of admissions (figure 3.1)—were forged during the directorship of R. Stewart Miller, who succeeded Watson Smith in 1934. Miller rightly spoke of an

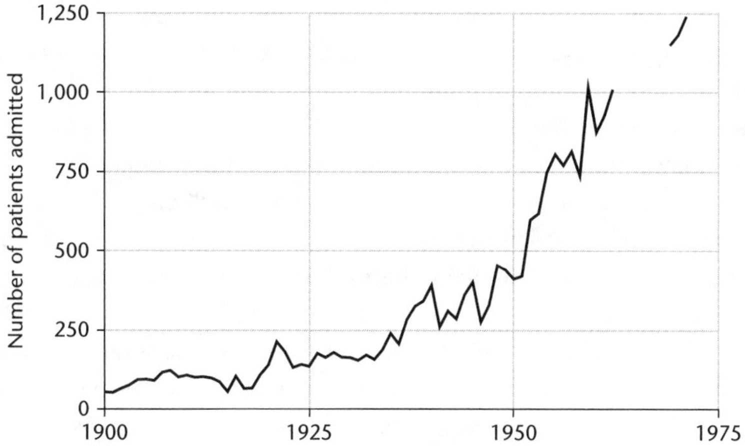

Figure 3.1
Number of patients admitted, 1900–1971. Data missing for 1963–1968.
Source: Data compiled from ARs.

"awakening."[17] It was under his directorship, on July 18, 1939, that the Royal Medico-Psychological Association recognized ʿAṣfūriyyeh as a training center for the certificate in mental nursing.[18] In 1941, the Lebanese Court of Appeal asked Miller, who was already a consulting expert for the criminal court, for advice on framing the new criminal code.[19] Until then the Ottoman Sanitation Act (*Irade-i seniyye*) of March 15, 1876, had governed the fate of those who were deemed insane.[20]

Indeed, a spate of laws in 1865–1885 (during the Tanzimat period) made the health-related professions (from physicians to druggists) more formally regulated.[21] Two new laws recognized the responsibility of the public authorities vis-à-vis the health of their citizens. The 1871 Ottoman Municipal Law (*Belediye Kanunu*) stipulated that a medical doctor should always be present in the municipality. Such doctors had to report epidemics and contagious diseases, provide vaccinations, serve as court experts when requested to do so, and offer free consultations to whoever solicited their services, rich and poor alike.[22]

The 1876 Ottoman Regulation for Lunatic Asylums (*Bimarhaneler Nizamnamesi*) was issued following the recommendations of Luigi Mongeri, the medical superintendent of the main lunatic asylum in Constantinople, who complained of arbitrary incarcerations by religious authorities.[23] According to the new decree, only the police had the authority to incarcerate people who were believed to be a danger to public order. In all other cases, a person who appeared at a lunatic asylum (either voluntarily or involuntarily) had to provide a medical certificate detailing the state of his or her illness over at least a fifteen-day period. This certificate had to be signed by two or three doctors (in the case of a public or private asylum, respectively) who were unrelated to the person. In cases of emergency, a signed declaration by the accompanying individual replaced the medical certificate. In all cases, within three days the hospital's director had to send a full medical report to the local civil authorities and (in the cases of non-Muslim patients) to the local religious authorities. In addition, every year the asylum's director had to send a report to the police on every patient who was being cared for.

The Ottoman Provincial Municipal Law of 1877 (*Vilayet Belediye Kanunu*) clearly stipulated the new duty the municipality had in terms of maintaining public health, including hygiene and the establishment of hospitals.[24]

Although these new laws were intended to prevent wrongful incarcerations, they were rarely, if ever, followed. Medical directors of ʿAṣfūriyyeh often complained about these laws being out of date and about the poor quality of the *billets d'hôpital* (medical notes for hospital admission) that the municipal doctors sent.[25]

Before joining ʿAṣfūriyyeh, Miller had been director of one of the largest Egyptian mental hospitals, El-Khanka Hospital—which had 1,700 beds and provisions for the criminally insane as well as those convicted of substance abuse.[26] This explains why one of Miller's major achievements during his tenure at ʿAṣfūriyyeh was to forge new institutional relations with the criminal justice system, despite the troubles of the Second World War.

These institutional links between the new experts of the mind and the law paved the way for a new approach to criminal insanity. The collaborative efforts with the government were widely hailed as the birth of a new era for psychiatry, one in which the law recognized psychiatry as a legitimate discipline that had authority over what counted as abnormal behavior, and one that would eventually change perceptions about the mentally ill. The new Lebanese penal code was eventually signed on March 1, 1943. Articles 231–236 of the code set new provisions for those who were deemed insane (*ḥālat junūn*), mentally deficient (*muṣāban bi-ʿāha ʿaqliyya*), or dependent on alcohol or drugs (*ḥālat tasammum nātija ʿan al-kuḥūl aw al-mukhaddarāt*).[27] The Syrian penal code, decreed on June 22, 1949, was a replica of the Lebanese version.[28]

This period of institutionalization of psychiatry was also marked by a new style of thinking steeped in mental hygiene and neuropsychiatry that characterized a generation of psychiatrists who had been trained in the 1930s and 1940s. According to one physician, it was clear that by the 1930s, an understanding of the fields of both neurology and psychiatry had become necessary to grasp the complexity of the nervous system, which now faced tremendous pressures from increasingly industrialized societies, an increasingly connected world, and an increasingly mechanized civilization.[29] In 1937, for example, the outpatient department clinic in neurology and psychiatry at the American University Hospital in Beirut was attracting an "ever-increasing number of patients," many of whom were hospitalized at ʿAṣfūriyyeh.[30] The psychiatric field was changing from one focused on the downtrodden and the forgotten to one that was of boundless reach, encompassing new types of people who were suffering from various mental ailments in their homes, in their schools, in their factories, and in the military.

After Miller's retirement, the first step that the new medical director, Robert Robertson, undertook was to open a neuropsychiatric clinic in Beirut in 1947. Ali Kamal, a Palestinian neurologist who had completed his training at the Hospital for Nervous Diseases at Queen's Square in London, became its director.[31] A year later, ʿAṣfūriyyeh opened its School of Psychiatric Nursing, the first of its kind in the Middle East. W. M. Ford Robertson (no relation to Robert Robertson) was responsible for these two major breakthroughs.[32] Ford Robertson, a key member of the LGC, succeeded Robert Robertson upon the latter's resignation in 1949, a mere two years after being appointed.

From National to Regional Influence

Ford Robertson's six-year tenure (1950–1956) helped transform ʿAṣfūriyyeh from a national institution to one with broader regional influence in the Middle East. The Hospital's regional sway, as well as its mental hygiene strategy and ideology, continued under the leadership of Antranig Manugian, who became medical superintendent in 1956 and medical director in 1962—a position he held until the closure of the Hospital in 1982.

What also helped sustain the urge for innovation, growth, and influence was the continuous rivalry between the American medical school and its French counterpart (explored in chapter 2). The conversion of Dayr al-Ṣalīb into a proper psychiatric hospital in 1950 was a result of the continuous competition between these two "styles of imperialism," to borrow the words of the historian John Spagnolo.[33]

Ford Robertson's Vision

For twelve years, Ford Robertson had worked as director of the West of Scotland Neuro-Psychiatric Research Institute, which served a dozen mental hospitals in and around Glasgow. He had also gained practical administrative experience at St. Andrew's Hospital in Northampton, England. He served as a member of ʿAṣfūriyyeh's LGC for nearly five years, and during this time, he acquired detailed knowledge of the Hospital—enhanced by a visit there in 1947.

Like the wife of ʿAṣfūriyyeh's founder, Robertson's wife was also invested in the work of the Hospital. As the daughter of a medical superintendent, she was familiar with life in a mental hospital, and she shared her husband's "sense of vocation in this pioneer work for the Near East."[34] Remarkably, this vocation was devoid of any reference to Christianity or missionary motives.

Ford Robertson believed that teaching and training were necessary before psychiatric knowledge could expand to the "home, the school and the hospital," key sites of the mental-hygiene strategy of which he was a fervent advocate.[35]

The School of Psychiatric Nursing, which opened in 1948, managed to attract eighteen students (ten women and eight men) in its first year and eighteen others the following year, with its numbers fluctuating between thirty and fifty students over the years. The majority were Lebanese, though many Palestinians, some Syrians, and a few East Africans also enrolled.[36] Students from neighboring countries started to be sent to the school through fellowships funded by the World Health Organization (WHO). The first three to come to ʿAṣfūriyyeh in 1953 were Sudanese women.[37]

More nursing students were also trained through collaboration with the School of Nursing at the AUB. (Founded in 1905, the school is the oldest of its type in the Middle East.[38]) A three-month course of lectures in mental health nursing for AUB nursing students had been in place since 1948, with further training in psychiatric nursing provided through either a two-month internship for graduates of AUB's School of Nursing or a one-year intensive course for graduates in general nursing from other Middle Eastern countries.[39] The WHO subsequently had specialized personnel trained at ʿAṣfūriyyeh to serve in the Eastern Mediterranean region. Students from all over East and North Africa and the Middle East attended the first session, in 1961.[40] By 1968, around eighty nurses, all trained at ʿAṣfūriyyeh, were working at the Kuwait Government Mental Hospital.[41] And by the 1970s, qualified psychiatric nursing graduates were staffing the nursing facilities of various Arab countries, including Iraq, Syria, Saudi Arabia, Jordan, Qatar, Kuwait, Bahrain, and Palestine.[42]

Manugian—the last medical director, to whom we will return below—had served as an expert member of the WHO since 1958. Like his predecessors, he also advised many neighboring nations (from the Gulf countries to those in the Horn of Africa) on their mental health strategies.[43] British officials repeatedly highlighted this recognition by the WHO and the status of ʿAṣfūriyyeh as a center of expertise in the Eastern Mediterranean region as a strong reason to continue supporting the institution financially over the years.[44]

The expansion of ʿAṣfūriyyeh's teaching activities also included AUB medical students, who had been regularly attending clinical demonstrations at the Hospital since 1926 (as mentioned in chapter 2). Ford Robertson became an associate professor of psychiatry at AUB in 1950.[45] By then medical students had a full curriculum from their first to their fifth years. First-year students were given a course on "normal psychology," second-year students an introduction to "abnormal psychology" and exposure to clinical demonstrations, third-year students were introduced to clinical psychiatry, fourth-year students spent a one month clinical clerkship at ʿAṣfūriyyeh, and fifth-year students had the option of doing a two-month elective internship on the premises of ʿAṣfūriyyeh with consultations at the AUB outpatient neuropsychiatric clinic mentioned below. During the period 1951–1952, six interns were given the opportunity to train at ʿAṣfūriyyeh. The Hospital's medical director was proud of this achievement in medical education. At the time, only a few universities in North America had this kind of full curriculum, and "none so far in Great Britain," according to him.[46]

Under Ford Robertson, the Hospital witnessed its largest financial surplus to date. It was growing steadily, with 415 patients in residence at its peak (the limit at the time was 420 patients).[47] More importantly, the Hospital saw an increase in the number of private patients—the main source of revenue to cover the costs of poor patients and to compensate for the inadequate payments of the assistance publique. The director reported a general increase in confidence and better social and recreational facilities. A social club for staff and patients was also developed, and a Ladies Auxiliary Guild was organized.[48]

The Ladies Guild of Help had been in existence since 1947, when the Ladies Committee, a group of notable women, had met at Mrs. Ford Robertson's home to organize themselves into a guild.[49] In turn, the Ladies Committee had been active since 1913, when the wife of Watson Smith—along Mrs. Baumkamp (the head attendant's wife), the Matron Miss Gibb, and "Sitt" (Arabic for Lady) Helene (a local woman who has been responsible for a long time for the sewing room and the laundry at 'Aṣfūriyyeh) started a Dorcas Society that provided garments for the poorer patients.[50] This group of women had been offering essential financial assistance throughout the history of the Hospital.

As part of the extramural strategy of spreading mental hygiene, neuropsychiatric clinics were established at four key strategic locations to cover the broadest swath of the population: two were opened in 1947, one at 'Aṣfūriyyeh (in Mount Lebanon) and one at AUB; and two more in 1957, one in Sidon (south Lebanon) and one in Tripoli (north Lebanon).[51] In addition, a "forensic unit" dedicated to the care of prisoners who suffered from mental illness was created in the early 1960s, following the Lebanese authorities' wish to create a program for the rehabilitation of prisoners and drug addicts.[52]

The aim was to provide expert advice and treatment, follow up on patients who had been discharged from the Hospital, and above all to raise awareness about mental illness in an attempt to destigmatize it. As the LGC reported, "The Beirut Committee believed a consulting clinic in the town would be very useful and would pay well.... It was unitedly felt that an immediate start should be made with this most necessary work, which ought not only to bring patients and funds to the Hospital but help in changing the outlook towards nervous breakdowns in general and Asfuriyeh in particular."[53] The aim in the 1950s thus moved from propagating what Bayard Dodge, president of AUB from 1923 to 1948, called the "gospel of the modern care of the insane"[54] (characteristic of the late nineteenth and early twentieth centuries) to one of prevention and early diagnosis.

Rather than resisting such sites of psychiatric proselytism (as some have suggested),[55] the public appeared to readily embrace these new forms of expertise and approaches to mental afflictions. The neuropsychiatric clinics were increasingly popular, as reflected by the impressively large turnover of patients over the years. Between 1949 and 1956, for example, one clinic in Beirut had between two thousand and three thousand consultations and between six hundred and almost nine hundred new cases per year.[56] Demand for neuropsychiatric clinics was increasing, Manugian suggested, because of the "growing cosmopolitan population and the increased stress and maladjustment to life."[57] People were increasingly visiting these clinics for personal and interpersonal counseling. It seems that both the "psychologization" of ordinary life and the conversion of the locals—especially those who lived in urban settings—to the gospel of the modern care of insanity were finally at work.

The neuropsychiatric clinics were part of the preventive strategy of the mental hygiene aspect of psychiatry, which Ford Robertson argued was an essential component of psychiatric practice.[58] As part of this strategy and the new way of understanding psychiatric burdens, students were invited to live on the premises of the Hospital to gain knowledge of mental illness and become able to act appropriately when faced with mental health issues in the community.[59] Under Ford Robertson's supervision, a new unit for nervous disorders called the Lebanon House was also built.[60] Indeed, it was during his directorship that the name of the Hospital was changed to the Lebanon Hospital for Mental and Nervous Disorders, though Robertson preferred the term "nervous" to "mental"—believing that the former covered "all mental and nervous troubles."[61] The new name of the Hospital was thought to be more hopeful, "one with wider scope for dealing with those early and slight cases for whom some provision has long been needed."[62] After all, as Ford Robertson wrote in his medical report for 1950, a name change was necessary because the old one had become loaded with pejorative connotations: "just as the word 'Bedlam' became synonymous with insanity in Britain, so has 'Asfuriyeh' in the Middle East."[63]

In 1950, after a visit by the minister of health and other high-level officials, who were impressed by ʿAṣfūriyyeh's modern facilities, about fifty patients were transferred from Dayr al-Ṣalīb to ʿAṣfūriyyeh.[64] The committee members decided not to interfere to avoid suspicion that ʿAṣfūriyyeh was taking patients away from Dayr al-Ṣalīb.[65] This was deemed a delicate matter, with the possibility that whatever was done would be misconstrued. Ibrahim Khairallah, a member of the BEC, suggested that they should "let the good deeds speak for themselves." He agreed with Joseph Hitti, the BEC's chairman, on the need to "avoid any friction with existing institutions" while maintaining close contact with the municipality of Beirut, which had a monopoly on triaging patients whose care was covered by the government.[66] Hitti suggested that ʻAṣfūriyyeh should concentrate on providing care for the new patients that it "was best fitted to treat."[67] In the end, the committee members stressed the complementarity of ʻAṣfūriyyeh and Dayr al-Ṣalīb.

At the jubilee celebrations of the Hospital that same year, Ford Robertson was awarded the Gold Medal of Merit from the first president of the Lebanese republic, Bechara el-Khoury, and in the following year, he received the Order of the Star of Jordan for civil services.[68] His wife received Lebanon's Gold Medal of Merit for her services in connection with the Ladies Guild a few years later.[69] Perhaps Ford Robertson's greatest (and final) achievement was to succeed in making the Royal Medico-Psychological Association recognize ʻAṣfūriyyeh as a training center for the prestigious DPM in 1956, for this was a sign of international legitimacy.[70]

Franco-American Rivalry

Foreign aid became a new weapon in the aftermath of the Second World War and its devastating economic consequences. The Cold War period saw an increased fear of communism, the rise of nationalism and pan-Islamism, and impending decolonization. Now the two influences that most threatened French interests were what the French ambassador in Beirut, Louis Roché, called "Americanism" (or Anglo-Saxon influence, with all the values it carried, such as individualism, materialism, and laissez-faire economics) and Arab nationalism or pan-Islamism.[71]

Postwar France was clearly in a disadvantaged position: it suffered from budgetary cuts and was unable to use foreign aid as a diplomatic weapon in the same way that the United States did.[72] Roché complained of disparities in aid that were not to the advantage of France.[73] The decision to grant significant funding through President Harry Truman's Point Four Program (a program of economic assistance to developing and underdeveloped countries)[74] to AUB rather than to the USJ vexed the French.[75] It also angered the Vatican, which in 1951 still considered AUB to be a Protestant missionary establishment.[76] Even the French chargé d'affaires still believed a few years later that AUB was anti-Catholic, echoing a sentiment that could be traced back to at least the nineteenth century (as we saw in chapter 2).[77]

The first Lebanese psychiatrist to teach the discipline at the Jesuit FFM in Beirut was Henri Ayoub. He was appointed in 1951, a year after Abūna Yaʻqūb's monastery had become a proper hospital that was recognized by the ministry of health as the Hôpital Psychiatrique de la Croix (Psychiatric Hospital of the Cross).[78] Ayoub, who would go on to pursue further studies in neuropsychiatry in Paris after graduating from the FFM, had assisted the doctor who occasionally provided medical consultations at Dayr al-Ṣalīb.[79]

It was the minister of health—Elias Khoury, who had visited ʿAṣfūriyyeh several times and was a graduate of the FFM—who advised Abūna Yaʿqūb in the 1950s to transform the monastery into a proper modern hospital that would specialize in nervous diseases as a way to compete with its rival, ʿAṣfūriyyeh (figure 3.2).[80] Mere altruism and charitable care were no longer enough to legitimize the care of those who were deemed to be insane. The

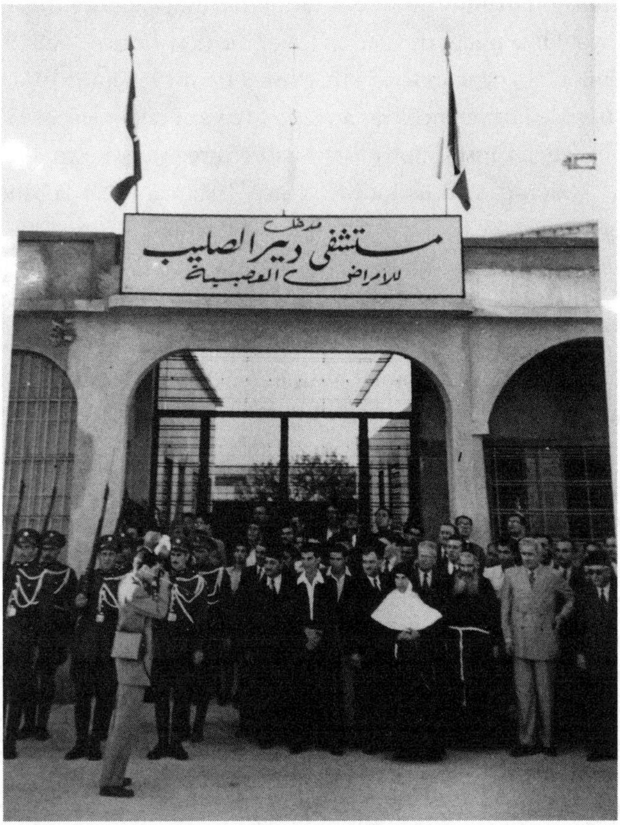

Figure 3.2
Inauguration of the Hôpital Psychiatrique de la Croix, November 13, 1951.
Source: Liban, Père Jacques, sous-dossier 3, côte: 685.13 Z54, ACF.

monastery had to modernize and transform itself into a proper hospital if it hoped to continue competing with ʿAṣfūriyyeh (a prospect that worried the Hospital's committees).[81] The "heathens" seem to have been converted to the "gospel of science,"[82] just as the intellectual elite of the Nahḍa had hoped a century earlier (see chapter 1).

In the 1950s, at the height of nationalism and pan-Islamism, Arabs and Islam became the new targets of French propaganda. The French became particularly alarmed when the Arab University was founded in Beirut, under the patronage of the Egyptian leader Colonel Gamal Abdel Nasser—an initiative they perceived to be politically motivated.[83] The French again became worried when in 1960 the Pan-Arab Congress of Medicine in Beirut adopted a recommendation to unify medical education in the Arab countries (a unification that would be under the patronage of the new United Arab Republic, a political union of Egypt and Syria that lasted from 1958 until 1961).[84]

What troubled the French was an earlier wave of nationalization and confiscation of French institutions that had occurred in Syria in 1945, a year before the nation gained its independence.[85] The fact that Lebanon had a much larger and more powerful Christian population reassured the French.[86] Nevertheless, they realized that AUB was better than USJ at attracting Muslims and other citizens of Arab countries. This was precisely what gave AUB strength, since its alumni were dispersed across the Middle East and often held influential positions—something the French regarded with much envy.[87]

In the postcolonial period that was beginning, it was urgent to find new "modes of influence," Roché wrote in a dispatch in 1959.[88] For him, the presence of a modern French hospital in Lebanon was "the best and most durable instrument of our [French] prestige."[89] Medicine, according to Roché, offered the great advantage of at least the appearance of disinterest.[90] The need to renovate and modernize the Hôtel-Dieu Hospital (the teaching hospital of the FFM) became an urgent issue because of the American competition that continued to intensify over the years. Roché lamented the continued growth of AUB "at the expense of our prestige and influence."[91]

At the seventy-fifth anniversary of the FFM in 1958, Roché was extremely pleased to find a totally "converted" (pro-French) audience, and it became clear that the renovation of the Hôtel-Dieu was of vital importance to preserve and sanctify the role of Beirut as a relay station or bastion of French influence within the wider Middle East.[92] It was no longer a matter of propaganda, as it had been a century before. Now the new elite formed at USJ showed absolute solidarity and loyalty to their school (as could arguably be said about AUB graduates).[93] Roché wrote that the new aim was to provide "support to the pro-Western elements in this country who remain the most attached to France"—a group that, according to the French, was being threatened with the rise of pan-Arab and pan-Islamist allegiances.[94]

When the Beirut-based newspaper *Le Jour* published an article in 1965 referring to the AUB medical campus as the "largest medical complex in the Middle East," Roché lamented the delays in financing the Hôtel-Dieu Hospital: delays that he believed would have irreparable consequences for French influence in the country.[95]

Manugian's Dream

Although Manugian was appointed medical director only in 1962, he had been making managerial decisions since the late 1940s, and he had become deputy medical director in 1949 and physician superintendent in 1956. An energetic physician and an aspiring politician (he was a member of the Lebanese parliament, holding an Armenian seat from 1972 until 1992),[96] he saw his ambitious plan of transforming the psychiatric hospital of ʿAṣfūriyyeh into a psychiatric institute vanish during the breakdown of the state of Lebanon amid chaos, instability, and the rise of a sectarian war that devastated the country for fifteen years (1975–1990), as explored in chapter 5.[97]

Born in 1910 in Turkey, Manugian came to Lebanon in 1921, as so many Armenian families had done following the genocide of Armenians during the collapse of the Ottoman Empire.[98] He graduated from AUB with a medical degree in 1935 and joined ʿAṣfūriyyeh as an assistant physician in the same year. From 1938 to 1939, he went on leave to the United Kingdom to gain more experience in the treatment of schizophrenia. He served as a clinical assistant physician at the Maudsley Hospital in London for several months and received the DPM in 1939, following clinical training at the Royal Edinburgh Hospital—and he was hailed as the first physician in the Middle East to have earned the DPM.[99] He returned to ʿAṣfūriyyeh but in 1941 became a medical practitioner with the Mediterranean Expeditionary Force of the British army.[100] In 1945, then a major, Manugian was granted British naturalization, and in 1970 he was awarded the Order of the British Empire for services rendered to the British forces during the Second World War.[101]

In 1947, along with Garabed Aivazian, Manugian was made an assistant lecturer in psychiatry at AUB.[102] In the same year, when the position of medical director of 'Aṣfūriyyeh became vacant, Manugian—who had worked full time at the Hospital since 1935 and who had been described as "indefatigable, reliable and extremely capable"—was not chosen for the position because members of the local executive committee thought it "unwise to consider appointing any Armenian, however good, as head of the Hospital" at that time.[103] Manugian was appointed physician superintendent a decade later, following the retirement of Ford Robertson in 1956.

The aim in the 1950s was to transform 'Aṣfūriyyeh from a psychiatric hospital into a psychiatric institute that would provide mental health services and expert advice and focus on short-term treatment.[104] Such was the faith in the therapeutic and preventive (rather than custodial) function of the hospital that Manugian wrote in 1957 that in the near future, "the 'chronic' wards will be a thing of the past in this Hospital. In fact, we can almost think that they are a thing of the past."[105] For the mental hygiene movement to succeed, it had to infiltrate every sphere of daily life—from the home to the school and from the factory to the courts. These were the sites that Manugian mentioned in the mental health hygiene manifesto he coauthored in 1950 with Aivazian, another Lebanese-Armenian psychiatrist at 'Aṣfūriyyeh.[106] They were also the sites of a much broader and more global mental hygiene movement at work in the rest of the liberal industrialized world.[107] Of course, this optimism and faith in the new biological psychiatry cannot be understood outside the context of a global mental hygiene movement, a style of thinking that came into prominence, especially in the aftermath of the Second World War.[108] The mental hygiene movement would influence a generation of psychiatrists at 'Aṣfūriyyeh, including the veteran Manugian.[109]

After Manugian had successfully established neuropsychiatric and outpatient clinics, he recruited the Hospital's first social worker to specialize in mental health in 1955: Selwa Firr, who had recently received her certificate in mental health from the London School of Economics.[110] The new psychiatric social-service infrastructure, which aimed at educating both patients and their families, was to facilitate the reintegration of mental health patients into society as a way to combat their marginalization and stigmatization.[111]

The 1950s also marked the intensification of the Hospital's provision of various extramural activities in different social forums to reach every segment of society.[112] The Hospital offered public lectures on mental hygiene, while AUB, the Lebanese Red Cross, and other schools (such as Makassed and the National School) used ʿAṣfūriyyeh's outpatient clinics to train students in psychiatric nursing.[113] ʿAṣfūriyyeh was also avant-garde in its "open-door" policy, which it launched in 1948 to make contact with the community. It sent invitations to journalists and students from across the country to visit the Hospital; it even dedicated a "hospital day" to the general public;[114] and it initiated a Psychiatric Advising Center in 1958. Located in the Gulbenkian Infirmary of AUB, the new center was popular because of its respect for people's anonymity.[115]

The new "Psychiatric Institute," which Manugian proposed in 1957, was meant to embody the idea of a total and totalizing mental health strategy for the country and the region. In his 1957 report, Manugian wrote, "This is a much wider field, and one which affects different strata of the community ... [including] social welfare, resocialization, child guidance, industrial medicine, training of psychiatrists and psychiatric nurses, etc." He continued, "this is an opportunity to make Asfuriyeh an Institute from which psychiatric service in its fullest sense can be given, thereby putting at the disposal of the communities it serves the experience Asfuriyeh has gained during its fifty-seven years of existence. It is a new sphere of activity outside and within the boundaries of a mental hospital with particular stress upon the extramural activity."[116] For Manugian, the need for such an institute in the Middle East was as critical as the need for a mental hospital had been in 1896. The institute was meant to be not only a hospital for acute treatment but also a place where people from the fringes of society who had behavioral and psychological issues could be mended—particularly delinquents and the growing population of drug addicts. Manugian envisioned a revamped forensic unit for the rehabilitation of prisoners. Forensic psychiatry, he argued, was essential for teaching purposes, making a profit, and maintaining good relations with the government.[117] This was a marked shift from the time when making contact with prisoners was viewed as being part of the reformist and humanitarian mission of ʿAṣfūriyyeh.

Members of the LGC did not share Manugian's opinion, however. While they did acknowledge the positive contributions the existing Hospital's forensic unit had made toward what they referred to as "the overall economy of the Hospital," they also decided to plan the new hospital without such a unit, for they felt that the mere existence of a forensic unit would have deleterious effects on the care of the remaining patients and was therefore undesirable.[118] The economic argument took over, however, notwithstanding the Hospital's commitment to the Lebanese authorities to build a new forensic unit. (There was no other alternative in the country at that time, or indeed in the Arab world.)[119] The goal of building a modern and better equipped forensic unit was never realized, however, due to the civil war and the ultimate financial collapse of the Hospital.

Manugian had even thought of a name for this new psychiatric institute that "would help dissociate itself from 'Asfuriyeh,' 'Mental' even 'Psychiatric.'" That name was the ʿAramūn Clinic, ʿAramūn being the new site where the Hospital (or rather the Institute) would be situated.[120] The name ʿAṣfūriyyeh had become too stigmatizing.[121] In addition, the institute's purpose was to focus on short-term or acute cases and hence Manugian envisaged sending all of the chronic patients elsewhere, for their management was becoming counterproductive. The "dead which cannot be buried" as Cornelius Van Dyck called them eight decades earlier (see Introduction) were no longer the worry or concern of the new preventive mode of thinking in psychiatry. Instead, they were the victims of a world that was becoming too demanding, hectic, and nerve-racking. These victims demanded immediate attention and management. In the new institute, the patients were not likely to stay more than a few months. The committee finally adopted the name the Lebanon Psychiatric Institute in 1976.[122]

Manugian's grand plans were destabilized by problems, complications, and challenges—the most unexpected and serious of which was the civil war that erupted in 1975. But even before the start of the war, the sociopolitical climate of the late 1960s had been tense for several reasons. These years of social crisis were marked by frequent strikes over increasing inequalities, the rising cost of living, a patronage system that privileged the few, and various political disturbances following the Six-Day War between Israel and its neighbors.[123]

The internal climate of the Hospital was also disrupted by internal power struggles, shifting political allegiances, and strikes by trade unionists and the syndicate of workers who were employed at ʿAṣfūriyyeh.[124] Manugian was generally perceived to be a very poor administrator, albeit an excellent psychiatrist.[125] P. W. Dill-Russell—the deputy medical adviser of the ODM, who had visited ʿAṣfūriyyeh in 1964—reported in his 1967 report a "deterioration in staff relations" since his last visit that was now compromising patient care.[126] This had to do with the fact that Dr. Haikal—the assistant director—was now controlling the Hospital, since he was more popular than Manugian among the staff.[127] Dill-Russell even suggested a possible "Armenian-Lebanese" conflict of interests between the medical director and the assistant director.[128]

Opinions on the cause of the deterioration of ʿAṣfūriyyeh differed, however. The British ambassador in Beirut, who served as ex officio president of the BEC, instead blamed ʿAṣfūriyyeh's ossified Victorian foundations. Dill-Russell found this argument implausible, retorting that many institutions in the country still provided excellent public services despite their obsolete foundations. Rather, the deterioration in the care of patients had to do, he believed, with the "antipathy" between the medical director and his deputy, and thus to the divided loyalties among the staff.[129] In 1969, the London committee appointed a new administrator under the British Technical Assistance Programme to resolve the issue and help plan the next stage.[130] Meanwhile, Manugian dismissed Haikal.[131]

On September 22, 1966, Hitti flew to London to discuss with the LGC the idea of selling ʿAṣfūriyyeh and building a more modern hospital on a new site.[132] Two years later, discussions were held with the Jesuits, who were interested in buying the land. Of course, it was no coincidence that the Jesuits seemed to have coveted all of the sites related to AUB. This was part of a long and continuous competition over epistemic and ideological influence. Nevertheless, the Jesuits' offer was deemed insufficient, and the plan fell through.[133]

In March 1973, after a short visit to Lebanon, Sir Geoffrey Furlonge, chairman of the LGC, signed a contract for the sale of the entire site of ʿAṣfūriyyeh and authorized the purchase of the land in ʿAramūn. According to Manugian, this was "an area of sectarian homogeneity": geopolitics, it should be remembered, had been a constant concern ever since the foundation of the Hospital.[134] Gefinor, a well-known investment firm, was contracted to build the new hospital, but the firm also ended up buying ʿAṣfūriyyeh's land for LBP 12.7 million.[135]

The new site at ʿAramūn was bought for LBP 12.7 million, and it was generally hoped that the new hospital would cost no more than around LBP 9.5 million, so that a sum would still remain for an endowment fund.[136] A groundbreaking ceremony on April 25, 1974, was attended by around three hundred people, including the minister of health (representing the Lebanese president, Suleiman Frangieh), the British ambassador, and the chairmen of the Beirut and London committees. An inscribed

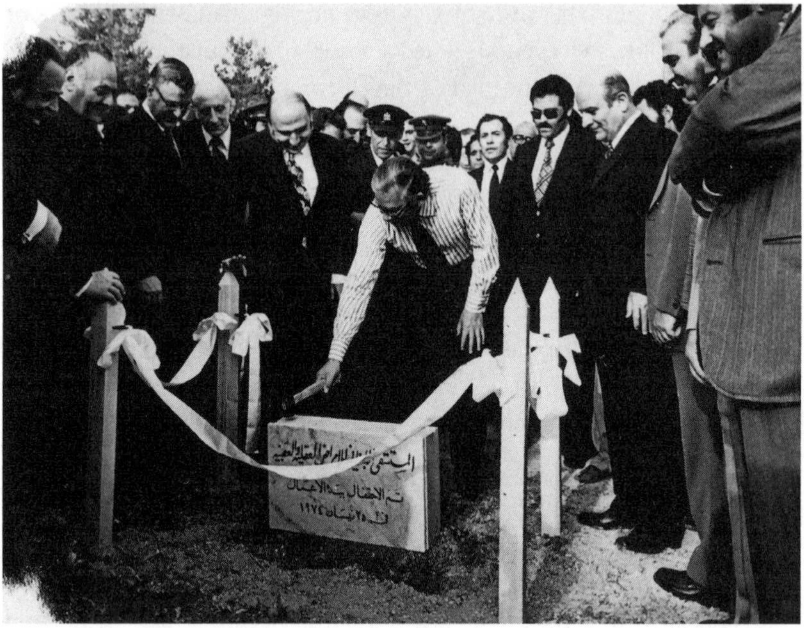

Figure 3.3
Groundbreaking ceremony in ʿAramūn, April 25, 1974.
Source: LH/11/03, box 16, LH, SOAS.

marble commemorative slab was placed during the ceremony (figure 3.3), and a cedar, the symbol of the nation's resilience, was planted.[137] Earlier that day, Furlonge—accompanied by the British ambassador, Raif Nassif (chairman of the BEC), and Manugian—had met with President Frangieh to show him an architectural model of the new hospital. The president then gave a luncheon party to celebrate this new milestone in the history of what had become a national institution.[138] In 1974 Manugian was able to confidently and optimistically write, "We are now at the threshold of a new area in the history of the Lebanon Hospital for Mental and Nervous Disorders. In fact it is a continuity of the mission of our hospital which has been pioneering in introducing the new developments in therapy, in architecture and in organisation."[139] A year later, however, two events that followed several months of bombings, assassinations, and other political troubles would plunge the country into an infernal civil war that would last for fifteen years.

On April 13, 1975, shots were fired from a car that killed a number of people during the consecration ceremony for a new Maronite church in ʿAyn al-Rummāna that was attended by Pierre Gemayel, leader of the Kataeb (Christian) party. A few hours later, Kataeb militiamen retaliated by massacring all the Palestinian passengers on a bus returning to the Palestinian refugee camp of Tall al-Zaʿtar from a commando parade in Beirut.[140] The events that followed plunged the country into darkness, chaos, and violence, with ʿAṣfūriyyeh caught between the different militias and political factions. This war delivered the coup de grâce to an institution that, perhaps miraculously, had managed to survive two world wars.

Conclusion

As this chapter has shown, ʿAṣfūriyyeh's mission, aims, and even character changed over time: from a home for forsaken and impoverished lunatics, it became a place for all the victims of modernization and civilization. Although the founding of ʿAṣfūriyyeh had initially been motivated by missionary zeal, the religious and missionary fervor quickly subsided with the general medicalization of the psychiatric discourse and the increasing number of people who sought services at ʿAṣfūriyyeh or its neuropsychiatric clinics. Indeed, the Hospital now represented this new modernist and positivist discourse of managing and treating mental pathology in a postcolonial world. Many medical doctors who had trained at ʿAṣfūriyyeh joined the ranks of the Hospital during their professional lives as professors of psychiatry and consulting physicians, sometimes taking over the directorship in the absence of the British medical director.[141] Some of these medical students ended up becoming influential psychiatrists elsewhere in the Middle East and beyond. For example, Abdul Rahman Labban, an AUB graduate (who is mentioned in chapters 5 and 6), served as a consultant to the Kuwaitis and Jordanians on mental health issues before he became Lebanon's minister of labor and social affairs in 1980.[142] Fuad Antun, an Iraqi medical doctor who had also graduated from AUB and trained and worked at ʿAṣfūriyyeh, became the head of the mental health program in Qatar in 1989.[143] Many more were trained in psychiatric nursing and later staffed major hospitals in the Arab world and East Africa.

The Hospital's character further shifted from a Protestant and British institution to a national institution (especially during the rise of the

Republic of Lebanon) and then one with regional expertise, producing a new breed of mind experts and influencing the framework of mental health policy from Palestine to the Gulf states.

To discount the agency of all those who contributed to the successes and failures of the Hospital in shaping these various agendas of modernity would be to distort the history of the complex professional and epistemological networks that were produced through ʿAṣfūriyyeh, which went beyond the narrow scale of colonialism or missionary work. After all, this was not the first time that the region had been colonized: empires have risen and fallen in this part of the world for millennia.

4 Patriarchal Power and the Gospel of the Modern Care of Insanity

> The relatives of hundreds of patients will spread the gospel of modern care for the insane in many parts of the Near East.
>
> —Bayard Dodge, Annual Report, Lebanon Hospital for Mental and Nervous Disorders

What did the "gospel of the modern care for the insane," as AUB president Bayard Dodge called it, consist of?[1] And who were its recipients? Where did they come from? Who brought them to ʿAṣfūriyyeh? What kind of pathologies did they suffer from? Were they coerced or treated voluntarily? And did they ever manage to get out of ʿAṣfūriyyeh? These are some of the questions that this chapter is concerned with.

It is difficult to describe any psychiatric patient population with a high degree of accuracy. Not only do diagnostic categories change over the years (indeed, each diagnosis has its own history), making comparative analyses problematic, but also in the case of ʿAṣfūriyyeh, the statistical data is sometimes incomplete. Yet despite these limitations, it is possible to form a reasonable map of major trends and shifts in the topography of mental illness.

Except for the emblematic case of Mayy Ziyādah—the famous poet whose hospitalization at ʿAṣfūriyyeh in the 1930s caused the first public outcry against involuntary incarcerations—and a few sporadic letters written by patients and other artifacts (such as an impressive collection of individual portraits of patients),[2] the patients' voices, personal narratives, and singular stories are buried in medical dossiers under the "tyranny" of their diagnosis.[3] To compensate for what Michel de Certeau calls "the discourse of the absent (*le discours de l'absent*),"[4] I have opted to use aggregate data as an indicator of mutations in mental disorders. Having a topography of mental pathologies over a long period of time (from 1900 through the 1970s), gives us a picture—even if just an impressionistic one—of the trends in mental illness and their relation to the various sociopolitical and economic changes, as well as allowing us to identify the ways in which mental afflictions were discerned (after all, diagnose, from the Greek *diagignōskein*, means to discern or distinguish) and the therapeutics that were deployed to treat them.

Notwithstanding the constantly changing names and causes of the various mental afflictions examined in this chapter, there are a few constants: the gendered distribution of mental disorders, the stigmatization of mental illness despite increasing demands for psychiatric services (which might seem paradoxical), and the impact of war and instability (social, political, and economic) on the phenomenology and prevalence of many psychosomatic ailments.

These trends in many ways reflect similar patterns in other contexts, but there are also a few glaring differences. First, at the level of the psychiatric discourse, an interesting shift is noteworthy. Whereas in the nineteenth century, oriental minds were widely considered to be more primitive than their Western counterparts (as we saw in chapter 1), in the twentieth century, they had become equal in their pathologies—thus, patients in both groups could be classified and analyzed using the same statistical and nosological grids. This is why, just as the lunatic asylum's socialization of the insane can be seen not necessarily as a means of social exclusion (as argued by Michel Foucault and others mentioned in the introduction) but as part of the French Revolution's inclusionary moment, considering the insane to be equal social actors who are potentially salvageable and amenable to social relevance,[5] one can similarily argue that the naturalization (biologization or medicalization) of mental illness inadvertently "democratized" minds of people from different religious and ethnic backgrounds.

Second, in contrast to many Western mental hospitals, at ʿAṣfūriyyeh until the mid-twentieth century, the majority of the patients admitted were active members of society. They had jobs, and most belonged to the working or middle class. In other words, they were able-bodied rather than dysfunctional and disabled individuals. Indeed, through selection bias upon admission and because of increased discharges, the medical directors avoided—albeit with great difficulty—turning ʿAṣfūriyyeh into a storehouse for the chronically ill. Therefore, many patients had to be turned away, for this was supposed to be a hospital and not a hospice; a place of cure, not one of internment and incarceration. In addition, male patients consistently outnumbered female patients, which is another reflection of sociocultural specificities according to which the family and the patriarchy play a conspicuous and determining role in triaging who gets to be sent for treatment.

Finally, three peaks are notable in patient admissions throughout the history of the Hospital, which reflect the wider sociopolitical context. Two were related to the First and Second World Wars, and the third occurred during a period of economic growth and prosperity in the 1950s and 1960s. This last period was marked by problems related to substance use—a consequence of the laissez-faire approach to the growing narcotic market that the fledgling Lebanese republic chose to pursue at that time.

While chapter 3 pointed to a decline in missionary fervor concomitant with an institutionalization of modern psychiatric practice, this chapter will show how it was the relatives of the mentally ill who in the end played a key role in not only propagating the new ways of understanding and demystifying mental illness but also (perhaps inadvertently) in reinforcing psychiatric power.

Paths into the Asylum

As we saw in chapter 1, it was almost unanimously believed in the nineteenth century that insanity was not prevalent in the Orient. Yet when the Hospital opened its doors in 1900, we are told that patients flocked in. "The presence and demand for admission is so great," noted the Quaker missionary and founder of ʿAṣfūriyyeh, "that we are obliged to refuse many."[6] For Otto Wolff, ʿAṣfūriyyeh's first medical superintendent, the causes for admission included domestic grief, poverty, untreated malaria, idleness, inbreeding, licentious living (among the rich), and emigration to "America and other places."[7]

Poverty, Neglect, Religiosity, and Violence

As Theophilus Waldmeier reminds his readers, the Hospital's original aim was to be a refuge for "those maltreated 'dead who cannot be buried' whose condition and brutal treatment defies description."[8] Indeed, the first patient taken in, on August 8, 1900, was a sixteen-year-old silk spinner named Wardiyyeh from the village of ʿAbadiyyeh, in Mount Lebanon. The cause of her insanity was said to be maltreatment. Waldmeier wrote: "She had been bound with iron chains and put in a dungeon, she had torn her clothes and her head was full of filth, and her body one mass of wounds and bruises, she was excited and beat everyone who came near her and she made a fearful noise and was more like an animal than a human being."[9] Seventeen other patients arrived in August 1900. Many suffered from emotional distress (the causes that were mentioned included maltreatment, grief, and unhappy marriages) and some from "religious excess," while still others suffered simply from poor socioeconomic conditions.[10]

While "religious insanity" had been described in the travel literature in the nineteenth century in the context of the figure of the wise fool (see chapter 1), "religious excess" was used in the records of the Hospital as an explanation for symptoms of religious grandiosity (a delusional belief in prophecy or religious power, for instance). Such was the case of B. H., a medical student admitted in 1900 with the diagnosis of "dementia praecox" caused by "religious excess."[11]

However, the clergy might also have used excessive religiosity as a way to dismiss any rebellious act that challenged religious dogma and authority. Asʿad al-Shidyaq, the first convert to Protestantism in the Near East and its first martyr is a case in point. Al-Shidyaq, an Arabic instructor, was accused of heresy and persecuted to death by the Maronite Patriarch Yusuf Hubaysh for daring to convert to the Protestant faith. He was declared *majnūn* (crazy) and perished after being tortured, chained, and abandoned in a cave in the Holy Valley (Wadi Qadisha), not far from the Monastery of Qoṣhayya (mentioned in chapter 1).[12] Waldmeier was very much aware of al-Shidyaq's tragic story, which he retold in his 1886 autobiography.[13]

While "religious insanity" might have been an excuse to dispose of al-Shidyaq, Paul, a Maronite priest (or *Būlūs al-khūry*, as he was called in Arabic), suffered from "manic-depressive insanity."[14] Unlike his predecessor Patriarch Hubaysh and in contrast to earlier ways of dealing with mental symptoms as demonic possession (see chapter 1), the Maronite Patriarch Elias Butrus Huwayek decided to send Paul and a number of Maronite preachers for treatment at ʿAṣfūriyyeh—a hospital that many Catholic missionaries considered to be a Protestant institution and thus proselytizing and to be avoided at all costs.[15] The times had clearly changed from 1830, the date of the tragic death of al-Shidyaq, to this point, in 1903. A visitor at

ʿAṣfūriyyeh recalled looking through a door and seeing Paul, noting "the terrible sight of a big, strong man lying quite naked in a heap of hygienic straw in the corner of a room. His shouting of disjointed fragments of prayers still seems to sound in my ear."[16] We do not know if the cause of Paul's insanity was excessive religiosity ("the cause of illness" in the patient records is blank). In any case, he seemed to have made a remarkable recovery, for he was discharged as cured six months later. The patriarch sent a letter of appreciation to the Hospital, grateful for the "wise treatment of the physician."[17] This is how Paul became the poster child of ʿAṣfūriyyeh's growing success and acceptance among the locals.

In his first medical report, Wolff wrote that a hundred chronic cases had been brought to him for consultation. This was a land, he wrote, where a great number of chronic cases were caused by neglect and maltreatment.[18] Many came with what he referred to as the stigma of violence marked on their frail bodies: cauterized heads and iron chains.[19]

Ever since the early days of the Hospital, the poor were treated free of charge, following a suggestion initially made by Cornelius Van Dyck, a medical missionary who served on the first executive committee of ʿAṣfūriyyeh.[20] But this service could not be sustained, despite the financial donations and funds allocated for that purpose. With the rise of a paying middle class and in the context of the financial struggles of the Hospital, the committee members decided that the wealthier patients would pay for the care of those who could not afford it. The idea came up in 1901 when the wife of an affluent merchant in Beirut sought assistance at the Hospital. The London committee hoped that this strategy "would open up the way for the better class of people to send their patients to the Hospital who by their fees may considerably reduce the cost of maintenance of those who cannot pay."[21] Private patients also helped improve the Hospital's reputation. The Hospital administrators saw the steady increase of private patients as indicating popular approval of and growing confidence in their institution.[22]

Interestingly, until the mid-twentieth century, patients who were active in the labor force always made up a greater share of the patient population than those who were jobless (68 percent versus 32 percent).[23] More than half of those who worked belonged to the middle or working class. More than a third were unskilled workers (peasants, laborers, and the like), artisans (such as tailors, shoemakers, carpenters, dyers, tanners, and weavers), or merchants (figure 4.1). Strikingly, 85 percent of the women did not work,

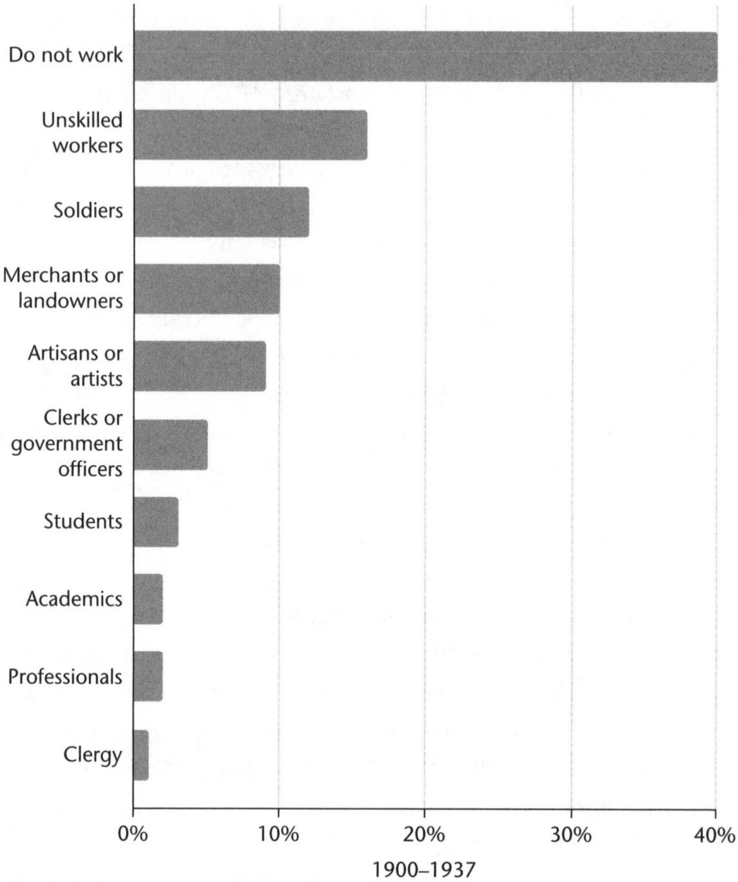

Figure 4.1
Percentage of patients admitted by profession, 1900–1937.
Source: Data compiled from ARs.

compared to only 18 percent of the men. This should come as no surprise, since men—as the main source of income in predominantly patriarchal societies, such as those found in the Middle East—sought care only when their illness seriously interfered with their productivity.[24] In other words, men's symptoms were tolerated until they became disabling.

Although the Hospital had been founded to serve the most vulnerable and neglected—the poorest of the poor—it quickly became obvious that chronic cases would defeat the original therapeutic purpose and make it impossible for the Hospital to survive financially. As Harry Thwaites, then the medical director, wrote in 1908, "Numbers of the hopeless class have been rejected owing partly to the fact that they are hopeless, and partly because they were unable to pay towards their maintenance."[25] Two decades later, his successor, Henry Watson Smith, admitted in the *British Journal of Psychiatry* that triage and "selection bias" upon admission was imperative to avoid overcrowding, thus turning the Hospital into a dumping place for the disabled.[26] Clearly, some patients had to be turned away, for this was supposed to be a therapeutic hospital and not a storehouse or a place of last resort.[27]

Emigration and Degeneration

As discussed in chapter 1, medical doctors in the late nineteenth century and even in the early twentieth century believed that civilization played a crucial part in the rise of madness. In line with the spirit of the time, the various medical directors of ʿAṣfūriyyeh believed that insanity was a tragic consequence of modernity. While they thought that what they called degeneration was the result of an inherent hereditary trait coupled with consanguineous marriages (which were frequent in the Middle East at the time), they also linked degeneration to civilizational forces.

Emigration to the New World became a major global social phenomenon in the late nineteenth and early twentieth centuries that dramatically affected the Levant, particularly *bilād al-shām*.[28] But it had such considerable social, economic, and political implications that the Inter-Departmental Committee on Physical Deterioration had to present a report to the British House of Commons in 1904 that discussed, among other matters, the correlation between emigration and insanity.[29] One of the committee's expert witnesses, a medical doctor from the University of Dublin named C. R. Browne, claimed that "the sound and the healthy—the young men and young women—from the rural districts emigrate to America in tremendous numbers, and it is only the more enterprising and the more active that go, as a rule." He concluded that "the less able bodied are left to reproduce themselves … and carry on the race."[30] Emigration was thus seen as a major cause of the decline or degeneration of the race.

Emigration as a cause of insanity—more specifically, the misfortunes of failed emigrants who had returned to the country penniless and desperate—was likewise a leitmotif in the records of the Hospital in the first decade of the twentieth century. Like Browne, Thwaites thought that emigration depleted the local population of its healthy stock, thus producing an "abnormal proportion of cases of mental degeneration."[31] Emigration was viewed as a source not only of the corruption of morals due to exposure to worldly vanities, but also of existential anxiety, nervous breakdowns, disillusionment, and hopelessness. The story is typically one of failed American dreams: "During the last thirty years or so more than 50,000 Syrians from Mount Lebanon and its plains have emigrated to America where they are mostly engaged in trade. Some get on well and gain much money, others have failed and lost what they had and have fallen into a destitute condition. Many of these Syrian emigrants have returned home to their country insane; for all they had done, seen, heard, and felt was too much for them, and some of them were brought as patients into our asylum in Asfuriyeh."[32] Indeed, among the first cases admitted to ʿAṣfūriyyeh in the early 1900s were emigrants who had returned to the country.[33] The reason that was provided as the cause of their insanity was the alienation resulting from the sophisticated way of life to which they had been exposed. As the *British Medical Journal* put it more explicitly, "in countries where life is more complex than in Syria they were exposed to a mental strain which they could not bear."[34]

Conversely, the lack of civilization was also believed to be a cause of mental degeneration. For Thwaites, the lack of exposure to more exciting forms of civilized life made weak-mindedness the most prominent type of mental disease due to "the secluded life ... [and] lack of education and development acting through many generations."[35] Particularly in rural areas, life was generally considered simple, unexciting, unintellectual, and uneventful.[36] To quote the *British Medical Journal* further, cases of acute mania were rare, "possibly due to the fact that the general life of the people is of an unexciting and primitive nature."[37]

There were other "degenerative" causes—such as malnutrition, misery, and general suffering—that caused mental afflictions.[38] For Thwaites, it was above all negligence and indifference that led to such chronic and untreatable forms of insanity.[39] As we saw in chapter 1, the oppressive socioeconomic and political climate of the region was widely deemed to stifle mental energy and thus lead to early forms of dementia. Thwaites agreed with this causal explanation of mental pathology: "In Syria, for generations the social conditions have been such as [to] obstruct the outlet of mental energy, with consequent damage to the producing machine; the impelling force, working from behind and demanding achievement in all directions, thus becomes weakened, and the country is stocked with an apathetic race, and the asylum with cases of dementia."[40] In the first decade of the twentieth century, dementia praecox (a term coined by Emil Kraepelin that was ultimately supplanted by schizophrenia)[41] accounted for the second most prevalent form of mental disorder in the Hospital, the first being the affective disorders: melancholia, depression, mania, and manic-depressive insanity (or alternating insanity).[42] For Thwaites, the abundance of early dementia—on average, 33.5 percent of male patients and 16.3 percent of females had this diagnosis each year in the period 1906–1908—was "a striking feature in the work of this asylum."[43] This was the case because, though dementia was found in a similar proportion of the US population (32.1 percent of all cases of insanity in the 1890 census), the rate was slightly higher among females there (32.23 percent) than among males (31.98 percent).[44] But then, there were more male than female patients at ʿAṣfūriyyeh.

Indeed, this was the case throughout the history of the Hospital (figure 4.2). The psychiatrist John Racy has suggested that the predominantly male patient population may have been due to a number of factors: a reluctance in patriarchal societies to expose women (which might bring shame),

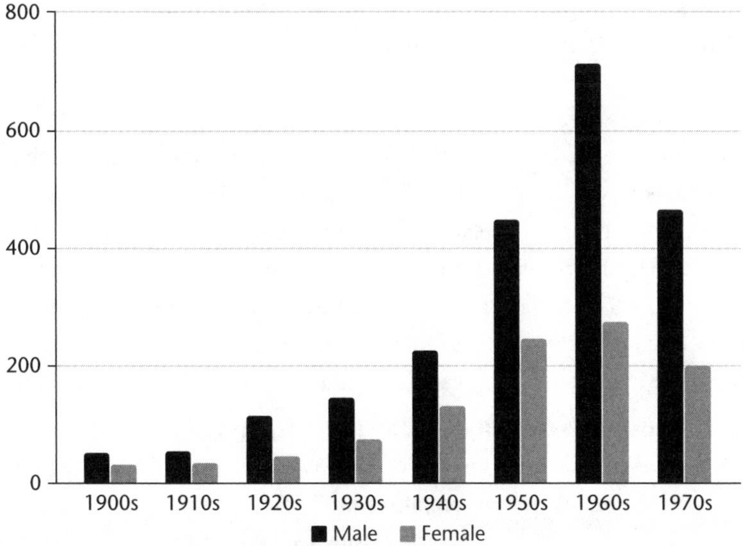

Figure 4.2

Average number of patients admitted by gender per decade using available years, 1900s–1970s.

Source: Data compiled from ARs.

the greater value attached to the well-being of males in such societies (which means they are higher-priority patients), or perhaps the belief that mentally disturbed men were a greater threat.[45] What is clear, according to Racy, is that this was not the case because mental illness was less common in women: studies have shown that the incidence of psychiatric symptomatology among females is at least as high as it is among males.[46]

While in the nineteenth century, the minds of the Orientals were widely considered incomparable to those of Westerners, by the beginning of the twentieth century, a globalization of the Western psyche was in the making. East and West appeared to be converging in terms of mental pathologies, and the same statistical grids and nosological categories were deployed to make sense of symptoms. Despite the fact that Thwaites believed in 1907 that "insanity in this country includes all the prominent European types and there is no type which is peculiarly Syrian," he still viewed it as peculiar to Syrian and similarly stifled minds that hereditary degeneration and early dementia far exceeded all other types of insanity.[47] Around 1910, however, the general view of the nature and incidence of mental illness began to shift in the direction of a universalization of mental ailments. Watson Smith, who succeeded Thwaites in 1909, was more assertive in his opinion than his predecessor. "Mental disease is mental disease all the world over," Watson Smith wrote.[48]

Male Maladies

Mental illness among the ʿAṣfūriyyeh patient population was distributed quite predictably along gender lines (see figure 4.3). While "puerperal insanity" and other childbirth-related psychoses were found exclusively among women and hysteria was predominantly believed to be a "female malady" (to borrow Elaine Showalter's memorable phrase),[49] there were exclusively male maladies: the psychopathic personality, war-related pathologies, and the so-called toxic insanities (specifically related to the use of drugs or alcohol).

The Psychopathic Personality By the time ʿAṣfūriyyeh opened its doors in 1900, the Ottoman Sanitation Act of 1876 was regulating the management of asylums as well as the incarceration process. As mentioned in chapter 3, the law was supposed to make admissions less arbitrary, more scientific, and better controlled by the Ottoman authorities.[50] The Ottoman governor of Mount Lebanon, Yusuf Pasha (ruled 1907–1912) seemed to value expert opinion on arbitrary incarcerations: "The Hospital at ʿAṣfūriyyeh is one of the most interesting and needful institutions of the country, and it does us

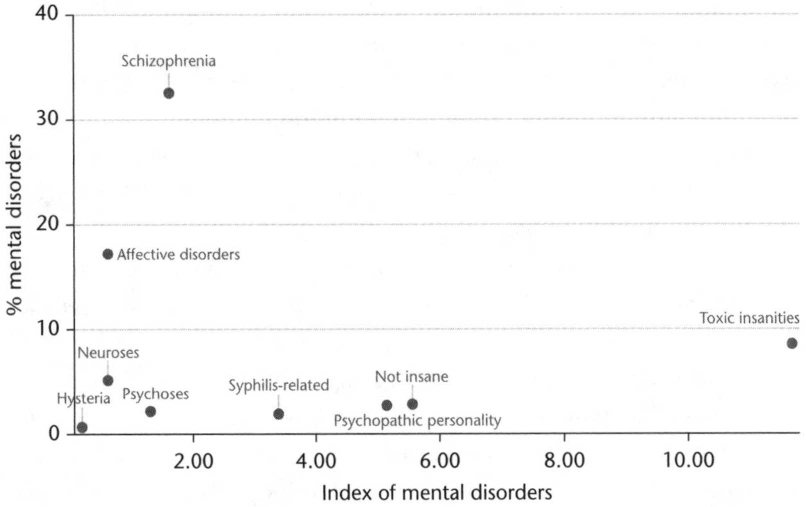

Figure 4.3
Ratio of male-to-female prevalence rates for the most prevalent mental disorders, 1900–1976 averages. When the ratio is 2, for example, the prevalence of the disease among males is twice that among females. When the ratio is 1, the prevalence is the same for both males and females.
Source: Data compiled from ARs.

a most necessary service as regards the criminal patients, whom we often send to your Asylum for examination and observation, and the Doctor's judgment is a sure guide to our Government for a final judgment. I will gladly do all in my power to be helpful to such a noble institution."[51]

In 1903, ʿAṣfūriyyeh received its first criminal case, a prisoner whom the local authorities had sent there to obtain an expert opinion on his sanity and mental soundness. The prisoner committed a criminal offense as the result of alcoholic intoxication.[52] This can be considered the moment when crime from an illicit act gets medicalized and transformed into an abnormal psychology that ought to be normalized and thus rehabilitated.[53]

Nevertheless, for the administrators and doctors at ʿAṣfūriyyeh, treating anyone who suffered from a mental disorder, including the criminally insane, was part of their humanitarian philosophy and mission. As the 1907 annual report put it, the "criminally insane" illustrated "one of the many directions in which the Hospital is of value to the country, and to those who, being irresponsible for their conduct, hardly merit the extreme measures dealt out to the ordinary criminal."[54]

For the ʿAṣfūriyyeh psychiatrist Garabed H. Aivazian, 1938 marked a change in the psychologization of crime and criminal behavior.[55] By this point, a team of psychiatrists rather than a single general practitioner was being appointed to assist courts in making decisions. As mentioned in chapter 3, ʿAṣfūriyyeh's medical superintendent, R. Stewart Miller, was consulted in the framing of the new criminal code (signed into law in 1943), which medicalized criminal insanity.

ʿAṣfūriyyeh's raison d'être had not necessarily shifted to the custodial care of the criminally insane. In fact, many of the prisoners who were sent for assessment or treatment were found to be not insane. In Aivazian's 1953 study of cases admitted to ʿAṣfūriyyeh during the period 1951–1953, 30 percent of the patients were found to have been discharged as "not insane," while the remainder were found to be mostly suffering from schizophrenia (about 22.0 percent) or to have a "psychopathic constitution" (18.5 percent).[56] In 1958, Vahé Puzantian (who had joined the Hospital a year earlier, as a full-time resident psychiatrist) began to visit prisons twice a week free of charge.[57] In 1961 the first unit for rehabilitating prisoners and drug addicts in the Middle East was opened at ʿAṣfūriyyeh, in part as a response to a request by the Lebanese authorities.[58] A report from the time predicted that this was "a venture with great potentialities with both scientific and national service value."[59]

Until the 1970s, ʿAṣfūriyyeh cooperated with the authorities and even initiated new policies that it believed were progressive and humane in the spirit of a mental hygiene strategy of reaching every sphere of society (including prisons). While in the 1960s and 1970s social activists, reformists, and critics in the West started to condemn asylums and psychiatric hospitals as incarcerating institutions,[60] ʿAṣfūriyyeh's role in the humanization and medicalization of criminal behavior and the nondiscriminatory treatment of prisoners and nonprisoners alike was widely considered by the locals and the medical elite to be liberal, visionary, and progressive.[61] This lack of critique of a growing psychiatric power is one of the striking contrasts between ʿAṣfūriyyeh's trajectory (and psychiatric practice more generally speaking in the Middle East) and the trajectory that psychiatric hospitals took in Europe and North America after the period of intense scrutiny and critique of psychiatric institutions in the 1960s and 1970s that led to their eventual demise.

War Psychopathologies The First World War and its aftermath spawned moribund conditions. *Seferberlik*, the Ottoman conscription, became remembered in the collective memory as a long journey (*safar*) across the land (*barr*) marked by famine, misery, and traumatic displacement.[62] Patients were brought to ʿAṣfūriyyeh starving and absolutely destitute. One woman who had been brought in nearly naked died at the gate of the Hospital before she could be admitted.[63] Many people suffered from dysentery and consumption, diseases of poverty and deprivation. The majority of the patients who were brought to the Hospital were insufficiently clothed or covered with vermin.[64]

In 1920, sixty-two soldiers, mostly from the Légion syrienne, were admitted for acute forms of mental illness.[65] The French Legion was multiethnic, composed of men from different colonies: Senegalese, Algerians, Egyptians, and Syrians. Some presented with the symptoms of shell shock—a term coined by British psychiatrists to describe a new condition that consisted of nervous exhaustion and other invisible wounds inflicted to the brain and nervous system that became visible on the battlefields of the First World War.[66] Several of the cases had to do with physical exhaustion, and some of these were associated with malaria-induced psychosis—which was to be expected, since malaria was endemic in the region.[67] A great number of soldiers from the French military were also brought in suffering from fatigue and strain following the multiple battles the French were fighting: against the Turks on the northern front of Syria and against the Arab rebels led by the sharif of Mecca in the east.[68] Upon their recovery, the French General Henri Gouraud sent a letter of appreciation to the medical director, as his British counterpart, General Edmund Henry Hynman Allenby, had done a few years earlier.[69]

Foreign and ailing troops occupied again ʿAṣfūriyyeh during the Second World War. At the onset of hostilities in September 1939, the British military sent 122 cases, most of whom were suffering from acute conditions. Some were also found to be "psychopathic" (39 percent), while 15 percent suffered from "exhaustion psychoses."[70] No real attempt was made to explain this tendency toward violence and psychopathy among the Allied soldiers. Miller, the medical director of ʿAṣfūriyyeh at the time, dismissed these men as "half mad, half bad—unhappy misfits of life."[71] The other notable diagnoses were alcoholic psychosis and weak-mindedness, each of which accounted for roughly 11 percent of the military cases. While one might have expected a high rate of syphilitic soldiers (as was the case in the American context),[72] such cases constituted only 6–7 percent of all military cases.

In 1941, the Free French Forces (*Forces françaises libres*) joined the British troops to oust the pro-Vichy forces that had taken over the administration of Syria and Lebanon concomitantly with the German occupation of France. This military operation came to be known as the Syria-Lebanon campaign. During the same year, the Australian forces and later the New Zealanders, both part of Great Britain's commonwealth army, were offered accommodation and treatment at ʿAṣfūriyyeh (figure 4.4).

The recollections of Frank Fenner, an Australian soldier who served as a physician at the 2/1 Casualty Clearing Station involved in the Syria-Lebanon campaign, are worth mentioning.[73] Fenner remembered that even in 1944 ʿAṣfūriyyeh was thought to be the "only mental hospital in the Middle East."[74] For someone who had traveled widely in the Middle East (including Jerusalem and Damascus), his glaring omission of both Ezrat Nashim and the Asile d'Avicenne de Damas is, if anything, an indication of the astonishing reputation ʿAṣfūriyyeh had attained. Fenner noted that the Australians had moved their field hospital from Nazareth (133 kilometers from Beirut) to ʿAṣfūriyyeh (about 20 kilometers east of Beirut) and remained there until the liberation of the land by the Allied forces six months later. He admitted that he felt "sympathy for the Palestinians ousted by the state of Israel,"[75] an exodus he witnessed firsthand. He also reminisced about befriending a microbiologist at ʿAṣfūriyyeh who worked at AUB and the Hitti family, which was involved in the Beirut-based committee of the Hospital.[76]

Another witness of the British occupation of ʿAṣfūriyyeh worth mentioning is the Palestinian physician Elias Srouji, who had studied at AUB and

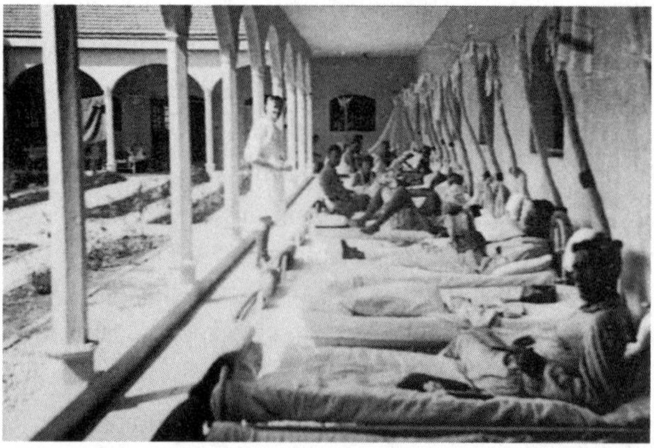

Figure 4.4
The courtyard of Webster House (built in 1937), occupied by the Australian army during the Syria-Lebanon campaign, 1941–1948.
Source: Photograph by Dorothy A. Vines, courtesy of the Australian War Memorial.

trained at ʿAṣfūriyyeh as a medical student in the 1940s. In his memoirs, he recalls the military physicians from the British Medical Corps lecturing on malaria and other tropical diseases. He also recalls how Sir Howard Florey, one of the discoverers of the effects of penicillin on war wounds, gave a lecture to a full auditorium at AUB during a visit to Beirut a year or two before he received the Nobel Prize in Medicine in 1945. Florey had been appointed Honorary Consultant in Pathology to the British Army and was at the time supervising the treatment of British Prime Minister Winston Churchill, who fell ill while on a visit to the British troops in North Africa.[77]

The Free French Forces also sent forty-eight soldiers for treatment at ʿAṣfūriyyeh.[78] Despite being reluctant to help what was widely considered to be a British institution (as we saw in chapter 2), the French continued to send their soldiers for treatment there, even after the opening of their own asylum in Damascus in 1923. By 1944, three hundred cases from the French military forces had been treated at ʿAṣfūriyyeh. The prevalent diagnostic category among French soldiers had shifted to alcoholic psychosis (36 percent), followed by schizophrenia (31 percent).[79] By 1946, the last year when the French military sent its affected soldiers to ʿAṣfūriyyeh, five hundred French soldiers had been treated and paid for.[80]

It is important to note that in contrast to the case in colonial asylum settings, such as India or Algeria, patients from the region were not separated from Europeans and other Westerners at ʿAṣfūriyyeh.[81] There were always a few Western patients (wives of missionaries, missionary workers, and the like) among the patient population, but most of these "foreign" patients mainly consisted of British and French soldiers recruited from colonized lands (Indians, Africans, and so on). Curiously either because they were not always numerous or because they were not considered fully "white" (as in the case of foreign troops), the question of separating "Westerners" from indigenous people was never raised. This is mere speculation, of course, but it is worth stressing the absence of such a concern at ʿAṣfūriyyeh. Other kinds of separations did exist, however, especially in terms of gender (women and men were separated), criminal history (those who had committed criminal acts were separated from those who had not), and state upon admission (those who were in an acute condition were separated from the chronic cases).

ʿAṣfūriyyeh also literally became a place of refuge, where distressed war refugees could seek assistance, shelter, and care. Armenian refugees from

Turkey were the first to arrive. In 1940, "some 20,000 Armenians fled from the Sandjak [of Alexandretta] when it was finally taken over by Turkey and were in camps scattered over Syria and Lebanon," and Miller, ʿAṣfūriyyeh's medical superintendent at the time, decided to welcome "the more urgent cases among them."[82] In 1944, the United Nations Relief and Rehabilitation Administration, in collaboration with British military forces, sent several refugees from Yugoslavia and Greece for treatment at ʿAṣfūriyyeh.[83] These refugees mostly suffered from schizophrenia and manic-depressive illnesses, though there were also cases of exhaustion psychosis and melancholia among them.[84] The following year, the Polish delegation of the government in exile sent fifteen patients.[85] More would follow suit. Among these could well have been Jewish Poles who had fled persecution and deportation following the invasion of Poland by the Nazis—especially considering that some of them were not mental patients but refugees seeking asylum.[86] From the onset of the Nakba (the Palestinian catastrophe following the creation of the State of Israel) in 1948 until the closure of the Hospital, it was now up to Palestinian refugees to seek mental refuge at ʿAṣfūriyyeh. Twenty-nine Palestinian refugees were admitted in 1948, and their number kept increasing with time—reaching eighty-three in 1960.[87]

When the Lebanese army was constituted in 1945 (two years after Lebanon was declared independent),[88] it started to send its affected soldiers to the Hospital, with the first cases being admitted in 1946.[89] In 1956, ʿAṣfūriyyeh's psychiatrists were asked to serve on the committee that selected candidates for the officer's training course of the Lebanese army.[90] Later, at the beginning of the civil war (as we will see in chapter 5), the premises of the Hospital were put at the disposal of the Syrian authorities so that they could be helped and advised on various psychiatric issues.[91] In 1977, the Hospital was occupied by the Arab Dissuasion (or Deterrent) Force, a peacekeeping army sent by the Arab League to put an end to the Lebanese civil war.[92] Even the new unfinished hospital in ʿAramūn was occupied for several weeks by the Israeli army during the invasion of Lebanon in the summer of 1982.[93]

Toxic Insanities As we saw in chapter 1, substance use is pervasive in the Orientalist literature on the pathogenesis of mental ailments, but the nature and scope of its related mental manifestations has changed dramatically over the years.

In 1907, alcohol became the second most common cause of mental illness (after heredity) at ʿAṣfūriyyeh. What could have accounted for the emergence of this new form of pathology, the so-called toxic insanities?[94] Although the region did not lack substances that could excite the nervous system—be it qat (*Catha edulis*) in Yemen, hashish (cannabis) in Egypt, hemp in Morocco, opium all over the Middle East, or wine—the Protestant missionaries blamed both the French for introducing absinthe and the locals for dramatically increasing the production of arrack (an alcoholic spirit).[95] In contrast to Thwaites—who, as mentioned above, tended to view people in rural areas as more prone to severe forms of mental degeneration—for Waldmeier it was the city that was the source of demoralization and degeneration, precisely because of the exposure cities provided to new and vicious habits, such as alcohol consumption.[96]

Initially behaviors that were only occasionally problematic, drug addiction and alcoholism became serious social problems starting in the 1950s (figure 4.5; table 4.1). This situation prompted the publication of several articles by two psychiatrists who had trained and worked at ʿAṣfūriyyeh, Herant Katchadourian and Vahé Puzantian, who highlighted the rise of what they believed to be a new socioeconomic scourge.[97] Cases of drug addiction, which were seven times as common as alcoholism at the Hospital, became

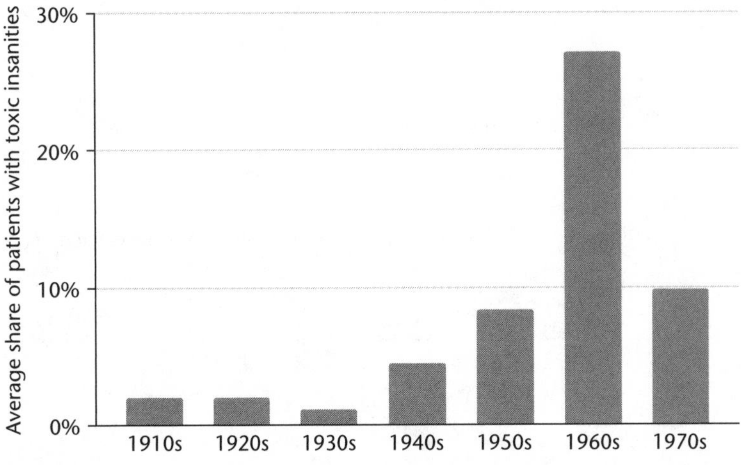

Figure 4.5
Average number of patients diagnosed with toxic insanity per decade using available data, 1900s–1970s.
Source: Data compiled from ARs.

almost sixteen times as common during the period 1958–1970 (table 4.2). A breakdown for 1959 shows that patients were mostly addicted to heroin, followed by morphine, opium, alcohol, and cannabis. The noticeable surge in admissions related to substance use during the 1950s and 1960s occurred during a period of economic growth, when Lebanon became known as the "Switzerland of the Middle East."[98] This was also the period when narcotic trafficking reached its apex.[99] This period should actually be considered a kind of Gilded Age, since underneath the socioeconomic prosperity were deep social divisions that threatened to throw the precarious republic into chaos.[100]

This period also coincided with a different trend in the nature of the patient population at the Hospital: for the first time in its history, the proportion of patients who did not work slightly exceeded those who did.[101]

This surge in substance use—coupled with increasing regional and international pressure, especially from Egypt, for which Lebanon was the main

Table 4.1
Gender distribution of toxic insanity diagnoses among patients, 1958–1962.

Year	Men	Women	% Men
1958	92	0	100
1959	241	8	97
1960	200	11	95
1961	276	11	96
1962	286	12	96

Source: Data compiled from ARs.

Table 4.2
Number of patients diagnosed with drug addiction or alcoholism, selected years in 1958–1970.

Year	Alcoholism	Drug addiction
1958	9	92
1959	10	249
1960	7	211
1961	13	287
1962	16	298
1969	20	210
1970	19	127

Source: Data compiled from ARs.

provider of hashish—[102] led to harsher sentences for selling hashish in the decree of 1960. In contrast to the laws of 1935 or 1946, a drug dealer could now be sentenced to up to fifteen years in prison.[103] For the first time, however, the law recognized that drug addiction was a disease that was potentially curable through rehabilitation. Consequently, people who were convicted of drug addiction were supposed to serve their sentences in a hospital rather than a prison, and if they were found to be medically cured of their disease, they could be exempted from serving the duration of their sentences.[104]

To avoid being apprehended by the police, some people voluntarily sought treatment at ʿAṣfūriyyeh, which operated a forensic unit for the rehabilitation of prisoners who had been convicted of criminal offenses, including substance abuse.[105] Only a minority turned themselves in, however; the majority were referred to the Hospital by the court or the police.[106] Interestingly, many American hashish smugglers (who did not suffer from drug addiction) ended up serving their sentences at ʿAṣfūriyyeh's Webster House (which housed the forensic unit) rather than at Beirut's central prison. Some had to pay for the transfer, while others used their connections to be sent to the Hospital.[107]

The police customarily questioned substance users for a few days before sending them to the central prison in Beirut. There a social worker would see them first, and later a psychiatrist would prescribe a tranquilizer to manage the withdrawal symptoms until the trial, which usually took place several months later.[108] If convicted, the person would be sent to ʿAṣfūriyyeh's forensic unit for further treatment and rehabilitation. The treatment generally consisted of controlling the withdrawal symptoms: psychotherapy or behavioral cognitive therapy was rarely provided.[109] Indeed, an American hashish smuggler, with whom I was fortunate to talk, complained that he was offered neither treatment nor counseling when he was brought to Webster House in the early 1970s. He did mention, however, that Reverend Romain Swedenburg, an American minister who had worked for the US consulate in Beirut, started to visit and counsel American smugglers at ʿAṣfūriyyeh's Webster House.[110] Antranig Manugian, the medical director, did not have much faith in recovery from drug addiction, and he even blamed the condition on drug addicts' irremediable psychopathic personalities. Psychotherapy was useless for presumably poorly motivated personalities.[111]

Who exactly introduced cannabis to eastern Lebanon's fertile Beqaa Valley is unclear: it may have been the Romans, the Ottomans, or farmers who were forced to find an alternative source of income to replace the collapsed local silk industry.[112] In any event, at the root of the surge of substance use problems from the 1950s through the 1970s were regional and local socioeconomic and political conditions. In a pioneering paper published in 1975, Katchadourian and Jeffrey Sutherland blamed this state of affairs on the Lebanese government's lenient laissez-faire capitalism as well as the widespread ignorance about the consequences of substance abuse.[113] More recently, the journalist Jonathan Marshall added to the complex and global network of narcotic trafficking influential local politicians who got rich in the process (some of them are still active in politics at the time of this writing).[114] Strikingly, what Marshall omitted to say is that while the drug profits benefited the ruling political classes, it was as Katchadourian and Sutherland showed it the lower and middle classes who suffered from the long-term consequences of drug addiction.[115]

The fifteen-year civil war that started in 1975 saw another boom in drug trafficking and use.[116] This time, however, in what the Lebanese psychiatrist Charles Baddoura has called "the democratization of drug addiction," most of the drug users were militiamen and youth from the lower or middle class.[117] The actress Darina Al-Joundi aptly described this phenomenon in her autobiography (co-written with the Algerian novelist Mohamed Kacimi). With remarkable candor, she discusses her drug experience during the civil war, how cheap and easily available drugs were, and the intoxicating effect drug addiction had on a pathological society that had normalized war and violence.[118]

In the 1990s, psychiatrists were better able to see in hindsight that the causes of substance use had shifted to the constant climate of insecurity and instability and the need for self-induced amnesia for those who participated in or hoped to overcome the atrocities committed during the war years—which saw the climax of what one psychiatrist called "toxicomania."[119] The sharp drop in the numbers of drug addicts at ʿAṣfūriyyeh during the civil war was due to the total chaos and lawlessness that had engulfed the country and made access to the Hospital not only difficult but also dangerous, as we will see in chapter 5. Lebanese psychiatrists compared the drugs-and violence-filled culture of the militiamen who took part in the civil war to that of the *hashashin*, the radicalized medieval Shiite sect that allegedly committed massacres while intoxicated on hashish.[120] The militiamen-cum-mercenaries of the civil war conducted similar atrocities, frequently under the influence of psychoactive drugs, and they often used drugged youths as human shields and informers.

Female Maladies

As for the exclusively female maladies, they include hysteria as well as the affective disorders, both examined in this section (see figure 4.6). The poet Mayy Ziyādah, also discussed in this section, is a case in point of how these female maladies were constructed as well as an illustration of how the history of madness and mental illness in the Middle East has been written.

Hysteria Although hysteria was not high on the list of prevalent mental disorders in the history of ʿAṣfūriyyeh, it tended to be more frequent among women than men. This so-called female malady, which came to prominence in Victorian England, was widely considered to be a marker of a more intense, neurotic, and refined civilized life.[121] This explains why Benoît Boyer, a professor of therapeutics and hygiene at the FFM, predicted in an 1897 report that hysteria was bound to surge with Syria's increasingly lenient customs,

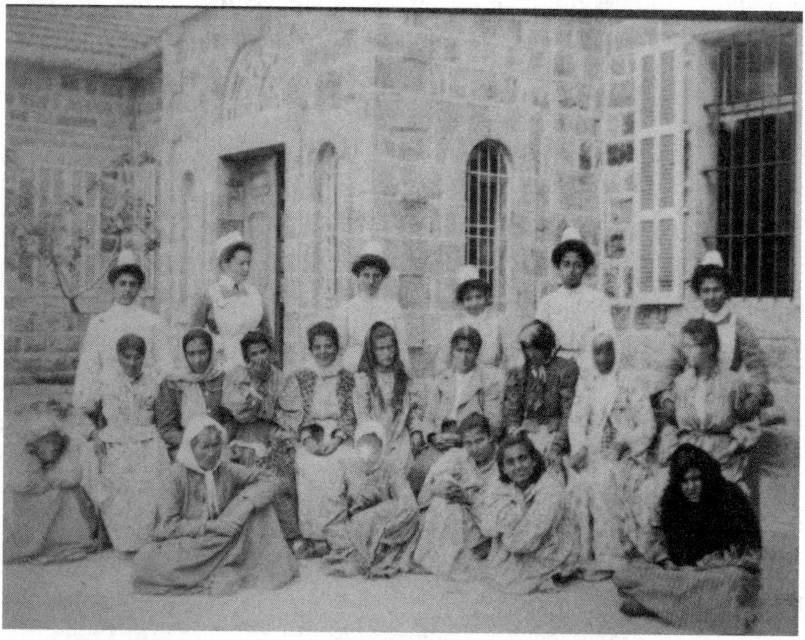

Figure 4.6
Female patients, nurses, and the British matron in front of the Philadelphia House, ʿAṣfūriyyeh, 1904.
Source: Album with pictures of ʿAṣfūriyyeh by Theophilus and Fareedy Waldmeier, LH/11/01, box 16, LH, SOAS.

women's whims and materialistic preoccupations, and the growing celibacy and futility of the new fin de siècle generation—even though in his comprehensive report hysteria accounted for only 2 percent of all diseases.[122]

This was not necessarily a specifically "orientalist" diagnosis as much as a sign of the times.[123] The few articles published in *at-Ṭabīb* (the Arabic medical journal mentioned in chapter 1) on hysteria are typical rehashings of contemporaneous understandings of this quintessential female malady. In one such article, a medical graduate of the SPC named Wadīʿ Effendi Rizʾallah Al-Barbārī wrote that the cause of hysteria was to be found in a woman's "reproductive organs" (*al-jihāz al-tanāsulī*), for they are the center of her physical and mental well-being.[124] Nevetheless, hysteria per se disappeared from ʿAṣfūriyyeh's statistical tables in 1936, most likely because it was conflated with the neuroses more generally speaking. (Indeed, the number of neurotic cases increased starting in 1937.[125])

While at the beginning of the twentieth century, the causes of hysteria and other female maladies were thought to be women's reproductive organs and other constitutional idiosyncrasies; by the 1960s, these causes had become socioeconomic and cultural in nature. In a 1967 report on the causes of hysteria in Lebanon, the psychiatrist Alexandre Habib discussed problems of social integration and adaptation as well as religious causes.[126] For Habib, it was less the biological constitution of women and more the socioeconomic and cultural context that was the source of hysteria. Christian women, he claimed, were more vulnerable because of their strict religious and moral education, which considered the discussion of sexual issues to be taboo. Sex was internalized and inhibited. Muslim women, in contrast, were oppressed and submissive, and their hysterical symptoms arose out of a need to either liberate themselves or totally submit themselves to male figures (husbands or fathers). As in other Western contexts, hysteria was often thought of as a form of disorderly conduct that reflected particularly repressive, normative, or conservative sociocultural and political conditions.[127] But women also resorted to such explosive behaviors out of despair or rejection of the roles ascribed to them. To quote the historian Carroll Smith-Rosenberg, "In all these ways, then, the hysterical woman can be seen as both product and indictment of her culture."[128]

Affective versus Psychotic Disorders While melancholia, depression, psychoneurosis, manic-depressive illness, and alternating insanity—in other words, disorders of the affect—were predominantly female maladies, schizophrenia was more prevalent among the male population (figure 4.3).

In 1969 two psychiatrists from AUB, Katchadourian and John Racy (both of whom had trained as medical graduate students at ʿAṣfūriyyeh)[129] examined the gender distribution of the affective psychoses and schizophrenic reactions.[130] They came to the conclusion that the distribution was clearly gendered, which was consistent with the overall gendered distribution of mental disorders at ʿAṣfūriyyeh over the years. Women's diagnoses were more likely to fall into the category of the affective psychoses, while men were more apt to suffer from schizophrenic reactions. They concluded that this gendered distribution was not merely the result of a differential use of psychiatric services and facilities (outpatient versus inpatient, for instance) but also to the true prevalence of these illnesses between men and women. To date, however, no one has found a consistent pattern of a higher incidence of schizophrenia among men than women, although there do appear to be marked differences between the genders in terms of the age of onset, prognosis, and expression of schizophrenia.[131] Symptoms seem to appear earlier in men, while clinical outcomes seem to be better among women.

The Case of Mayy Ziyādah The case of the hospitalization of Mayy Ziyādah at ʿAṣfūriyyeh shows that the history of madness and gender is an object of fascination susceptible to various interpretations and mythologies. Her case also illustrates the way in which the current postcolonial and poststructuralist reading of medicine in the Middle East has become parochial.

Ziyādah was an influential and prolific poet and novelist, as well as a feminist of Lebanese and Palestinian origins who took part in the intellectual renaissance of the late nineteenth century, enlivening a famous literary salon in Cairo.[132] Ziyādah was hospitalized at ʿAṣfūriyyeh in the 1930s following a period of personal losses and grief marked by the successive passing of her parents and the lover she never met, the celebrated writer Gibran Khalil Gibran.[133] The Hospital's records show that Miller, ʿAṣfūriyyeh's medical superintendent at the time of her hospitalization, had advised Ziyādah's uncle (himself a physician) to hospitalize the writer after she was found to act erratically, refusing to eat, and neglecting her person.[134] A close friend of hers, the Egyptian writer Salāmah Mūsa, documents the changes he witnessed in Ziyādah's personality, her persecutory delusions and paranoia, her conflicted internal dilemmas, and nervous breakdowns "clouding her reason"—a multitude of symptoms that, according to Mūsa, became apparent only when Ziyādah reached the age of forty-nine exactly one year before her hospitalization.[135]

The Hospital records show that Ziyādah was indeed hospitalized, as a private patient with the diagnosis of "involutional melancholia," not for several years as Mūsa and others have claimed, but from May 16, 1936, to March 22, 1937.[136] As Ziyādah had attested in her own writings, and as her friend Mūsa confirmed in his memoirs, she was prone to bouts of mania and depression following long periods of emotional distress.[137] Two incidents at ʿAṣfūriyyeh were particularly painful and traumatic for Ziyādah: the time she was force-fed after refusing to eat and when she was forced to wear a straitjacket, which is quite remarkable given that the Hospital claimed to have used straitjackets only in certain extreme situations.[138] There may have been other painful and traumatic memories of her hospitalization, but unfortunately the unpublished book in which Ziyādah related her recollections, "Layālī al-ʿAṣfūriyyeh" (ʿAṣfūriyyeh nights), has never been found.[139]

As soon as Ziyādah was hospitalized, her circle of friends (which included influential intellectuals, journalists, and politicians) launched a campaign to get her out of the Hospital. They were ultimately successful, by order of the attorney general.[140] They claimed that Ziyādah had been confined by relatives who were eager to silence her and get their hands on her inheritance. Indeed, her stay at ʿAṣfūriyyeh had provoked fierce criticism of the Hospital for the first time in its history. (As shown in chapter 5, the second time would be during the civil war.) According to Ziyādah's friends and despite Mūsa's testimony to the contrary, she "had never been anything but sane and had become mentally ill in the hospital because of what she saw and suffered," and "Dr. Miller had been (perhaps unconsciously) implicated in a plot to keep her there"—influenced by Mayy Ziyādah's malicious uncle, a doctor who was well connected politically.[141] To prove her mental and functional competence to her detractors after she was discharged from ʿAṣfūriyyeh, Ziyādah delivered a public lecture at AUB a year later.

The attorney general (who is described in the archival records as "an ardent Maronite" and therefore presumably anti-Protestant) intervened, demanding to see the Hospital's permit to operate and Miller's permit to practice in the country.[142] The issue of the legality of the Hospital was then raised in the Lebanese parliament, when a member accused the Hospital of confining people against their will and making them insane. And the press exploited the issue by making a variety of accusations against "this foreign institution" (meaning ʿAṣfūriyyeh), ignoring the fact that ʿAṣfūriyyeh had been considered a "Lebanesse bimaristan" since its inception. Ultimately, the British consul had to intervene, warning the Lebanese prime minister that he would be forced to take the matter up with the French High Commissioner (this all happened during the French mandate) and the Foreign Office in London if this "abusive tirade" did not stop.[143]

The threat seemed to have worked, since the next day the prime minister read in parliament a statement by the British consul in which the latter asked for the suspension of a committee that had been illegally appointed to investigate the Hospital. (Indeed, according to the law, such investigations were supposed to be conducted by a court rather than a parliamentary commission.) An official statement was then published in the press "with wonderful words about Asfuriyeh."[144] According to the Beirut-based newspaper *Le Jour*, the government praised ʿAṣfūriyyeh for being the premier institution for the treatment of the insane in the Orient, recognizing its valuable services to Lebanon and recommending an increase in the government's financial support of the Hospital.[145] But the parliament also took the opportunity to reinstate the Ottoman law of 1876 that governed the management of the insane—an action that ʿAṣfūriyyeh dismissed not just because the government itself had undermined the law but also because the law was obsolete.[146]

At the root of the public outrage over Ziyādah's hospitalization was the persistent stigmatization of mental illness in general and of ʿAṣfūriyyeh in particular as a dreadful place of incarceration. The label *majnūn* had pejorative implications, and despite ʿAṣfūriyyeh's efforts to combat the stigma of mental illness, the Hospital had become a symbol of madness. In its coverage of the Ziyādah case, the Beirut-based newspaper *L'Orient* felt the need to clarify that ʿAṣfūriyyeh treated not only the insane (*les aliénés*) but also those who were afflicted with a range of mental illnesses: "neurasthenia, neurosis, a whole range of physical or intellectual burnout and exhaustion who like the insane need a special treatment to recover."[147]

Several medical directors of ʿAṣfūriyyeh as well as numerous committee members were acutely aware of the stigmatization of mental illness. They had also suggested several policies to try to change popular misconceptions. In 1914, the hospital administrators removed the word "insane" from the original name of the hospital.[148] The following year the Hospital was again renamed, this time as the Lebanon Hospital for Mental Diseases. The administrators were also aware of the exploitation of vulnerable patients, which is very likely why 'Aṣfūriyyeh's medical directors were eager to mention in their annual reports people who were found to be "not insane." This included prisoners and other civilians whom the authorities sent for assessment or admission.[149] Every effort was made to make the Hospital's procedures as transparent, and its practice as scientific, as possible (according to the general practice of the time). Reports that included statistical data and analyses of the patient population were published annually and distributed to subscribers. As early as 1938, the committees had suggested renaming 'Aṣfūriyyeh the Lebanon Hospital for Nervous and Mental Disorders to "better express the spirit of the times."[150] Local and foreign personalities, officials, and members of the press had regularly visited the Hospital since its earliest days, and starting in 1947, those visits were recorded in a visitors' book.[151] As we have seen in previous chapters, these efforts continued well into the 1950s, with an open-door policy used in an effort to further destigmatize and demystify mental illness.

Of course, there were stories of forceful confinement of unwanted or problematic relatives, but these must be examined with care.[152] Similarly, one cannot deny the stories of abuse and neglect, such as the 1955 strangulation of a patient by two attendants (who were eventually sentenced to prison).[153] What is clear, however, is that 'Aṣfūriyyeh at least strove to be transparent by investigating incidents of violence, suspicious death (by drug overdose), or suicide and by punishing the perpetrators.[154]

In contrast, the reputation of Dayr al-Ṣalib—'Aṣfūriyyeh's competing institution—is tainted with rumors and stories of forced confinements. And because that hospital remains closed to researchers, it is hard to draw broader conclusions. Still, one poignant story is that of Darina Al-Joundi, the actress who was mentioned above in the context of drug addiction during the civil war. Al-Joundi revealed how she was hospitalized against her will at Dayr al-Ṣalīb for daring to live as a sexually liberated, secular-minded, and emancipated woman.[155] She also disclosed that she met other women there whose family members had hospitalized them against their will.[156] Unsurprisingly, Al-Joundi considered Ziyādah's forced hospitalization at 'Aṣfūriyyeh similar to her own experience with the dominant and domineering patriarchy.[157]

The term *majnūn*—especially in the 1930s, the time of Ziyādah's hospitalization—implied a total loss of mental competence. As a result, people in this category could be stripped of their legal rights and their decisions made invalid.[158] Thus, it is understandable why one would see Ziyādah's hospitalization and her tragic story as symptomatic of the abuse and exploitation of vulnerable women, and especially the forced silencing of defiant feminists. Nevertheless, it is curious to note how commentators, historians, and other "second-order critics" (as Jürgen Habermas might have called them)[159] have interpreted Ziyādah's tragedy and used it to make broader claims about mental institutions in the Middle East.

Some of the factual errors that have been made could be evocative of the dark side of asylums and mental hospitals—such as the claim that Ziyādah died in ʿAṣfūriyyeh at the age of fifty-five.[160] This is not true: as the records show, Ziyādah was discharged from the Hospital in March 1937, four years before her death. (This is also confirmed in the memoirs of her contemporary, Salāmah Mūsa). As it turned out, she died not in Beirut but in Cairo a few years later, where she was buried in an old neighborhood of the city.[161]

Others have tried to debunk the myth of Ziyādah's insanity in ways similar to those others have used in attempts to debunk the madness of another famous writer, Virginia Woolf.[162] In a two-volume book, the Syrian writer Salma al-Ḥaffār Al-Kuzbarī, who has unraveled materials (especially medical reports) that supposedly disprove Ziyādah's insanity, spends an entire chapter arguing why a nervous breakdown does not amount to junūn (insanity). Al-Kuzbarī, who understandably has tried to protect Ziyādah from popular misconceptions and the stigma of insanity, ironically ends up perpetrating another myth of what mental illness is or ought to be. For, according to Al-Kuzbarī (and Rose Ghorayeb, another feminist scholar who defended Ziyādah and attempted to debunk the myth),[163] madness was a death sentence and a dreadful thing, and a mental hospital was a madhouse where those deemed insane are confined against their will and abused. In contrast, a nervous breakdown for Al-Kuzbarī was a reaction to life's miseries and injustices and thus was a sorry state of affairs that could be remedied in a normal hospital—or, ideally, resolve on its own.[164] But that is precisely what ʿAṣfūriyyeh's medical doctors were trying to do: convince the general population that mental illness was, like any other disease, treatable and even curable in some cases.

It was important for Al-Kuzbarī to argue that to suffer from a nervous breakdown or a neurosis did not mean losing one's mental competence. It is also clear that, contrary to what Ziyādah's relatives have claimed to get their hands on her possessions (as they generally are thought to have done), she was not mentally incompetent. Nevertheless, she did go through a very difficult period of grief, anxiety, and guilt (accompanied by solitary confinement and suicidal ideation), which were feelings she never recovered from. Yet Al-Kuzbarī seems to refuse to believe that Ziyādah suffered from a mental illness that should have been treated somehow.

The sociocultural and historical contexts are of course important in understanding this common resistance to acknowledging Ziyādah's emotional, personal, and mental vulnerability. Al-Kuzbarī and Ghorayeb belonged to an early generation of feminists who were leading the fight against a domineering patriarchy. Conceding anything that might have been perceived as "weakness" was seen as defeatist. Their fight consisted in directly confronting the dominant patriarchy or "neopatriarchy" as Hisham Sharabi has described this modernized form of patriarchal structure that emerged in the post-independence era in the Arab world (1950s–1970s).[165]

In addition to sharing Al-Kuzbarī's view of ʿAṣfūriyyeh as a "dumping ground for unwanted and uncontrollable family members," the historian Jens Hanssen uses Ziyādah's tragic story to support his claim within the Foucauldian narrative of grand confinement and state control.[166] He claims that the "Ottoman Government happily supported the hospital ... to cleanse Beirut's streets from unwanted and unaccountable elements of society."[167] While the first half of his claim is true, the second half is not supported by the historical evidence. A more careful examination of the patient population shows that admissions varied between 52 (for the year 1900 when ʿAṣfūriyyeh opened its doors) and 213 (for the year 1920–1921) with an average of 113 patients over the 1900–1930 period and out of a population of roughly one million for Beirut and Mount Lebanon combined (see figure 3.1 in chapter 3).[168] Moreover, most patients came from Mount Lebanon and not Beirut.[169] While it is true that many of them were poor, these people were generally brought by their families, not by municipal or other public authorities.[170]

In fact, the number of municipality patients at ʿAṣfūriyyeh was never very significant, for example they accounted for only 15 percent of all admissions over the period 1930–1936 (figure 4.7). Indeed, the majority of admissions were regular hospitalizations. If we look at the overall admissions of non-government-related patients—what I call "regular patients" (i.e., mostly private patients and some of the poor covered by the Hospital

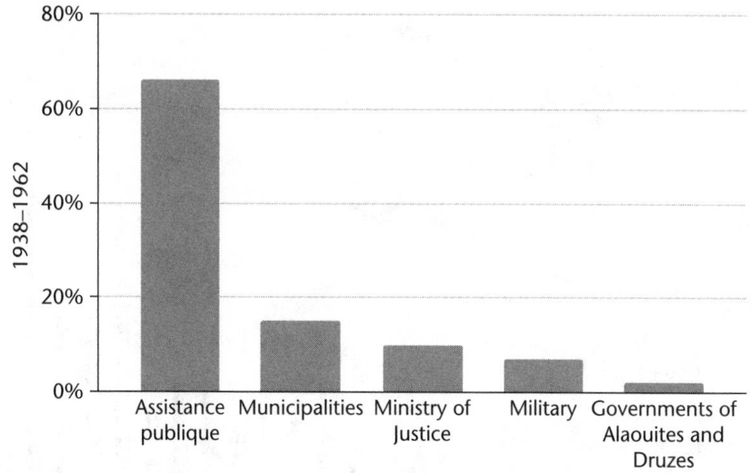

Figure 4.7
Percentage of patients sent by government agency, 1938–1962. The governments of the Alawites and the Druzes, created during the French Mandate, lasted from 1920 to 1936.
Source: Data compiled from ARs.

or benevolent associations)—then the number of private patients consistently exceeds that of the government-related patients (paid for by the assistance publique, municipalities, military, or Ministry of Justice), except at two key times (figure 4.8).

The first such occasion was 1959, the year after what became known as the year of crisis (or the first civil war). Strikingly, it was the Ministry of Justice that sent ʿAṣfūriyyeh most of the government patients during this period. The second occasion was in 1962, when the number of patients covered by the assistance publique nearly tripled. This is a legacy of the social welfare policy during the administration of President Fouad Chehab (1958–1964). That period witnessed a surge in patients covered by the assistance publique and a more generous coverage that was widely hailed as a turning point in the history of the Hospital.[171] Not only did Chehab finally meet the demands for an equitable ethic of care, but his government also provided ʿAṣfūriyyeh with a substantial grant—thus relieving it of years of financial problems.[172]

However, the fact that a large share of the patient population at ʿAṣfūriyyeh (66 percent of government-related admissions) depended on the assistance publique does not mean that they were incarcerated involuntarily by

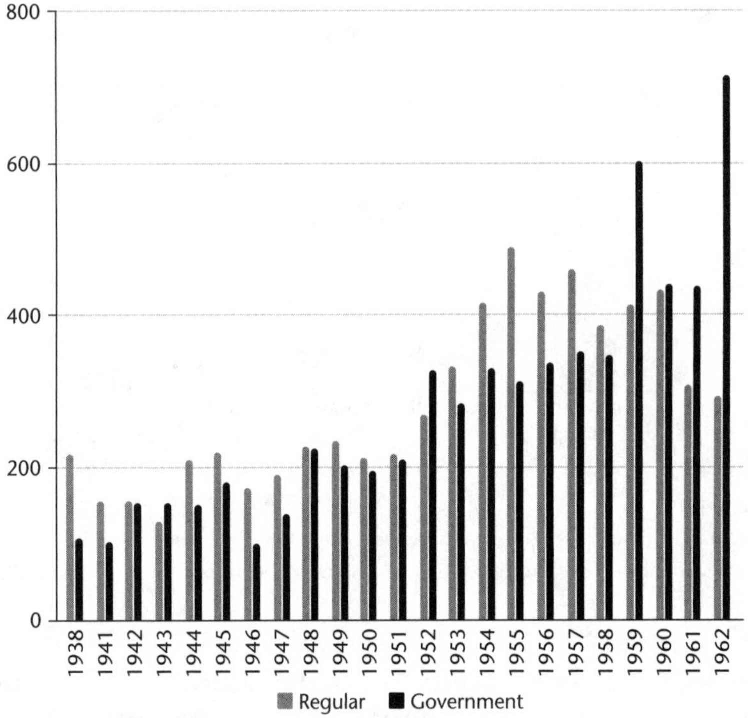

Figure 4.8
Number of regular and government patients admitted, 1938–1962.
Source: Data compiled from ARs and statistical tables irregularly published in the minutes of the BEC and LGC.

government orders. The assistance publique is a safety net for people who cannot afford the cost of their hospitalization. In contrast, patients who were incarcerated against their will by government agencies were sent by the Ministry of Justice, the military, or a municipality. Of course, as the case of Ziyādah or Al-Joundi illustrate, one cannot deny the coercive means that families (not only law enforcement agencies) could deploy.

Unlike the case with many Western public asylums, 'Aṣfūriyyeh was supposed to be a voluntary hospital that depended on voluntary donations and not public funds. As we will see in chapter 5, however, one reason for the demise of the Hospital in the late 1970s was the increasing number of patients who were dependent on public funds at a time when the government was barely meeting its financial obligations.

Therapeutics

Moral treatment was the approach and philosophy that distinguished ʿAṣfūriyyeh from other institutions, and such treatment put it on a par with what were considered reformed and modern lunatic asylums in the nineteenth century. Although Waldmeier was skeptical of mental alienists, in the end it was the alienists and their new means of managing insanity—from physical treatments to chemical cures—that transformed ʿAṣfūriyyeh into a pioneering institution where the spiritual means in which the founder had put so much faith eventually became footnotes in the Hospital's annual reports.

Moral Treatment

ʿAṣfūriyyeh was widely praised for being the first asylum in the Near East to have unchained the insane and liberated them from the caves in which they had once been abandoned, long before French psychiatrists were said to have done the same in the Maghreb.[173] The chains were not only physical ones—as were pictured from time to time in the annual reports and publicity materials of the Hospital—but also metaphysical ones: the results of the brutality, superstition, and ignorance of the clergy, who had monopolized the power of curing madness through exorcism and demonization.

As mentioned briefly in chapter 2, Waldmeier nonetheless had little faith in the power of the alienist. "I had a very exaggerated idea of the powers of a specialist of mental diseases," he wrote in his autobiography, "and expected rather too much from him."[174] Time and experience had taught him that medicine could be of very little value in the recovery of the insane: "What is most disheartening is that there is no effective medicine or remedy, nor is any medical doctor in the world at large able to say, 'I can cure the insane.' Medical men with all their modern attainments, experiences, science and skill still stand as helpless before insanity as before a cancer, general paralysis or epilepsy, etc."[175]

For Waldmeier, the best remedy consisted of "kind and good open-air treatment, long walks, good food, plenty of light and space, and true Christian care without restraint."[176] In addition to Quaker values and the Christian spirit of brotherly love and charity, Waldmeier mentions several reformers who inspired his own work: Philippe Pinel at the Bicêtre in Paris; William Tuke at the York Retreat; and the German Princess Pauline of Lippe, who reformed the treatment of the insane in a lunatic asylum she founded in the Principality of Lippe in 1811.[177] However, Waldmeier mainly turned to the German physician Johann Christian August Heinroth for inspiration. Heinroth, who had introduced the term "psychosomatic" (from the German term *psychosomatisch*) in his 1818 *Textbook of Disturbances of Mental Life*, promoted a combination of spirituality and medicine for the treatment of mental disturbances.[178]

Spiritual healing was practiced at the Hospital not as an act of proselytism, as has been claimed, but as complementary (though voluntary and optional) to the physical healing process. All patients, regardless of denomination, were invited (but never forced) to participate in the ecumenical Sunday services held in the John Cory Hall.[179] The founder held these services in Arabic for the first few years after the opening of ʿAṣfūriyyeh.[180] After his death, the service was taken over by members of the American Presbyterian mission and theological seminary in Beirut.[181] Patients of all faiths regularly attended these spiritual meetings and seem to have appreciated what they offered.[182]

Nevertheless, spiritual healing was quickly marginalized as a potential core therapeutic approach, relegated to a secondary role in the arsenal of therapeutics deployed to treat mental ailments. During the first decade of the Hospital's existence, the founder mentioned the healing power of these religious meetings in his reports. Then the meetings were briefly and inconsistently mentioned in the medical director's reports—and always toward the end of the reports, which were generally devoted to administrative issues. The meetings may have been of interest to subscribers and donors, but they were clearly not the concern of the medical director, unless they were of some clinical value.[183]

Moral treatment—which excluded restraint and seclusion treatment (although those were used in some cases) and included work therapy—was used in the first decade of the Hospital's existence.[184] Work and occupation therapy necessitated what was known as the cottage system (discussed in chapter 2): an architectural arrangement of the hospital into different villas separated by arable land.[185] In 1900, the premises of ʿAṣfūriyyeh had two villas: the Swiss House, for "quiet men," and the American House, for "quiet women."[186] Four decades later, twenty such villas collectively accommodated up to five hundred patients.[187]

Until the 1920s, a type of therapy consisting of useful occupation was the only treatment that was followed at ʿAṣfūriyyeh. As in other contexts, occupation was highly valued for its therapeutic effect.[188] Every patient had an occupation, whether indoors or outdoors. While women did needlework, embroidery, or laundry, men helped by doing more laborious manual work.[189] According to the founder, "The occupation of the insane men and women in an asylum is one of the most important means of physical and mental improvement, and many doctors say that it should be a leading feature in the management of every asylum according to the inclination and physical condition of the patient."[190] Thwaites, the medical director at the time, shared this faith in the curative effects of work therapy. He often quoted the prominent English alienist David Yellowlees (who was an early supporter of the Hospital, as mentioned in chapter 2) for whom "manual work [was] better than medicine for the lunatics."[191] A hall that was fully dedicated to occupational therapy and named after Lady Scott-Moncrieff—a longstanding committee member of ʿAṣfūriyyeh—was inaugurated in the summer of 1938.[192]

Innovative Cures

The new specialists of the mind did not share Waldmeier's skepticism of medical cures. Almost all the new therapeutic discoveries and approaches that became widely used in Europe and North America were transplanted to the East (as the psychiatrist John Racy has put it), although sometimes with reservations about the hype regarding certain new procedures.[193]

Blood examinations for malaria and the use of "Wasserman reactions" to detect syphilis (which is associated with psychotic symptoms) are mentioned as early as 1929.[194] The shock therapies—including insulin-induced coma therapy and Cardiazol- or Metrazol-convulsion therapy—were introduced at the Hospital in 1937 for the treatment of schizophrenia, only a few years after these therapies were first used in Vienna.[195] Miller, the Hospital's medical director at the time, had observed the insulin-induced coma and Cardiazol-convulsion therapies performed in Vienna, and he was cautiously hopeful about the positive outcomes that might ensue. These therapies were "far from pleasing to witness," he wrote in 1937, but "that must not deter us if only some success follows in its wake."[196] Of the schizophrenic patients who received insulin-induced coma therapy at ʿAṣfūriyyeh in 1938, he reported that "no dramatic recoveries have taken place in this group."[197]

Electroconvulsive therapy was initiated in 1944 at ʿAṣfūriyyeh for the treatment of depression, schizophrenia, and hysteria, six years after it was first performed in Rome.[198] Prefrontal leucotomy, or lobotomy, was first performed at ʿAṣfūriyyeh in 1948. The procedure consisted of destroying parts of the frontal lobes and was purposefully omitted from the list of memorable therapeutic achievements at the Hospital.[199] This is to be expected since the practice ultimately fell into disgrace. Two patients underwent lobotomy operations—both performed by an AUB physician named Jidijan—only a year before the Portuguese neurologist Egas Moniz received the Nobel Prize "for his discovery of the therapeutic value of leucotomy in certain psychoses."[200] This was not the first time that such a procedure had taken place in the Middle East (as the Hospital claimed), since by then at least four such operations had already been conducted in mandatory Palestine by an émigré Viennese neurosurgeon.[201] In his medical report of 1954, Manugian joined a number of scientists who by then had started to challenge Moniz's procedure. As Manugian complained, "The leucotomy operations have not shown very satisfying results."[202]

In the mid-1950s, the impact of new chemical cures was beginning to be felt, which precipitated the demise of psychosurgery and the birth of a new chapter in the history of psychiatry: the psychopharmacological revolution.[203] Stabilizing drugs such as reserpine (an antipsychotic drug) were found to dramatically improve symptoms in patients who suffered from schizophrenia, to the extent that Manugian hailed the drugs as "instrumental in producing the generally improved social atmosphere of the various wards."[204] Chlorpromazine (marketed as Largactil in Europe and Thorazine in the United States) was used for the first time at ʿAṣfūriyyeh in 1952, barely two years after its synthesis in the French pharmaceutical laboratories of Rhône-Poulenc, and only a year after the French psychiatrists Jean Delay and Pierre Deniker published their results from using the drug on a number of psychotic patients at the Hôpital Sainte-Anne in Paris.[205] Patients could now be easily pacified by the new benzodiazepines (such as Valium) and other tranquilizers that were made available in the 1960s. Patients were becoming less noisy, less aggressive, and hence more manageable. What moral treatment had striven to achieve, according to Foucault—namely, to "reduce madness to silence"[206]—was now spectacularly possible with drugs.

These observations were startling for the medical personnel at ʿAṣfūriyyeh. For one thing, a greater number of patients could now be successfully managed with neuroleptic drugs. Not only were wards becoming quieter, but the management of outpatients was also becoming more satisfactory, as Manugian noted in his 1958 medical report.[207] Imipramine (a tricyclic antidepressant) was first tried at ʿAṣfūriyyeh for the treatment of depression in 1959, before being prescribed in the outpatient clinics.[208] Unlike the experimental nature of French psychiatry in colonial Algeria—the peripheral colony that served as a laboratory for the French metropole[209]—ʿAṣfūriyyeh served as an experimental setting for "the growing cosmopolitan population" whose members lived outside the institution with their ever-increasing "stress and maladjustment to life," as Ford Robertson put it.[210] These symptoms of modernity would be supplemented by the stress and trauma of war, as we will see in chapter 5.

Nevertheless, nonchemical treatments (such as electroconvulsive therapy or psychotherapy) continued to be popular because psychiatrists at ʿAṣfūriyyeh believed in the superiority of combined therapies.[211] The 1950s saw the emergence of a concern for patients' social recovery and environment and the initiation of psychosocial work. For Manugian, this new rationale of socially rehabilitating patients was on a par with neurochemical therapies. He wrote that psychosocial work yielded dramatic results in the "general improvement in the atmosphere of the Hospital."[212]

Finally, the Hospital's open-door policy, which it initiated in 1956, was both an attempt to fight the stigma of mental illness by demystifying it and an opportunity for patients to resocialize and reintegrate themselves into society.[213] Perhaps above all, the medical doctors at ʿAṣfūriyyeh were acutely aware of the importance that local culture played in understanding and managing mental pathologies. "It is a well-known fact," wrote Manugian in 1961, "that a thorough knowledge of the local culture is an indispensable element for the understanding and management of psychiatric patients."[214] The doctors never preached a pure neurochemical approach, though psychotherapy and cognitive behavioral therapy were limited in scope, and psychoanalysis was rarely if ever mentioned in the written records of the hospital.

Paths from the Asylum

Several paths existed for leaving ʿAṣfūriyyeh. Patients could be considered cured and socially recovered, relieved of their symptoms, or discharged with the label "not improved,"[215] and these people were often removed by their relatives.[216] Some committed suicide or died from natural causes or endemic diseases due to the poor economic conditions of the time.[217] Others were discharged as "not insane," and a few escaped. In some cases, escape posed legal problems. An example is the case of R. C., who in 1957 ran away from ʿAṣfūriyyeh, went back home, and murdered his wife in a state of frenzy. The case was taken to court, and the family's lawyer asked for a hefty indemnity.[218]

Because the Hospital was intended to be a place of cure rather than a dumping ground for the chronically ill, massive discharges of inpatients and increased turnover of patients occurred starting in the 1940s, which coincided with the development and expansion phase of the Hospital.[219] In 1957, those deemed to be socially recovered or otherwise symptomatically relieved accounted for around two-thirds of the discharged patients.[220] A few surviving vignettes describe those who recovered and went back to work. These vignettes always begin with a sectarian label and end with an affirmation of the patient's reintegration into his or her ordinary life and routines. For instance, B. A. was a Muslim woman who became addicted to morphine after undergoing an abdominal operation. The 1931–1932 annual report stated that she was "in a very wretched condition when admitted," but she was discharged after treatment, "quite cured."[221] R. A., a Maronite woman, was admitted for severe depression and a suicide attempt via self-immolation. She recovered and found employment as a servant. L. G., a Turk who had converted to Christianity, was very suicidal on admission but recovered and went back to his work as a chauffeur. S. W., a psychotic and excited young Armenian man, was cured and became usefully employed as a mechanic in Beirut.

Conclusion

By sketching a landscape of mental ailments at ʿAṣfūriyyeh, the aim of this chapter was not to be exhaustive but to highlight salient findings on the different mutations in the understanding and management of mental illness over the years.

ʿAṣfūriyyeh strove not to be a place of last resort, even if it was stigmatized as such in the popular imagination. Laws were put in place in the Ottoman Empire to avoid wrongful incarcerations. Even though successive medical directors of the Hospital dismissed the Ottoman law of 1876 as obsolete and useless, they were mindful of the vulnerabilities of their patients. They did not rush to admit anyone who presented with the symptoms of mental illness (including those who had been sent by local authorities), and Hospital administrators expressed a constant desire to make contact with the community.

What is also clear from this history is the growing faith among ordinary people in "the gospel of modern care for the insane" (to quote the epigraph), to the extent that medical doctors started to complain in their annual reports about the excessive confidence the common people showed in the infallible curative power of treatment for mental afflictions.[222] Although the Hospital managed to propagate and demonstrate the values of progress and enlightenment, it did not do so as a way of converting the locals to the Protestant faith. Not only was religion always invoked in an ecumenical spirit, but it also became irrelevant. The gospel of modern care for the insane was a secular tool that was in the hands of a new group of experts (the psychiatrists), many of whom were now drawn from the ranks of the locals, and their new site of influence was the psychiatric hospital. These new experts on the mind undermined Waldmeier's authority (as we saw in chapter 2) and very early on began to disregard his preference for spiritual healing.

5 The Downfall of ʿAṣfūriyyeh and the Breakdown of the State

> We have escaped like a bird from the fowler's snare; the snare has been broken, and we have escaped.
>
> —Psalm 124:7

> When the country itself went insane, the doors of the Asfourieh were opened and the birds flew.... Forty years later the Asfourieh I knew was an empty shell in the no-man's-land between the two halves of the divided city.
>
> —Charles Glass, *Tribes with Flags: A Dangerous Passage through the Chaos of the Middle East*

This chapter chronicles what it was like to live in, and especially manage, a psychiatric hospital during the sectarian civil war that erupted in Lebanon in 1975 and lasted through the Israeli invasion of the country in 1982, which coincides with the official closure of ʿAṣfūriyyeh.[1] The chapter is also a testimony to those who lived and perished on the premises of ʿAṣfūriyyeh during the Lebanese civil war, whose stories we will never fully know—much like the stories of the several thousand people who disappeared during the war and are still missing.[2] Indeed, their stories remain impressionistic because of the archival material—which in this chapter consists chiefly of the reports and correspondence of Antranig Manugian, the Hospital's medical director during the war. The chapter is intentionally detailed for two reasons. First, this story has never been told before, since many of the actors involved in the violence that was perpetrated on patients and staff are still active in Lebanon and elsewhere in the Arab world. Second, in detailing the shift in the nature of political violence over the years, I tried to highlight a new form of violence that deliberately targets medical hospitals as a tool of war—which is perhaps more conspicuously seen today in Syria and Yemen.[3]

Adnan Mroueh, ʿAṣfūriyyeh's current *mutawallī* (trustee or overseer of the *waqf*), rightly diagnosed the final period of the history of the Hospital as "a reflection of the dissolution of the state of Lebanon and the civil disturbances that started in 1975."[4] This chapter charts the breakdown of the state and the downfall of an institution that had managed to survive several critical geopolitical turning points after the fall of the Ottoman Empire, including the two world wars and the civil war of 1958.

The chapter also provides a major counterargument to studies of missionaries that condemn them as conveyers of sectarianism.[5] As the long history of ʿAṣfūriyyeh shows, the Hospital remained faithful to its nonsectarian credo until the end, despite the raging sectarian war that surrounded it. Nonsectarianism was not mere propaganda or "public relations," as Eugene Rogan has claimed, but a genuine belief—almost an ideology—in addition to being a politics of survival.[6]

Life under the Bombs

In contrast to the 1950s (a period of economic growth), the mid- to late 1960s were a period of economic and social stagnation and the beginning of political turmoil. This period also saw the rise of a Palestinian military presence whose guerrilla activities against Israel prompted frequent clashes between the Palestinian fedayeen and the Lebanese army. The first significant attack by the fedayeen against Israel occurred on June 14, 1968, a year after the spectacular Arab defeat in the Six-Day War.[7] Israel's retaliation was painful. Lebanese villages were shelled by heavy artillery, and thirteen civilian aircrafts at the Beirut airport were destroyed.[8] For a long time, Lebanon had attempted to stay neutral in the Arab-Israeli conflict, while welcoming more than two hundred thousand Palestinian refugees by the mid-1950s. Consequently, it had become a "de facto confrontation state."[9]

The 1969 Cairo Agreement, signed under pressure from various Arab countries and the supervision of Egyptian president Gamal Abdel Nasser, further reinforced and legitimized the military presence and activity of the Palestinian Liberation Organization (PLO) in Lebanon.[10] In time, this agreement gave the PLO free reign to develop a "state within a state."[11]

By April 10, 1973, when ʿAṣfūriyyeh's LGC agreed to purchase a new site for the Hospital in ʿAramūn, a town overlooking the Beirut airport, Lebanon was starting to descend into an infernal cycle of violence accompanied by the increasing deterioration of Palestinian-Lebanese relations. On the same day, an Israeli commando exacted revenge for the massacre of Israeli athletes a year earlier at the Munich Olympics by a Palestinian group that called itself Black September.[12] The Israeli commando murdered three of the key PLO leaders who were living in Beirut, along with nine bystanders. Despite Lebanon's national mourning in solidarity with the Palestinians, the situation quickly deteriorated amid a growing number of Palestinian operations, which undermined Lebanese sovereignty while provoking Israeli wrath and thus prompting further clashes between the Lebanese army and the Palestinian factions.[13]

As early as April 1973, Manugian was documenting in his reports to the LGC and his correspondence with the committee's chairman, Sir Geoffrey Furlonge, the violence that was starting to erupt in his country. Starting in May 1973, ʿAṣfūriyyeh, which sat on a hill just above two Palestinian refugee camps (Tall al-Zaʿtar and Jisr al-Bāshā), was caught in the middle of severe fighting between the Lebanese army and armed Palestinians.[14] On one day alone, Manugian reported, a rocket had fallen near the Hospital, and stray bullets had flown everywhere. "We have a lull today," he noted, "but I feel we still have to go through a rough patch before the more lasting call comes."[15] Indeed, perhaps the most violent chapter of the civil war for ʿAṣfūriyyeh was the period known as the Two-Year War (also commonly referred to as the Christian-Palestinian War), which lasted from early 1975 to late 1976.[16]

In fact this was more than a Christian-Palestinian war, since Christians and Muslims were fighting on both sides of the conflict. It was an ideological war against the idea of Lebanon as an independent nation and about the role that Lebanon should play in the region, given the hemorrhagic wound the Israeli-Arab conflict had inflicted ever since the creation of the state of Israel in 1948 and the ensuing Palestinian exodus. On one side were the members of the Lebanese National Movement (the Islamic-progressivists), a left-wing coalition that was led by the Druze leader Kamal Jumblatt and various Arab nationalist parties and that supported the Palestinian resistance.[17] On the other side were the members of the Christian Nationalist Front (the Christian conservatives), who believed that allowing Palestinian guerrilla fighters to launch their attacks on Israel from Lebanon was a violation of Lebanese sovereignty and the root of the lawlessness that had engulfed the country—not to mention Israel's costly punitive retaliations.

On October 13, 1975, Michel Zeidan—a psychiatrist at ʿAṣfūriyyeh who played a key role in enhancing psychiatric training at AUB—was kidnapped and taken to the Tall al-Zaʿtar camp, which had become a zone of regular conflict between the Kataeb (Christian) militiamen and the fedayeen.[18] As was the case with many of the other random abductions, executions, and other forms of violence that were perpetrated on civilians before the Lebanese civil war (and more intensively during the Two-Year War), Zeidan's kidnapping was most likely because he was Christian. Although he was released unharmed through the help of influential friends of the Hospital, the kidnappings and violence toward patients and staff did not stop. In fact, they increased both in intensity and in frequency.

Muslim staff and students, especially the Palestinians among them, now feared reprisals and executions. "There is an increasing feeling of insecurity amongst the Moslem staff," Manugian reported.[19] This feeling of insecurity had increased since the recent wave of sectarian-based abductions and murders, and especially after "the Moslem staff of a neighboring factory were asked to leave the factory by the Christians of this region." One should remember that the Hospital was located in a predominantly Christian area controlled by right-wing Christian militias, and in this sectarian war being a Christian or a Muslim in the wrong place could be fatal. Not surprisingly amid this sectarian-based conflict and the sectarian purges that were common on both sides of the conflict, people felt more allegiance to their communities than they had before the conflict.[20]

On November 5, 1975, armed and masked men from the Kataeb militia forced their way through the Hospital barrier and kidnapped several Lebanese and Palestinian Muslim students. This, Manugian reported, was a "severe blow to the dignity and neutrality" of ʿAṣfūriyyeh, a charitable hospital and national institution that prided itself on its status as a nonsectarian establishment.[21] The militiamen were avenging the kidnapping of three Kataeb partisans the day before. The students were released the following day, after negotiations among the various parties. One Palestinian student suffered lacerations to the head, various bruises and cuts, and a broken arm—injuries that were to become an all-too-common manifestation of the brutality that was regularly inflicted on innocent civilians trapped on both sides of the conflict.[22]

Staff and students were kidnapped, as well as the "prisoners" from the Hospital's forensic unit—the majority of whom were being treated for substance abuse. On January 21, 1976, following a relatively quiet day, a group of several armed men disarmed the gendarmes who were guarding Webster House (which housed the forensic unit) and took away eight prisoners, leaving the prisoners who were of the opposite religion in a state of panic.[23] But as it turned out, these prisoners had been kidnapped by their own relatives. Ironically, the (now former) prisoners called the Hospital to express their gratitude for the medical care they had received and to apologize to Manugian for "letting [him] down for reasons beyond their control."[24]

These inmates were considered lucky compared to the many others who, despite being convicted of substance abuse, had been sentenced to terms in regular prisons.[25] As we have seen in previous chapters, ʿAṣfūriyyeh's successive medical directors engaged with the authorities on several occasions to try to convince them of the medical nature of drug addiction and the psychiatric dimensions of "criminal insanity"—and hence the need to treat those ailments in a medical (rather than a carceral) setting. Unlike the social critics of the 1950s and 1960s, the progressivists of that same period (for instance, the mental hygienists who included among their ranks many of the successive medical directors of ʿAṣfūriyyeh, as we saw in previous chapters) did not conflate the clinic and the prison. On the contrary, they saw themselves as reformers and viewed mental hygiene as a means of emancipation and of freedom as well as a technique for shaping the troubled self and "governing the soul"—a style of thinking that emerged in the 1940s and crystallized in the 1970s.[26] During the war, Manugian had even discussed with the attorney general the possibility of transferring these chronic patients from prison to ʿAṣfūriyyeh for treatment. As was the case in many other parts of the world in the 1970s, the state of prisoners' mental health was starting to come under scrutiny.[27] Alas, Manugian lamented, every time the Hospital was close to making more radical reforms to prisons, events in Lebanon delayed or prevented such actions.[28]

On the morning of March 14, 1976, armed men—among them former patients of the prison section of ʿAṣfūriyyeh—took away four prisoners from the forensic unit after disarming the gendarmes.[29] It is not clear if they had come to release friends and relatives or to exact revenge. Two days later, several armed men again attacked the prison section, this time freeing thirty prisoners. Later that day, still another group of armed men came and asked for the release of three prisoners whom they named. The gendarmes (who by now were both helpless and hopeless) handed the prisoners over without any resistance. Several of the prisoners who were taken away that day were suffering from serious mental disorders. Two of them, Manugian noted, were "very dangerous."[30] Manugian informed the authorities, who replied that they could no longer prevent prisoners from Roumieh Prison (the largest prison in the country) from being released by gangs of armed men. The country had plunged into total lawlessness.

The same group of armed militiamen who had attacked the Hospital on March 14, 1976, visited the next day, saying that they wished to release another prisoner who was seriously ill as well as three of those whom they had returned the day before. Again the gendarmes presented no opposition. Manugian tried to reason with the armed men, but again to no avail. Their intention was clear: they were releasing Christian men who were being treated for drug addiction as a favor to the men's families, and they were frequently kidnapping and killing Muslim patients in retaliation for similar violence that had been perpetrated against their own partisans in Muslim-controlled areas. On March 18, 1976, three of the prisoners who had been released by the armed men were found dead.

On March 19, the atmosphere outside the Hospital was so hellish—with bombings, heavy shelling, and machine-gun fire—that Manugian had to increase the prescription of tranquilizers to calm both patients and staff. On March 20, one of the prisoners who had been taken away by the armed men came back, wanting to be readmitted to the forensic unit. The world outside the Hospital seemed more insane to him. Utterly baffled by this turn of events and unwilling to take any unnecessary additional risks, the gendarmes refused to readmit him. Nevertheless, Manugian decided to admit him to the general ward, given "the miserable condition in which he was."[31]

In the early morning of March 25, a shell burst in front of the forensic unit, causing substantial damage.[32] The next day, heavy shelling injured a patient, and two days after that, a patient was killed when one of the shells damaged the roof of the Scottish House. By March 29, every one of the Hospital's buildings had been hit at least once (figure 5.1). The gendarmes, now desperate, handed the keys of the forensic unit to the medical director and walked away. A few days later, armed men came to the gendarmes' offices in the forensic unit and took away several items, including their safe and several of their machine guns. Manugian, who was known to be overly optimistic even under duress, noted with a bit of pride that, given the total lack of security in the country, it was quite remarkable that

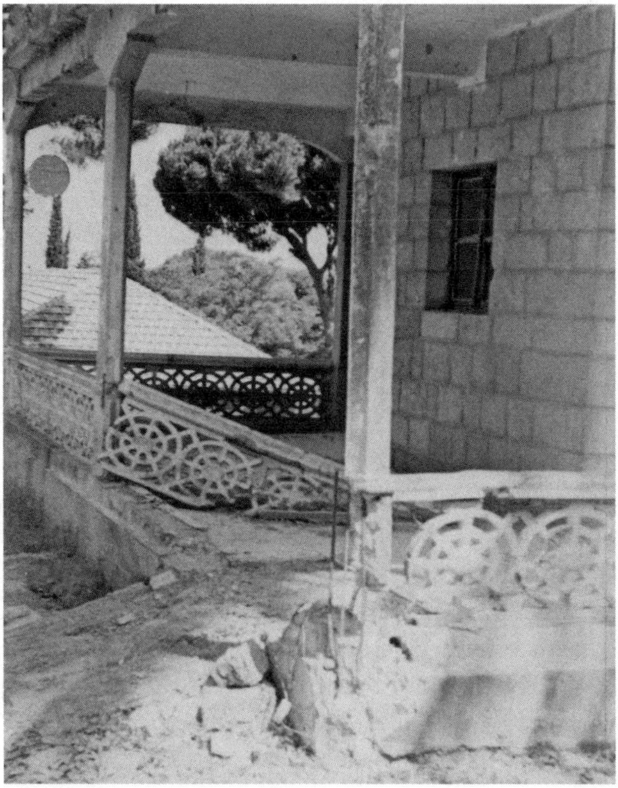

Figure 5.1
The damaged Khairallah House (named after Asʿad Khairallah, a member of the original Beirut committee), March 1976.
Source: LH/08/08, box 11, LH, SOAS.

any prisoners were still left at ʿAṣfūriyyeh.[33] The continuous shelling and explosions caused heavy damage to the Hospital, and the physical violence against the patients continued unabated, with more patients being killed, injured, or kidnapped.[34] The militiamen had also violently assault female patients. Two of them were "ill-treated" by armed men, Manugian reported, and "had evidence of trauma on their bodies."[35] Sexual violence remains a pervasive, if often overlooked, occurrence in modern armed conflicts.[36]

On April 6, three patients were injured and one killed amid intense shelling and bombing.[37] A ceasefire later that day allowed the Hospital to discharge a few of the remaining patients for their own protection, since it was becoming too dangerous to stay on the grounds. The patients' transport was a delicate affair. The Muslims among them had to be safely transferred to Muslim-controlled areas and the Christians to Christian-controlled areas.[38] In addition, patients who identified themselves as Druze, Jewish, Buddhist, and atheist also had to be transferred.[39] This moment marks the beginning of the disintegration of the pluralistic community that had managed to provide a model of harmony and peace in which "diverse races, creeds, temperaments and social conditions" had coexisted for almost eight decades.[40]

The Arab League created the ADF in 1976 as a peacekeeping army to put an end to the civil war. However, since the ADF was mostly composed of Syrian troops, it ended up legitimizing Syria's presence in Lebanon. This "pax Syriana," as scholars and journalists have called it, lasted until the withdrawal of the Syrian army in 2005.[41] On December 21, 1976, the ADF occupied two buildings at ʿAṣfūriyyeh.[42] The Hospital matron made sure to note in her report the sympathy that these Syrian soldiers showed toward the patients and their illnesses by keeping them entertained during the occasional curfews.[43] Perhaps she was contrasting their compassion with the erratic and violent behavior of the militiamen who frequently visited the Hospital and showed no empathy toward the vulnerable men and women who were caught up in a violent and senseless conflict.

On February 7, 1978, fighting with heavy machine guns erupted between the ADF and the Lebanese army in the vicinity of ʿAṣfūriyyeh. The fighting initially lasted for several minutes. Then sporadic fighting of increasing intensity took place for the next twenty-four hours, with several shells falling on the Hospital's grounds. On February 21, a patient attempted to escape, but the Syrian soldiers brought him back.[44] On the same day, three staff members attempted to leave but had to return, since it had become too dangerous to pass the barricades.

A few months later, renewed fighting erupted between the ADF and the Lebanese army. This time the Hospital was under siege, with heavy artillery installed in its vicinity.[45] The Hospital staff used all basic commodities (fuel, food, and medicines) with caution, and because of the acute shortage of staff it became necessary to appoint patients to look after the Hospital's wards at night. "I am pleased to report [that the patients] did well and no incidents occurred," the matron reported.[46] She extolled all the patients—"even the prisoners," for their courage and, perhaps paradoxically, their sense of responsibility when the need arose.[47] Manugian even had a term for this new bond of solidarity among patients and staff: a "therapeutic community."[48]

Manugian often underlined what would become a recurrent theme in his war chronicles: the solidarity expressed by his staff and patients in the midst of a sectarian war. In his medical report for 1976, he wrote, "In our hospital of many races, nationalities as well as religious and political affiliations both amongst patients and staff, we did not have any reason to worry about possible emotional tension. This, we must agree, indicates a high level of Team Spirit devoted to the care and welfare of suffering human beings."[49] He also frequently invoked the cooperation and camaraderie among staff of different religious backgrounds: "We are in a Christian dominated area. But our non-Christian staff continues working."[50]

This unity and harmony across sects, which were eroding on the national level, managed to remain intact throughout the war, though they were increasingly being tested. Anonymous callers made repeated phone calls to the Hospital in which they threatened various members of the staff.[51] When Kamal Jumblatt, leader of the Progressive Socialist Party, was assassinated on March 17, 1977, some of the Druze staff decided to leave.[52] Sectarian tensions had become especially high by July 1978, when the Hospital was under a state of siege.[53] Manugian frequently met with staff and students to reduce their anxieties and fears.[54] He also wrote letters of appreciation and gratitude in the Hospital's newsletter in which he praised their ethic of care, which placed the welfare of the patients "above all personal, religious and political considerations."[55] Remarkably, the Hospital continued to offer psychiatric counseling at its dispensaries in Ḥazmiyyeh (the city where ʿAṣfūriyyeh was located).[56] ʿAṣfūriyyeh's medical staff braved bullets and shells to provide these services free of charge to an increasingly nervous, anxious, and traumatized population that lived outside the Hospital walls.

AUB, with which the Hospital had long-lasting ties (as we saw in previous chapters), also lost a large number of students and staff during the civil war. In February 1976, two AUB deans were assassinated: Raymond S. Ghosn, dean of the School of Engineering and a former member of ʿAṣfūriyyeh's BEC, and Robert Najemy, dean of students.[57] The fates of at least another thirty AUB students and staff who were abducted during the war remain unknown.[58] Acting president David Dodge was kidnapped in June 1982 and held for more than a year before being released, and Thomas M. Sutherland, dean of agriculture, was seized in June 1985 and was not set free for another six years. Perhaps the greatest blow to the cosmopolitan and liberal ethos of AUB—and of similar institutions such as 'Aṣfūriyyeh, where people from different creeds and cultures, be they foreigners or locals, worked and lived together—was the assassination of AUB president Malcolm Kerr in 1984 by an unidentified gunman who fired two bullets into Kerr's head while he was walking to his office.[59]

Although occasional shortages of food, electricity, and water occurred, the Hospital managed to survive throughout the war without facing a serious crisis. However, Manugian had to be escorted outside the grounds by the military on several occasions, so that he could bring flour to the Hospital.[60] A year later, militiamen confiscated the flour, and a tank of heating oil had to be escorted by the military because of earlier attempts by armed men to steal it.[61] It seemed as if little had changed since Ottoman times, when Watson Smith, 'Aṣfūriyyeh's medical director at the time, had had to cooperate with the Ottomans to secure a supply of vital commodities to the Hospital as well as the safety of the patients and staff. One radical departure from Ottoman times, however, is the deliberate violence perpetrated against both patients and property and the total disregard for the Hospital's neutrality. It is worth remembering that during the First World War, the Ottomans recognized 'Aṣfūriyyeh as a charitable hospital. And although the medical director and the matron were British subjects, and thus citizens of an enemy country, the Ottoman authorities did not arrest them. On the contrary, the authorities allowed them to remain and work on the premises of the Hospital. By November 1976, the number of patients and staff had dropped precipitously, and in addition to the injuries and death the staff and patients suffered, many staff members had lost relatives.[62]

The Hospital now had to cope with one of the few times when it was attacked in the press. As we saw in chapter 4, the first time 'Aṣfūriyyeh was attacked was when the famous poet and feminist writer Mayy Ziyādah had been hospitalized there. Now rumors were circulating that patients were being massacred, and these rumors insinuated that the Hospital had failed to protect its patients from sectarian abductions and assassinations.[63] It is true that Manugian and the Hospital staff felt helpless: the belligerents rarely, if ever, took their opinion into consideration. But, as Manugian tried to explain to the LGC, despite the killing and abductions of several patients, some had returned unharmed, and some had been safely returned to their families. Manugian also tried to reassure the committee that all the patients had been taken away without their identity papers, since these could have been a liability for anyone who was caught on the wrong side of the conflict.[64]

Despite the intensive shelling and shooting, the patients in general did not seem to be disturbed. "On the contrary," Manugian noted, "they seem to be calmer than usual ... this is a known phenomenon at times of crisis: the counter reaction of excitement often comes when the social tension is relaxed."[65] This line of reasoning is curiously in agreement with a prevalent nineteenth-century belief that idleness and insouciance were predisposing factors of madness, and thus they needed to be overcome through work and other occupation.[66] But of course Manugian was referring to the long-term psychological effects of war that are not necessarily visible during the war itself, when one's primary concern is survival.

As Manugian predicted, these psychological impacts were unleashed once the hostilities ceased. Indeed, the first few studies of the effects of war on the Lebanese civilian population published in the 1980s (before the category of post-traumatic stress disorder took hold in the 1990s onwards) were conclusive about the rise in post-traumatic psychiatric complaints—most notably anxiety and depressive symptoms.[67] In addition, as we saw in chapter 4, significant increases in substance abuse and alcoholism were also noted. And psychiatrists found themselves loaded with patients.

For Abdul Rahman Labban, a psychiatrist who worked at ʿAṣfūriyyeh during the civil war as well as supervising a home for the elderly that was transformed into a morgue in that period, it was not the people he cared for who were insane, but the so-called normal people who were participating in the armed conflict, killing other people arbitrarily and inflicting horrific violence on others. In transferring the diagnosis of abnormality to those engaged in violence, Labban was in line with a generation of psychiatrists who described political disturbance, disorder, and violence in terms of psychiatric pathologies.[68] For example, he reported seeing "sophisticated, educated, professional people—one of them I know to be an exceptionally fine doctor—standing on balconies with snipers' rifles killing almost at random with seeming pleasure."[69] And in postmortem examinations at the morgue in the former home for the elderly, Labban saw wounds that he believed could only have been perpetrated by what he called a psychopathic surgeon.

A few decades later, the first study to examine the mental health of soldiers who had taken part in the civil war concurred with Labban's observations. Charles Baddoura, chief psychiatrist at Dayr al-Ṣalīb, found militiamen who took part in the civil war to have "antisocial personality disorders,"[70] echoing the "psychopathic personality" diagnosis that was found among soldiers who fought in the two world wars, as we saw in chapter 4. In contrast, soldiers from the Lebanese army were found to be more likely to have situational and affective personality disorders. Perhaps Baddoura wanted to differentiate between the behaviors of soldiers who belonged to what was generally perceived to be a legitimate institution and those of militiamen who were accused of corruption and sectarian cleansing.[71]

One criminologist described the collective state of mind of people during the short periods of respite during the 1975–1976 round of civil war as psychopathology.[72] This disordered and regressive cognitive anomie seemed to challenge the observation that group cohesiveness and solidarity increase when people are faced with a common threat. What used to be attributed to the lax morals of Orientals in the nineteenth century (as we saw in chapter 1) was now attributed to their predilection for internecine warfare. Unlike in the nineteenth century, however, in the twentieth century these pronouncements were made not by missionaries or Western doctors but by a generation of new mind experts who were attuned to the cultural, political, and behavioral markers of their own communities.

In contrast, other psychiatrists emphasized the resilience and "high morale" of people during war, noting the emergence of what they called a "psychological mindedness"—especially in the 1980s, when people seemed more eager to express their political and personal distress.[73] It appeared that by the mid-1980s the Lebanese people had become "more psychologically aware," and they frequently used in the media "psychological and psychoanalytical concepts in discussing both their political and personal difficulties."[74]

Patients who died in the Hospital could not be buried properly. Because of the dangerous roads and the shelling and bombing of the area until at least 1978, it was difficult for the relatives of the deceased to attend burials, which were conducted hurriedly and under dangerous conditions.[75] It is not even clear where the patients who died on the premises of 'Aṣfūriyyeh were buried. We do not know if they were laid to rest on the premises or in a nearby cemetery, nor do we know the fate of the bodies of the non-Christians among them. We have a few indications, such as the story of a female Shiite patient from Baalbek who died of natural causes but, because of the raging war, could not be buried near ʿAṣfūriyyeh. Instead, her body was sent back to her village in the Beqaa Valley under dangerous conditions.[76] This brings to a tragic full circle the claim by Cornelius Van Dyck that these dispossessed and abandoned people at the margins of life and the city were indeed "the dead which cannot be buried."[77] Now they could literally not be buried.

Other stories are even grimmer, such as the unclaimed bodies that eventually ended up in AUB's anatomy department. This history has yet to be written, but it will suffice for now to sketch how this situation came to be. Because dissection was forbidden under Ottoman law, bodies (which were sometimes stolen from cemeteries) were smuggled to the SPC (renamed AUB in 1920).[78] Unclaimed bodies at ʿAṣfūriyyeh were also sent to the basement of the college's School of Medicine, where dissections took place. In 1921, during the French Mandate, the faculty informed the French authorities that the unclaimed bodies of ʿAṣfūriyyeh patients were among those that had been preserved at AUB for the purpose of teaching anatomy.[79] Other cases of unclaimed bodies were recorded in the 1950s.[80] One cannot exclude the possibility that the unknown victims of the Lebanese civil war met similar fates.

The Downfall

While three distinct periods of crisis took place in the history of the Hospital, the civil war that began in 1975 was the fatal one.[81] It is true that the two world wars left the Hospital struggling financially, but after the First World War, the Hospital was steadily moving toward self-sufficiency and scarcely needed to make public appeals.[82] In the aftermath of the Second World War, however, ʿAṣfūriyyeh was on the brink of closure because of a number of factors, including inflation; new and taxing labor laws, which led to dramatic increases in salaries and wages; the withdrawal en bloc of patients paid for by the government (who were sent instead to the much cheaper Dayr al-Ṣalīb, as discussed in previous chapters); and a decrease in the number of private patients, who had formerly traveled from neighboring countries to seek the specialized treatment offered at ʿAṣfūriyyeh.[83]

But a 1944 emergency appeal initiated by Fadlo Hourani (father of the historian Albert Hourani), a Protestant from south Lebanon and an active member of the London committee since the 1920s, successfully managed to raise the amount needed to salvage the institution, with the largest donations coming from local people.[84] On his visit to his native land (he had been living and working in Manchester),[85] Fadlo Hourani pleaded the case of ʿAṣfūriyyeh to the first elected president of the independent Republic of Lebanon, Bechara el-Khoury, and a few days later el-Khoury invited Hourani to his palace in Beirut to announce the government's decision to grant his request.[86] Hourani recounted how other local funds from "all sections of the population" had poured in following his appeal.[87] The largest sum was raised by the Friends of the Lebanon Hospital (i.e., ʿAṣfūriyyeh), a group made up of local notables such as Albert Pharoun (the Lebanese consul in Haifa) and Omar Bey Daouk (president of the municipality of Beirut). In 1944, Hourani also made an appeal in Arabic on the BBC that raised additional money from Great Britain and its colonies in West Africa.[88]

This historic bailout is noted in the records of the Hospital as a moment of "national awakening" and shared responsibility in institution and nation building: a first in the history of the Hospital and perhaps in the history of the country.[89] Hourani also suggested adding a Muslim member to the BEC during that period and hailed what he called a "new spirit of cooperation" among the Lebanese.[90] His suggestion was approved. A Syrian Muslim medical doctor named Hamsy had also joined the medical team of ʿAṣfūriyyeh during that period and was appointed second assistant to R. Stewart Miller, the medical director.[91] As President el-Khoury put it, this was "the dawn of a new era."[92]

A more sustainable financial basis for the Hospital was put in place in 1947–1948 that enabled a number of renovations and improvements.[93] In the 1950s, the Hospital became what was described as an exemplary manifestation of how foreign and national efforts could be "synergistic."[94] The Hospital continued to grow in the 1950s and 1960s, building new facilities to ease the increasing overcrowding in wards and units.

The fatal crisis started in the early 1970s. At this point, foreign donations, especially from Quaker groups, had been in decline for some time. The Quaker founder's granddaughters had promised to raise funds, but these had never materialized.[95] With the decline of missionary donations, a new charitable economy, driven by its own interests and ambitions, was starting to emerge in the modern Middle East. This new economy supplemented and increasingly supplanted that of the old imperial powers. As we have seen in previous chapters, these powers had played a profound role in shaping education and the health care system of the region. The chief stakeholders in the new moral economy—Saudi Arabia and Iran—were reluctant to invest in a country that was in the midst of a civil war, with seemingly no prospect for peace or stability in sight.[96]

Another reason for the crisis was the emergence of new and competitive markets in these oil-rich nations. After a visit to the Saudi city of Ta'if following an invitation to advise the Saudis on their mental health care system, Manugian noted the possible threat that the growth of the psychiatry field in that country posed to the viability of ʿAṣfūriyyeh.[97] To continue enjoying Saudi confidence and money, ʿAṣfūriyyeh had to be able to keep providing high-quality know-how and advanced teaching facilities, services that were becoming compromised by the civil war. The rapid development of Saudi Arabia's own infrastructure for mental health care was also becoming a threat, since ʿAṣfūriyyeh could lose the highly valued private patients from the Gulf. And indeed it did. During the civil war, income from private patients diminished, and the bulk of the inpatients' expenses became dependent on a government whose payments were continually in arrears.[98] The government debt to the Hospital was estimated in the mid-1970s to be over LBP 1 million.[99]

Furthermore, the British, who had long-standing ties to the Hospital, were now becoming increasingly attracted to the rich petrodollar economies and thus were reluctant to continue to support an institution that had become burdensome.[100] In 1972 this position of the British administration exasperated the British ambassador to Lebanon, Paul Wright who, in contrast to his predecessor—who viewed ʿAṣfūriyyeh as an obsolete Victorian institution—still valued the Hospital. In a confidential letter to Sir Geoffrey Furlonge, chairman of the London committee of ʿAṣfūriyyeh, Wright (who also served as ex officio president of ʿAṣfūriyyeh's Beirut committee and an informant to the London committee) made the case for pressing the British government for financial support if the existence of the Hospital were in jeopardy. Wright believed it was worth "preserving what is after all an important British concern and an institution of great value in the Middle East."[101] In a letter addressed to the British Ministry of Overseas Development, Paul P. Howell (head of the Middle East Development Division in Beirut) likewise lamented the lack of assistance to ʿAṣfūriyyeh, calling it a "most depressing story" that had made him pessimistic about the Hospital's future.[102]

Nevertheless, the Hospital ended up receiving substantial help from the British government. The British government sent a group of architects (who advised on planning the new hospital) and donated new equipment.[103] Rather than referring to the historic tie that linked ʿAṣfūriyyeh to Great Britain, as Ambassador Wright articulated it in his confidential letter to Sir Furlonge, the architects justified the British government's interest for such an investment as being merely self-serving. They explicitly mentioned three reasons: "publicity for the British government and industry," the "further expansion of trade in areas in the Middle East and parts of Africa," and the enhancement of "goodwill towards Britain."[104] More significantly, the British government made a major donation in 1978, which the Hospital used to pay staff salaries.[105] Still, this was not enough to save the Hospital from insolvency.

Though the Lebanese government's payments were chronically inadequate, that alone was not a fatal blow to the Hospital's financial situation. Far more detrimental was the period of inflation preceding the onset of the civil war in 1975, followed by governmental decrees that increased wages to appease public anger.[106] Under pressure from the Labor Federation, which called for a general strike in May 1971, the government approved a 5 percent increase in wages in both the public and the private sectors. A year later, with inflation still high and the global oil crisis well under way, the price of commodities skyrocketed, and the government had to increase wages by another 5 percent. In 1973, the year when the original estate of ʿAṣfūriyyeh was sold in exchange for the ʿAramūn site, inflation increased to 10 percent, and again the government had to increase wages—and so on for most of the first half of the 1970s. These increases in wages, salaries, and indemnities put a tremendous strain on the Hospital's finances. (Under a new law passed in 1963, the Hospital also had to pay for social security, which kept increasing with every new labor law passed in the 1970s.)[107] One should remember that ʿAṣfūriyyeh had grown in terms of both patient admissions and staff appointments: the Hospital had 231 staff members in 1974, compared to only 12 in 1941.[108] The increase in expenditures was substantial, and given the chronic deficit, the impact of that increase was considerable. Indeed, all of the funds raised during that period (especially from Great Britain as well as Saudi Arabia) were used to cover staff payments and indemnities.[109]

The financial losses during the civil war were in fact the largest the Hospital had incurred in its long history. In addition to the old Hospital premises (which, as mentioned above, sustained damage in the war), the new hospital at ʿAramūn was also substantially damaged, as an album of photos inventorying the destruction clearly shows (figure 5.2). Construction work

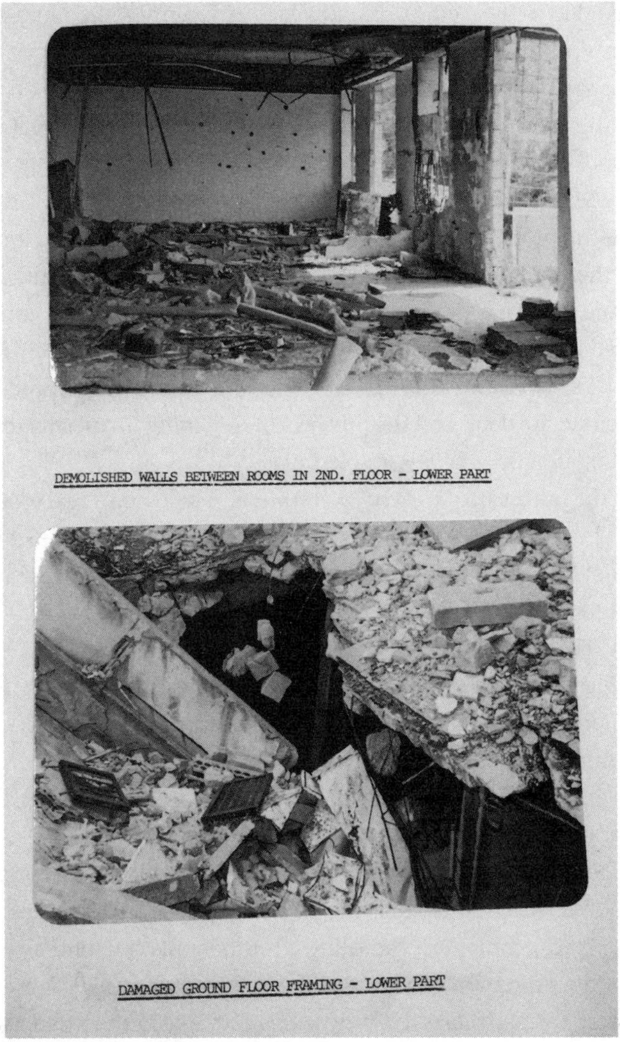
DEMOLISHED WALLS BETWEEN ROOMS IN 2ND. FLOOR - LOWER PART
DAMAGED GROUND FLOOR FRAMING - LOWER PART

Figure 5.2

Photographs taken from an album inventorying the damage of the hospital in ʿAramūn, by D. G. Jones and Partners Chartered Quantity Surveyors, October 1991. *Source*: LH/12/01, box 16, LH, SOAS.

was halted due to blocked roads and a lack of security.[110] In addition, it was becoming very difficult to continue the fund-raising campaign that was crucial for saving the Hospital from imminent financial collapse, given the political disturbances and donors' general distrust. "We are in real financial trouble both for completing the project and running it the way it should be," wrote Manugian to Sir Geoffrey Furlonge in June 1975.[111] In addition to damaging the property, militiamen also stole essential construction materials.[112] Further looting of the new material and damage to the infrastructure added more cost to a project that now seemed impossible to complete.[113] War-related losses at the new site were estimated at well over LBP 15 million (equal to US$3.5 million in 1982).[114] As the years passed, the Hospital continued to accumulate debt, and the prospect of becoming financially rescued by a major donation became less and less likely.

Before the outbreak of the civil war, Lebanon had seen a real estate boom thanks to petrodollar investments.[115] This had encouraged the committee to sell its old site and build a new hospital on new land—which, in their view, would be more cost-effective than upgrading the old facilities and buildings. The money that was raised by selling the old premises would have enabled the upgrading of hospital care (which was necessary to attract wealthier private patients) while also creating an endowment to make the Hospital financially sustainable.[116]

However, the civil war wrecked this modernization program on every level. The number of private patients dropped by half, while enormous debts—around US$8 million in 1982 or US$22 million in current purchasing power—accumulated at the new construction site because of war-related damage. (Staff salaries accounted for the other half of the remaining debt.)[117] A major loan from the Lebanese government in 1979 was insufficient to stem the Hospital's looming insolvency, given the financial weight of expenses from salaries, indemnities, and investment in the new site.[118]

On December 16, 1980, the Beirut and London committees passed a resolution to cease all activities at the Hospital.[119] The remaining funds were exhausted a few days later, and construction at the new site was halted.[120] The Hospital officially stopped functioning on April 10, 1982, two months before Israel invaded Lebanon and occupied the new site in in ʿAramūn, leaving the property even more damaged.[121] Like the original ʿAṣfūriyyeh site during the First World War, the ʿAramūn site was strategic, since it overlooked the Beirut airport. Following the Israeli withdrawal from Beirut in 1983 (Israel continued to occupy south Lebanon until 2000), the new occupying Syrian army built military barracks on the site, which then made it the target of the Lebanese artillery of General Michel Aoun during his Liberation War (1989–1990) against the Syrians and resulted in further damage.[122] To quote the anthropologist Shannon Lee Dawdy, not only does politics produce ruins but likewise "ruins produce politics."[123]

By the end of March 1981, the London committee had decided to transfer all rights and responsibilities to the BEC.[124] The LGC deemed it to be "no longer appropriate that an institution in an independent sovereign state should continue to be governed from London."[125] The London committee's decision seems to have been more of a pretext to abandon its responsibilities rather than a genuine rejection of a neo-colonial bond. First, the Lebanese members of the BEC approved of—in fact, valued—the London connection.[126] Second, although the "Lebanization" of the staff and personnel had occurred in the 1950s when Manugian joined the managerial staff, the relegation of power from the London committee to the Beirut committee was not an issue at the time.

The Hospital staff did not remain idle, however. Tension was rising, with several incidents reported.[127] Members of the Hospital staff syndicate were becoming frustrated and disappointed by the Beirut committee's inability to pay their salaries. But the committee attempted to clarify that, unlike other institutions that depended on the support of foreign governments, ʿAṣfūriyyeh had always been an "independent, non-profit-making establishment controlled by its own committee."[128] In other words, ʿAṣfūriyyeh was the responsibility of neither the British nor the Americans, despite the longstanding ties of both to the Hospital. This was not entirely true, as we will see in chapter 6—since the American and British embassies were next in line in the succession of trusteeship of the Hospital (and therefore of responsibility).

When the Beirut committee suspended activities at ʿAṣfūriyyeh on December 31, 1982, the employees held Manugian against his will as a way to pressure the committee for their pay.[129] One month later, all the employees decided to march to the presidential palace to protest the decision to close the Hospital, and they were supported in this action by the remaining patients and prisoners.[130] Nevertheless, their activities did not change the course of events, and employment contracts were effectively terminated ten days later. All liabilities to staff and employees (amounting to LBP 6.5–7.0

million) were covered by the sale of a land parcel (which was not waqf land and therefore could be sold) to Gefinor, an investment firm. [131]

On February 17, 1982, the chairman of the Beirut committee, Muhammad Shukayr, reported that the foundation of Rafiq Hariri (a businessman who had made a fortune in Saudi Arabia and would later become prime minister of Lebanon) was willing to finance the completion of the new hospital at 'Aramūn.[132] Although this financing never materialized, a company named Solidere ended up owning 'Aṣfūriyyeh. Founded by Hariri in 1994 and marred by scandals ever since, Solidere was a joint stock company for the redevelopment and reconstruction of Beirut.[133] Gefinor, which had "bought" (technically the land was exchanged as will be explained in chapter 6) the original estate in 1973, sold the property to Abdallah Tamari—who, according to one newspaper, was the front man for Solidere, in which the Hariri family had a major stake of "$100 million dollars."[134]

As of this writing, the plan is to turn the 130,000 square meters of green space, which includes forty-six buildings of historical and architectural significance, into a residential development site. From a space where the "dead which cannot be buried" constituted the sacred link to the eschatological missions of the fin de siècle, 'Aṣfūriyyeh may be en route to becoming an anonymous, amnesiac, and sterile site of consumerism.

Conclusion

The history of 'Aṣfūriyyeh (including its tragic downfall) departs from the trajectory and fate of nineteenth-century psychiatric hospitals in the West. In contrast to the wave of deinstitutionalization and the antipsychiatry movement that swept across Europe, Great Britain, and the United States starting in the 1960s (which led to the dismantling of overcrowded and underfunded psychiatric institutions), in Lebanon it was a civil war that aborted a grand vision of social reform and the expansion of mental health care. The dream and underlying philosophy of 'Aṣfūriyyeh of serving in the vanguard of progressive medicine was overly optimistic in a country that was taking risky bets on its own future.[135] The greatest blow came from the damage incurred during the civil war, which included direct damage to property and life as well as various kinds of indirect damage: the dramatic decrease in the number of private patients, the low incentive for donors to invest in the country, the increasing debt of the government, inflation, the decreasing influence of Great Britain as its interests shifted toward the Gulf, and the new challenges brought about by the rise of petrodollar economies.

Furthermore, from a longue durée perspective, it becomes clear that the Hospital's interdenominational reach and resoundingly nonsectarian philosophy were not mere propaganda efforts to attract Muslims but a natural strategy of survival, given the sectarian tensions that had not waned since at least the 1840s. Dismissing this politics of inclusion as mere publicity misses the point. The terminology that focuses on internationalism was in a sense a reflection of the mentality of the time, but it was also necessary, both politically and financially. ʿAṣfūriyyeh could have been promoted as a Christian hospital, but instead the founding committee and successive committees chose to present it as nonsectarian and hence nonpartisan. This turned out to be a boon throughout the Hospital's history. In times of crises as in times of peace, the Hospital managed to garner support from an international body of donors, local political authorities across sects, and various foreign governments that were sometimes at odds with one another. Most importantly, nonsectarianism became the Hospital's raison d'être. But the sectarian civil war took its toll. The national institution that ʿAṣfūriyyeh had become over the years disintegrated simultaneously with the Lebanese state. Along with them both went the dreams and aspirations of an entire generation.

6 The Politics of Health, Charity, and Sectarianism

And if a house be divided against itself, that house cannot stand.

—Mark 3:25

In 1983, a year after the official closure of the Hospital, the chairman of the BEC, Muhammad Shukayr, became mutawallī of the waqf.[1] He was the first Muslim and first Sunni to hold such a position. As noted in chapter 5, the LGC approved of this transfer of power, which it deemed necessary. But Shukayr, who was also a diplomat and political adviser to President Amin Gemayel and critical of the politics of Damascus, was assassinated in 1987.[2] What followed until the appointment of Adnan Mroueh in 1991 is not entirely clear. Mroueh, who at that time was dean and vice president for health at AUB, was elected chairman in 1991 by a committee made up of the following people: Raif Nassif (a previous chairman of the BEC), Nadia Khlat, Raja Shabshab, Antranig Manugian, and himself.[3] Although the London committee had advised the Beirut committee to draft a new constitution, it seems that the latter was following the 1965 constitution—which stipulated that a quorum of three was enough to make decisions, including elections of members to key positions.

Today, Mroueh claims to be the de facto mutawallī of the hospital, but the Supreme Council of the Protestant Community in Syria and Lebanon contests this claim.[4] The conflict arose when Mroueh struck a deal with a Canadian government–funded consortium of universities and insurance companies to rebuild and rehabilitate the damaged hospital in ʻAramūn while maintaining the historical academic affiliation with AUB. Not only did the Supreme Council contest Mroueh's trusteeship, but it also claimed that it owned ʿAṣfūriyyeh.[5] Since the Supreme Council also considered the waqf to be unequivocally Protestant (which as this chapter will show is not an obvious assertion), it also argued that the mutawallī should be the president of the council. Before any legal arbitration could be made, the Supreme Council appointed and recognized its president, Reverand Salim Sahiouny, as mutawallī of ʿAṣfūriyyeh.[6] The case is still in court as of this writing.

The first part of this chapter challenges the claim that ʿAṣfūriyyeh's nonsectarian character was deployed merely for propaganda purposes. It shows how from a longue durée perspective, using this otherwise anodyne feature as an analytical lens reveals its polysemic uses and various implications. Local supporters across all faiths as well as committee members were eager to promote this distinctive character of the Hospital to garner national support, especially in times of crisis. It is this particular feature that allowed ʿAṣfūriyyeh to be perceived as a national institution and to survive for so long. The Hospital staff and administrators' resilience and their rejection of threats to abandon this distinctive feature when the political climate was full of sectarian hatred and violence—as was the case during the Lebanese civil war (explored in chapter 5)—is testimony to this deep faith, almost an ideological commitment, in the nonsectarian philosophy of ʿAṣfūriyyeh as a therapeutic community in which coexistence and tolerance prevailed at a time when these two notions had eroded outside the Hospital.

The second part of the chapter argues that the downfall of this influential institution marks a shift in the configuration of health care in Lebanon, what I call the birth of the sectarianization of health—that is, the monopoly of health services by the various religious and political stakeholders, with mental health care being a case in point.

An International Hospital

Political scientists and economists have shown in recent years how welfare services in Lebanon and other similarly pluralist (yet weak) states are allocated along sectarian or ethnic lines.[7] These studies have tended to focus on the period after the civil war, which is generally agreed to have commenced a year after the Ta'if Accords were signed, on October 22, 1989.[8] But this sectarian configuration of health and welfare services has not always been the case. It is true that under the Ottomans, different religious groups provided some of these basic services (specifically related to education and health), with the Sublime Porte subsidizing its own Muslim charitable institutions. But the decree of 1839 that began the Tanzimat era (see the introduction) initiated what we could call more secular forms of health care services. For the first time it was decreed that municipalities, a nineteenth-century invention, would play a key role in health care provision.[9] These more secular or nonsectarian forms of health care provision were not necessarily created because of egalitarian concerns. Instead, they were a necessary by-product of the internationalization of public health care that had become necessary to cope with the new pandemics and other public health threats that had stricken the Mediterranean and beyond during the nineteenth century.[10]

Unlike the ethnic (i.e., sectarian or religious) nineteenth-century European and American hospitals or the so-called minority hospitals in Constantinople, ʿAṣfūriyyeh was from the outset open to people from all sects and denominations. (Minority and ethnic groups often felt compelled to found such hospitals to promote their own needs and protect themselves from experiencing intolerance or being forced to convert.)[11] The Hospital prided itself on being an ecumenical institution in which Jews, Muslims, and Christians of all kinds found shelter and sought care.[12] In all its official and unofficial documents and publications, ʿAṣfūriyyeh emphatically presented itself as nonsectarian, either interdenominational or nondenominational and international—although it did occasionally evoke its Britishness to garner financial support. The religious backgrounds of the patients were always published in the annual reports as proof of the interdenominational character of the Hospital. Patients came from all kinds of Christian denominations (Greek Orthodox, Maronite, Catholic, Protestant, and so on), and they also included Muslims, Druzes, Jews, Buddhists, and even atheists. And while Theophilus Waldmeier's original motivation for founding the Hospital came from his Christian and Quaker principles, not only was religion quickly sidelined and subverted (as we have seen in previous chapters), but starting in the mid-1950s onwards, Muslim patients began to outnumber Christian patients.[13]

One must ask if this emphasis on nonsectarianism was, as the historian Eugene Rogan argues, merely a show of public relations that was performed to gain the trust of the local population and of religious and official figures.[14] Of course, there may have been attempts to attract nominal Christians and Muslims by publicizing the cure of priests (like Paul, the Maronite priest, who is mentioned in chapter 4) or a prominent Muslim *sayed* (a title denoting descendants of the Prophet Muhammad). Nevertheless, these patients were often sent to 'Aṣfūriyyeh because of its reputation and not its nonsectarianism. This is shown by the letter of gratitude sent by Patriarch Huwayek, who sent Paul for treatment at the Hospital, and by the comment to the medical director from the family of the *sayed* that they had chosen 'Aṣfūriyyeh because "after inquiry they had come to the conclusion that this Hospital was the best."[15]

Moreover, something of a rationale or strategy of survival certainly had to be at work if the institution were to survive in a society that was divided along sectarian fault lines. Not only were the sectarian tensions still fresh in people's minds (notably the 1840 and 1860 massacres, which the missionaries frequently invoked), but suspicions of Protestants' intentions to secretly proselytize the locals by seducing them with their charitable activities were equally pervasive and a cause of concern to many sects.[16]

It would be simplistic to say that the Hospital used its nonsectarian cachet merely for propaganda purposes, however. The international character of the Hospital had been inscribed in its constitution as early as 1896. Article 1 stated, "This Institution is designed for the benefit of the insane of all classes, denominations and nationalities without distinction, but preference shall, as a rule, be given to the natives of the country."[17] This was an age of increasing international awareness and sensibility, as well as of intense humanitarian intervention and evangelical philanthropy.[18] It was also a time of increased connectedness around the world, whether in terms of cooperation and conflict, of flow of capital and labor, or of creativity and innovation.[19] Ignoring or underestimating the impact of this international context would necessarily lead to interpretating the recourse to nonsectarianism as being merely a self-interested effort to gain acceptance and support.

Was the Hospital's emphasis on nonsectarianism, then, a way to present a progressive and unified Christian (Protestant) faith above the "morass of sectarianism 'inherent' in the local population," as missionaries are thought to have believed and acted upon?[20] In other words, was nonsectarianism another tool in the armamentarium of the missionaries' "gentle crusade"?[21] This is a paradoxical claim, for Western Christians were far from being unified in the East. As we saw in chapter 2, Protestants and Jesuits constantly competed with and fought against one another along ideological and religious lines. If anything, then, theirs was a crusade within a crusade. In a typical characterization of the clerical battle for power and legitimacy in the Levant, Waldmeier wrote: "On the appearance of Protestantism in Syria in the year 1823, by the American Missions to the Oriental Churches, the Jesuits, well aware of the power of Evangelical teaching, lost no time in instructing the Maronite patriarch, bishops, and priests, and all other Popish Christians to oppose the missionaries by counteracting and neutralizing their influence by every possible means."[22] Indeed, while it is true that missionaries often complained about the "prejudices of a deep-rooted character" and the active fanaticism they encountered in the locals, mass conversion was never expected, and the reasons for this went beyond the missionaries' belief in an inherent kind of sectarianism.[23] Waldmeier recognized how difficult it was to come up with statistical figures for conversions, since many people did not publicly convert from fear of persecution.[24] The missionaries were acutely aware of the fate of people who had vocally and openly converted to Protestantism, especially (but not limited to) the Muslims among them.[25] But, perhaps more interestingly as the American Presbyterian missionary Howard Bliss (who succeeded his father, Daniel Bliss, as president of the SPC in 1903) argued, ecclesiastical statistics were not a measure of missionary success, nor were they an end in themselves.[26]

During the founding or missionary phase of the Hospital, various people invoked at least three different reasons for emphasizing the nonsectarian nature of ʿAṣfūriyyeh. Thomas S. Clouston, superintendent of the Edinburgh Royal Asylum, was of the opinion that this emphasis concerned humanity writ large. He reported being particularly moved by the "human neglect, misery and cruelty" faced by the insane in the East, which he had witnessed firsthand.[27] For him, nonsectarianism entailed humanism. For David Yellowlees, superintendent of the Gartnavel Royal Asylum near Glasgow (who had also traveled in Syria and was an early supporter of the Hospital, as discussed in chapter 2), the international character of the Hospital conferred on it political immunity, "away from Turkish interference or control."[28] Far from inciting sectarian divisions and sentiments, the founders of ʿAṣfūriyyeh were acutely aware of the need for inclusion and consensual politics. As article 10 of the 1896 constitution clearly put it: "In order to increase the general interest in this enterprise and to commend it to the confidence of the public, the Committee will invite a number of prominent men, representing the various nationalities and religious denominations, and the commercial and civil interest of the country, to constitute a Corps of Honorary Members, who shall meet with the Committee on special occasions to listen to reports as to the condition, progress and needs of the Institution, and to offer such suggestions for the consideration of the Committee as they may deem desirable."[29] If this statement were mere public relations, then the recommendation would have stayed at the consultation level. Instead, the committee's official members (who had voting privileges) included Protestants and Quakers as well as Muslims and Jews.[30] Well into the 1970s, the committee included leading figures from across faiths. Through this strategy of political survival, the Hospital benefited from the endorsement of all the major political forces it had worked with throughout its history, from the different Ottoman governors of Mount Lebanon to the American, French, and British authorities and the successive Lebanese governments that frequently bestowed national medals of recognition on its personnel.

The Hospital even maintained cordial relations with the warring militias during the civil war. In 1976, a year after the war broke out, Manugian wrote to the BEC: "[We] continue to keep our good relations with all organizations irrespective of religion, political affiliation or social status. This policy has served us well in the past and we have tried to continue in the same policy successfully during the present crisis."[31] While the terms "international" and "nondenominational" had characterized the Hospital's rhetoric in the late nineteenth century, nonsectarianism, inclusion, and solidarity across sects became the raison d'être of the Hospital during the civil war.

Economically, too, it made sense for ʿAṣfūriyyeh to be as international and interdenominational as possible in an age of internationalism and humanitarianism. The Hospital frequently received financial and material donations from foreign donors throughout its history, not only from different Quaker groups but also from various auxiliary committees and governments in Europe, Great Britain, and North America.[32] Commodities were flown in: linen came from Amsterdam, an American-made pump was used to supply water as early as 1899, the lighting of the entire Hospital (initially by gas) was made possible thanks to Swiss financial and technical support in 1910, and medical equipment was sent from London.[33] As we have seen in chapter 5, an important donation from the Rockefeller Foundation made teaching and research at ʿAṣfūriyyeh possible in its first years, while major Saudi and British grants in the late 1970s made the Hospital's closure more palatable by covering many expenses including its indemnities toward its

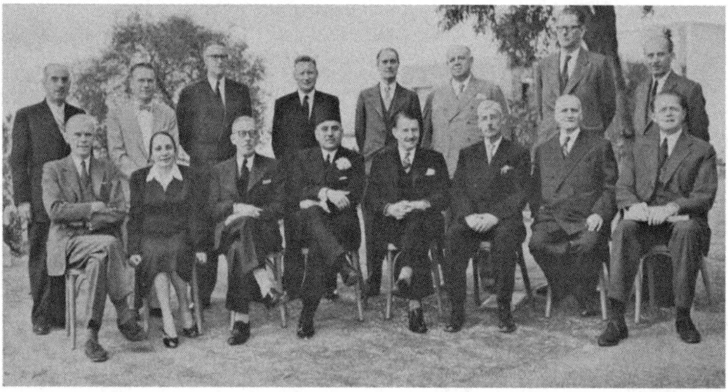

Figure 6.1

The Beirut Executive Committee, 1954. Standing: Professor S. Himadeh (AUB), Professor J. J. McDonald (AUB), E. P. Southby, H. C. Lees, Dr. J. Hitti. Seated: W. F. Gosling, Mrs. E. Cortas, K. Joly, Saeb Salam (prime minister in 1953), Sir E. Chapman-Andrews (British ambassador in Beirut), H. W. Glockler, Dr. A. Khairallah (AUB), and R. J. D. Belgrave.

Source: AR, 1953–1954, n.p., LHMND, AUB-SML.

staff. ʿAṣfūriyyeh was in fact the product of international efforts and generosity, as attested to by the different buildings that were erected over the years and named after the various nationalities of their donors.[34]

More importantly, local notables and ordinary citizens alike from across the different sects that make up modern Lebanon financially and politically supported ʿAṣfūriyyeh (see figure 6.1). As mentioned in chapter 5, in 1944 the Committee of the Friends of ʿAṣfūriyyeh, which was responsible for a critical fund-raising campaign to save the institution from bankruptcy, included Christian and Muslim notables.[35] Even secular organizations such as the Grand Lodge of Freemasons in Beirut and the Iraqi state oil company sent financial contributions.[36] As also mentioned in chapter 5, a major grant from the Lebanese government helped the Hospital make the transition during the difficult financial crisis of the Second World War. And President Fouad Chehab's firm support was the largest boost the Hospital had received from a Lebanese government. This was possible precisely because these different actors (much like the intellectuals of the Nahḍa period before them) considered ʿAṣfūriyyeh to be a national institution.

The LGC also firmly believed that the international cachet of ʿAṣfūriyyeh was the key to its success. The Hospital surely benefited from various political endorsements in terms of publicity as well as of protection, support, and legitimacy, especially during economic hardship and political turmoil. (As we saw in chapter 3, however, these relationships were occasionally fraught, given the growing competition with other institutions that had similar aims and aspirations.) The committees also believed that the French Mandate authorities were somewhat friendlier toward 'Aṣfūriyyeh than toward other Anglo-Saxon institutions in the country—such as AUB, for instance—precisely because of its more explicit international character. "They are our debtors," the LGC reported, "for 'Aṣfūriyyeh serves a great purpose to them ... the facet of the Hospital being international and interdenominational is a great advantage over other institutions."[37]

The British Connection

Though long lasting, the British connection mutated over the years. During the Hospital's early stages, the connection was through Quaker missionaries. It became more formalized by having the LGC oversee the BEC and the British ambassador in Beirut serving as ex officio president of the BEC. As the large volume of correspondence attests, the British ambassador's position essentially allowed the LGC to keep an eye on the BEC's decisions. Sir Geoffrey Furlonge, the last British mutawallī of 'Aṣfūriyyeh before it closed its doors, served as the British consul in Beirut from 1934 to 1946 and regularly corresponded with the British ambassador to Beirut.[38]

The interest that the British officials took in saving 'Aṣfūriyyeh from imminent bankruptcy in the 1970s had a different motivation than earlier interests in the institution (as we saw in chapters 2 and 3): It was a last-ditch attempt to salvage what remained of British influence and reputation in a crowded territory of foreign penetration. During the Lebanese civil war, when 'Aṣfūriyyeh, then on the verge of bankruptcy, asked for financial help from the British government, the Foreign Commonwealth Office and the British ambassador to Lebanon argued that failing to provide it would be damaging to Britain's reputation in Lebanon, especially at a time when other Western powers were being more generous.[39] As the minister of overseas development argued at the time, "The French have made a special contribution of over 1 million British pounds for 'their' hospital [the Hôtel-Dieu de France] in the Lebanon. There would be unfavourable publicity for the UK if the 'British' Hospital had to close."[40] In a telegram sent on February 11, 1977, Sir Peter Wakefield—the British ambassador to Lebanon and ex officio president of the BEC—complained about the low-key nature of the British response compared to that of the Americans and the French.[41] He then proposed that the British government should offer technical assistance to the Lebanese government to avoid accusations of being interested only in business and not in philanthropy. His predecessor, Cecil King, had likewise argued a few years earlier that because 'Aṣfūriyyeh was "the most substantial manifestation of British interest in this country," its failure would have "unfortunate repercussions on [the British] position."[42]

Nonetheless, the British link was also through the Hospital's therapeutic philosophy and its ethic of care. As we have seen in previous chapters, since the founding of the Hospital in 1896, professional links had existed with British institutions in terms of personnel training and the exchange of expertise and ideas. And although each of the Hospital's directors was a British subject (with the exception of the Swiss Otto Wolff), and generally the matrons were British,[43] Manugian—'Aṣfūriyyeh's last medical director—was the product of different cultural and genealogical lineages. Of Armenian descent, he has been described as a "cultural Protestant."[44] He had earned British citizenship while serving in the British army, but he was also a Lebanese minister who took part in the Ta'if Accords. These different characteristics made him the living embodiment of the mutation of Lebanese institutions from their colonial to their postcolonial stages.[45]

From a longue durée perspective, it thus becomes clear that instead of being part of a civilizing strategy, the nonsectarian institutional governance of 'Aṣfūriyyeh made the Hospital a model of intercommunal coexistence and "human cooperation," as Camille Chamoun, president of Lebanon in 1952–1958, put it in his endorsement of the Hospital on the occasion of its fiftieth anniversary.[46] Over the years, the patient population included people with up to thirty-four different religious affiliations.[47]

The paradox in this model is the Hospital's colonial superstructure. Starting in 1907, when its constitution was written, the London committee retained overall authority over the Hospital, overseeing its administration and finances and appointing its personnel.[48] Even its land and premises were under British and American consular protection, as stipulated by the waqf deed.[49]

The Sectarianization of Mental Health

Between the Ottoman Empire's *millet* system[50] and the politicized communalism of post-civil war Lebanon (where political parties displaced the state as providers of welfare services),[51] the country went through a period in which a more nationally and secularly oriented vision took hold. This new vision was visible during the national bailout of ʻAṣfūriyyeh in the mid-1940s under the presidency of Bechara el-Khoury and in the 1960s within the framework of a social security system during the Chehab presidency.

As we saw in chapter 2, the assistance publique, which was put in place by the French, was expanded under Chehab. Within that welfarist paradigm, the president's major achievement (one that became the emblem of his regime) was the establishment of the National Social Security Fund (*Caisse nationale de sécurité sociale*).[52] The fund was intended to provide health insurance and a pension program for employees and their family members who worked in the formal private sector, as well as contracted employees and wage earners in the public sector.[53] After a period of gestation that lasted more than two decades, Chehab had to create the Social Security Code (*Code de sécurité sociale*) by presidential decree on September 26, 1963, since the parliament had failed to vote on the bill (or even discuss it, despite having been invited to do so since 1956).[54] This, wrote the French ambassador in Beirut, reflected the "wide gap in political consciousness" between the parliamentarians and Chebab.[55]

ʻAṣfūriyyeh strove to offer a model that was publicly and unapologetically nonsectarian. First, from the Hospital's founding phase until the First World War, this model was justified by the Hospital's ecumenical Quaker values as well as its strategy of survival in what was widely perceived to be a precarious and hostile milieu. This period was followed by a nationalistic drive from the 1940s until the 1960s. The Hospital again clung to its model of nonsectarianism as a survival strategy during the civil war. The case of mental health care, and how it developed in Lebanon after the downfall of ʻAṣfūriyyeh, is a particularly striking example of what I call the birth of the sectarianization of health care, which marks a departure from a service that is emphatically not sectarian based. This configuration became visible only with the downfall of ʻAṣfūriyyeh and its closure in 1982.

As we saw in chapter 3, Dayr al-Ṣalīb, which was founded by a Lebanese Capuchin priest, became a proper psychiatric hospital in the 1950s as a way to compete with the increasingly influential ʿAṣfūriyyeh—which the Catholics perceived to be a Protestant institution. This move paid off, since Dayr al-Ṣalīb continued to grow after the decline of ʿAṣfūriyyeh and eventually became the largest provider of mental health care in Lebanon and the second largest in the Arab world (after Egypt's ʿAbbasiyya). Today it is the only psychiatric hospital that offers training in clinical psychiatry in Lebanon under the academic leadership of the faculty of USJ, while it is still managed by sisters from a local branch of the Franciscan order that was founded by Abūna Yaʿqūb.

The second-largest psychiatric hospital in Lebanon is Dār al-ʿAjaza al-Islāmiyya (the Islamic Asylum for the Elderly). Initially conceived of as a house for the elderly (much like Dayr al-Ṣalīb), this Muslim charitable asylum was founded in 1952 by prominent Sunni notables and philanthropists to cater to the needs of "the Muslim community" (*al-mujtamaʿ al-islāmī*) in Beirut.[56] The asylum is sustained by donations, particularly the annual *zakat* (the alms tax, which is one of the five pillars of the Muslim faith). Similar to the situation of Dayr al-Ṣalīb, the asylum was soon converted to a psychiatric hospital in 1959, although it continued to provide health care to the elderly. Interestingly, it was Abdul Rahman Labban—who in the early 1950s had trained as a psychiatrist at ʿAṣfūriyyeh—who founded its psychiatric department.[57] The hospital, which is situated in the Shatila Palestinian refugee camp in the southern suburbs of Beirut, currently has six hundred beds, of which about 400 are for psychiatric cases (and the rest are for elderly patients with neuropsychiatric issues), as well as four outpatient clinics.[58]

The third large psychiatric hospital, which in contrast to the previous two has no religious connotation (neither Christian nor Islamic) in its name, was the Al-Fanār Psychiatric Hospital. Like ʿAṣfūriyyeh, it sits on a hill, but it is situated in the south of Lebanon in a predominantly Shiite area. Al-Fanār (Arabic for "the lighthouse") was founded by Labban in 1965 and, until 2019, was managed by three generations of secular-minded women from the Labban family who claimed to follow the philosophy of the influential Italian psychiatrist and social critic Franco Basaglia—who is known for having revolutionized psychiatric practice in Italy and for taking part in the antipsychiatry movement of the late 1960s.[59] Their appropriation of Basaglia's philosophy translated into an unfettered treatment of those who sought care or shelter at the hospital. Until the forced closure of the Al-Fanar Hospital recently, there was (allegedly) no recourse to straitjackets or other means of physical constraints, even for the most violent of patients, nor did the hospital administer electroconvulsive therapy.[60] Patients were called "residents," for their care was supposed to be community based.[61]

Strikingly, the Labban women resisted local pressure to turn the hospital into a Muslim institution. (A political party, which they declined to name, offered them financial assistance on the condition that they wear the veil in public.)[62] In the end, the Al-Fanār hospital was renovated with the support of the Italian embassy, perhaps in a symbolic nod to Al-Fanār's embrace of Basaglia's philosophy of care.[63] This resistance to the sectarianization of health care is telling, particularly given Labban's association with ʻAṣfūriyyeh: after graduating from AUB's medical school in 1948, he trained and worked as a psychiatrist at ʻAṣfūriyyeh in the 1950s before going to Edinburgh to attain his DPM—just as Manugian and the other Lebanese psychiatrists who trained at ʻAṣfūriyyeh had done before him.[64]

When ʻAṣfūriyyeh had to close its doors in 1982, most of its patients were sent to Al-Fanār or to Dār al-ʻAjaza al-Islāmiyya (the latter was referred to in the annual reports of ʻAṣfūriyyeh as the "Moslem Asylum").[65] Strikingly, none went to Dayr al-Ṣalīb, though a few were sent to a minor asylum run by nuns. However, one cannot exclude the possibility that some of the patients who had been discharged during the civil war ultimately ended up being admitted to Dayr al-Ṣalīb. Nonetheless, it is quite revealing that the discharge policy during the final years of ʻAṣfūriyyeh avoided favoring its rival institution.

In February 2019, the minister of health ordered the closure of the Al-Fanār hospital, after it appeared that conditions there had drastically deteriorated to the point that the minister of health had declared the hospital a "moral, social, and sanitary tragedy."[66] An exposé caused nationwide outrage and prompted the arrest of its owner, Labban's widow. She was later released because of her advanced age. Instead, her daughter, who was the hospital's general manager, and an employee at the Ministry of Health were taken into custody. They have been accused of corruption and fund mismanagement.[67] The case is pending at the time of this writing.

The Sectarianization of Charity

The other issue related to the sectarianization of health care has to do with the waqf institution. ʻAṣfūriyyeh was made a waqf on April 17, 1912, in a civil court in the Matn district of Mount Lebanon.[68] Under Islamic law, a waqf is an endowment for a pious cause that sets aside a nontaxable source of revenue to finance the endowment in perpetuity. This can be done for religious institutions (such as mosques) or charitable institutions (such as hospitals).[69] As emphasized in the wording of ʿAṣfūriyyeh's foundation deed (*waqfiyyah*), this was to be a charitable and not a religious endowment. The waqf was registered in a civil rather than a religious court, further giving credence to the benevolent and nonsectarian purpose of the Hospital.

Non-Muslims and even foreigners who resided in the Ottoman Empire could create a waqf for personal or public benefit.[70] In addition to being a conduit for *zakat*, the waqf was predominantly a sociopolitical tool.[71] It brought prestige to its patrons and empowered the clergy. Like the millet system (mentioned below), the waqf also came to reflect the pluralistic charitable economy that had started to impinge on the power of the state.

The centralization of the waqf administration started during the Tanzimat period under Sultan Mahmud II—who by 1826 had consolidated most of the imperial endowments into a ministry for imperial *evkaf* (the plural of waqf in Ottoman Turkish).[72] Muhammad Ali Pasha followed suit in Egypt to reassert state control, and a ministry of *awqāf* (the plural of waqf in Arabic) was established for that purpose. The rationale for these actions was that they would undermine the growing power both of ulemas (Muslim legal scholars) and other local notables while also reducing corruption.[73]

Just after their Mandate over Syria and Lebanon had begun, the French created the *Contrôle général des wakfs musulmans* (General Governing Body of Muslim Awqāf), which—though composed of influential ulemas and other Muslim leaders—was under the direct control of the French authorities.[74] The aim was to dismember the waqf system and to find financial resources for the maintenance of the Mandate by profiting from an otherwise dead capital (what the French call *mortmain*). But this takeover by the French authorities was met with strong opposition from those ulemas who perceived this seizure as an attempt to weaken their power, prestige, and privilege. In Greater Lebanon, the French reached a compromise: the religious and communitarian rules would continue to govern any *waqf* that was a religious institution, while waqf properties were to be given more flexibility, thus resuscitating the dead capital.[75] This is how, for instance, the old premises of ʿAṣfūriyyeh were "sold" in 1973; as will be mentioned below, technically the land was "exchanged" (rather than sold) for a different land on which the new hospital of ʿAramūn was eventually built.

Confessionalism

Before we proceed to observing how the waqf centralization took different paths in Lebanon and Syria, it is important to understand the genealogy of the confessional system in Lebanon. Confessionalism is a type of consociationalism, a term used by political scientists to describe a state in which groups share power along ethnic or religious lines, with no one group commanding a majority.[76] The Arabic word for sectarianism, *ṭā'ifiyya,* derives from the term *ṭā'ifa* (plural *ṭawā'if*). In contemporary terms, this refers to power sharing among the different sects that make up a country's population (as in the case of Lebanon or contemporary Iraq). Although the term *ṭā'ifiyya* was not common in the Ottoman Empire, the Turkish term *ṭā'ife* was commonly used to refer to non-Muslim communities. According to the thirteenth-century Arabic dictionary *Lisān al-ʿArab,* the word *ṭā'ifa* means a "piece of a whole" (*quṭʿa min al-shay'*)—or, within the context of the Quran and Hadith (the sayings and actions attributed to the Prophet Muhammad), "a group of people" (*jamāʿa min al-nās*).[77] Strikingly, the term *ṭā'ife* was frequently used by the Ottoman authorities in their official documents to refer to the different religious groups, communities, or nations—all of which were usually considered to be minorities, at least from the seventeenth century on.[78]

The more frequently used term in the literature is "millet," which has similar connotations. At the risk of being overly simplistic, the very fabric of Ottoman society could be said to have been a conglomeration of millets living side by side in an overwhelmingly Sunni population under the authority of an Islamic caliph whose rule differentiated between Muslims and dhimmis (the "People of the Book"—i.e., Jews and Christians). One's religion (or sect) was thus an important feature of one's identity. Not only were groups defined primarily by their religious affiliations vis-à-vis the law—*dhimma* people had to pay poll and land taxes, for example, and the various religious communities had the prerogative to manage their own internal affairs through their different communal courts—but they were also considered inferior to their Muslim fellow subjects (to whom the penal code, for instance, applied differently). Even people's attire was demarcated by their religious affiliations.[79]

This configuration is arguably a protoform of sectarianism because, despite the preeminence of religion in organizing the social and political life of the empire's subjects, state power was still monopolized by the ruling Sunni Islamic millet (*millet-i ḥākime*).[80] In contrast to this religious sectarian configuration, the institutionalization of sectarianism as a political system—where political (rather than merely judicial) power is shared proportionally among different religious groups—goes back to the division of Mount Lebanon in 1842 into two self-governing districts (*qāimaqāmiyya*): one under a Maronite district governor (*qāimaqām*) and the other under a Druze district governor. Wary of Ottoman ambitions to rule Mount Lebanon, several foreign consuls (French, British, Russian, Austrian, and Prussian) had pressured the Ottomans to create this precedent.[81] In 1861 these two *qāimaqāmiyya* were merged into a *mutaṣarrifiyya*, a semiautonomous province ruled by an Ottoman Christian governor appointed by the Sublime Porte.[82]

The French Mandate further institutionalized sectarianism, but it was the newly independent Republic of Lebanon that sanctified it.[83] In the law of March 13, 1936 (decree no. 60/LR), High Commissioner Damien de Martel recognized the "historical communities" (*les communautés historiques*) of Lebanon as legal entities.[84] The radical development here was not the recognition of these communities as well-delineated and autonomous groups.[85] Instead, it consisted of stripping the religious groups' of their monopoly on power by supplanting the Sunni sultan with the secular and republican French high commissioner.

Ṭā'ifiyya, in the sense of an independent, sectarian system of governance—that is, independent of either Ottoman or French tutelage—starts to emerge with the National Pact of 1943 that made Lebanese sovereignty (and hence independence) ironically conceivable.[86] All the different religious sects formulated their family laws during the postindependence phase—in 1951 for the Christian and Jewish communities.[87] The Sunnis had a decree legislated in 1942 that reactivated the Ottoman family law of 1917, but it was the law of 1962 that organized the Sunnis' jurisdiction. The Shiites organized their own code in 1967, while the Druzes' family law is subject to both the Ottoman family code of 1917 and the law of 1948.[88] As for the Protestants, while their family law had to be organized by the 1951 law, their religious courts and laws were further expanded only in the 1970s.[89]

The term *ṭā'ifiyya* crystallizes in the sense of a sect-based system of governance in the 1970s within the context of the Lebanese civil war and the rise of Islamist movements, alongside the repression of the Copts in Egypt.[90] Therefore, although sectarianism as both "practice and discourse" may have been more pronounced during the rise of nationalistic sentiments at the end of the Ottoman Empire (as Ussama Makdisi argues),[91] sectarianism actually became commonplace during the era of pan-Islamism and pan-Arabism.

It is important to note at this stage that while the 1936 decree opened up the possibility of civil status for those who did not wish to belong to a particular religious sect (the so-called *communauté de droit commun* [community of common law]), articles 14–21 were never enacted by the Lebanese state, since they were met with opposition from all religious sects. The strongest opposition came from the Muslim community.[92] When President Elias Hrawi tried in 1998 to uphold the decree of creating a civil personal status after the signing of the Ta'if Accords, Prime Minister Rafiq Hariri vehemently refused to sign the new bill, under pressure from his conservative Saudi allies and the influential Sunni cleric Mufti Qabbani.[93]

Hence instead of nationalizing its *awqāf*, as neighboring Syria had done after Husni al-Zaʿim's coup d'état in 1949 or Egypt after Gamal Abdel Nasser's 1956 revolution (both also created ministries of awqāfs),[94] Lebanon clung to its sectarian social contract and even expanded it to cover new aspects of sociopolitical and economic life.

In 1973, when the LGC and BEC decided to sell the old ʿAṣfūriyyeh to build a new hospital on a new site, a court order was needed. Because the property and land could not be sold but only exchanged according to the waqf deed, such an order was required to exchange the land and to ensure that the money would be used for the construction of the new hospital.[95] Whereas before the 1970s, decisions on a waqf were obtained from either a civil or sharia (Islamic law) court, this time it was obtained from a Protestant court. In a way, the law, of April 2, 1951, defining the "competencies of the confessional authorities [*al-marājeʿ al-madhhabiyya*] for the Christian and Jewish communities"[96] marks the beginning of the sectarianization of charity in contemporary Lebanon. In 1971, the court of appeal notified the BEC that the final authority in approving the alteration of the waqf property was the Protestant religious court though, as will be mentioned later, in 1968 the London committee consulted the sharia law for the interpretation of the waqfiyyah.[97] Since the Protestant sect (which had been given millet status in 1850) was the last to be recognized by the Ottoman Empire, one could say that by the 1970s, the institutionalization of sectarianism in Lebanon had been fully implemented and was now being reproduced.[98]

The clash of the Protestant religious court with Mroueh—who, as noted above, considered himself to be the legitimate mutawallī of the Hospital—is closely related to the sectarianization of the waqf. Before the fall of the Ottoman Empire, the Hospital was regarded as a nonreligious charitable waqf that was registered in the name of an American citizen, but the Protestant court appropriated ʿAṣfūriyyeh in the 1970s as a Protestant waqf. However, both the Protestant court's challenge to Mroueh's trusteeship and its forced sectarianization of the waqf are problematic for the reasons I will now turn to.

Challenging ʿAṣfūriyyeh's Waqfiyyah

The original articulation of the waqfiyyah is unequivocal: the *waqīf* (the founder of the waqf) is a foreign resident in Beirut. Despite being a missionary himself, the deed introduces Reverend Dr. Franklin Evans Hoskins—the waqīf—as "an American citizen living in Beirut in the Vilayet of Beirut, a division of the Ottoman Empire ... in full health of mind and body."[99] The first beneficiary of the waqf is listed as the "General Committee of the Lebanon Hospital for the Insane, well-known and testified-of whose centre is 35 Queen Victoria Street, London, E.C., England."[100] Hoskins entrusted the waqf to Robert Fortescue Fox, who is introduced as "a British subject, Chairman of the General Committee of the Lebanon Hospital for the Insane."[101] Fox, named as the mutawallī, was a Quaker physician associated with ʿAṣfūriyyeh.[102] He had been stationed for seventeen years in Zahleh (in the Beqaa Valley), where he had been the director of one of the missionary schools. In 1900, he moved to Beirut to take over the Protestant Missionary Press from Henry Harris Jessup. Fox also served as president of SPC's theological faculty from 1911 until his death in 1920.[103]

Curiously, however, the waqf deed left out all the religious backgrounds and affiliations of the waqīf and the mutawallī. The first beneficiary, the London committee, appears as a secular entity based in London. Generally, however, in religious awqāf (whether Christian or Jewish), the mutawallī is either a member of the clergy (the head of a monastery, a priest, a religious functionary, or the like) or a representative of a religious community (the president of the Jewish community, for instance). In other words, even if the waqīf or mutawallī were a layperson, the waqf deed typically mentioned the relationship of the waqīf to the religious community in question.[104] More importantly, the *ṭā'ifa* (communal affiliation) of the first beneficiary is usually also mentioned. Unusually in this waqf deed, however, Hoskins and Fox are introduced as private persons, not as representatives of the Protestant—or, more relevant in the history of ʿAṣfūriyyeh, Quaker—community.

The only time the "Protestant Evangelical community" (*al-Ṭā'ifa al-Protestantiyya al-Injīliyya*) is mentioned is in connection with the succession of trusteeship or beneficiaries. To guarantee the smooth continuity of the trusteeship—given that the waqf is a trust in perpetuity—the mutawallī was appointed in the following way: If the London committee had to be dissolved for any reason, then it was the chairman of the Beirut committee who "shall have the right to take charge of the management and administration" of the waqf or to appoint a mutawallī. Strikingly, the faith or religious background of the chairman is not mentioned. After the Beirut committee, the right passes to the "Embassies of England and America in Constantinople," and after these bodies to the "best qualified" (of any faith) from among the "poor of Mount Lebanon." Here we find the only reference to the Protestant community: a representative from among the poor is to be appointed by the religious leader of the Protestant community in Lebanon if the leader of that community declines to manage the waqf. Presumably, the leader of the Protestant community comes before the "representative from among the poor" in the ranking of trusteeship. Significantly, the waqfiyyah also mentions the following scenario: "If the original committee in London or the executive committee in Beirut is again brought into being after being dissolved, then the position in respect of the administration and management shall revert to the state mentioned before."[105]

This thorough wording of the waqfiyyah thus makes it more of a waqf for the benefit of people of "any faith" (as is plainly stated) who suffer from mental and nervous disorders than an a priori "Protestant waqf," as claimed by the Protestant court. In 1967 when the LGC requested a *fatwa* (legal decision) on the identity of the waqīf (the chairman or the board members of the London committee, i.e., a person or a group of people) to "dispel any possible doubt," on the trusteeship of the waqf, ʿAṣfūriyyeh's designated lawyer, Ibrahim Khairallah, approached Hassan Khaled, the mufti of the Lebanese Republic.[106] The mufti's verdict was very clear, "the sharia law permits the designation of a Board of Directors" of a waqf as mutawallī if the waqīf has designated "the board" as mutawallī.[107] As mentioned earlier, the waqfiyya did indeed recognize the "General Committee of the Lebanon Hospital for the Insane" based in London as first beneficiary of the waqfiyya. Interestingly, the mufti did not make any allusion to religion or the Protestant sect in his two-page judgement.

Nevertheless, even if we assume that this is a Christian waqf because both the original mutawallī and the waqīf were Western foreigners (presumably Christians) or because we know that the waqīf was a Quaker, or simply because the Protestant community is mentioned (even if only once) in the succession of trusteeship, the claim remains problematic. It remains problematic even more so if we assume that the Protestant court has the power of adjudicating any issue related to this particular waqf. The reason is this: when the LGC delegated its power and authority (including its rights and responsibilities related to waqf and non-waqf property) to the BEC in 1981, it was following the prescriptions of the waqfiyyah.[108] And when Mroueh was elected as mutawallī after the death of Shukayr (the designated and approved mutawallī following the dissolution of the London committee, as mentioned earlier), the Beirut committee was also following to the letter the prescriptions of the waqfiyyah. This leads us to wonder if the Protestant court contests Mroueh's trusteeship because he is not Protestant or because the circumstances of his election were unclear. These will remain open questions until the court's judgment on the issue.

Conclusion

With the downfall of ʿAṣfūriyyeh, a sectarian pattern of mental health provision started to become more visible. The two largest providers of mental health care in Lebanon today are Dayr al-Ṣalīb and Dār al-ʿAjaza al-Islāmiyya. This does not mean that these institutions are inherently sectarian or that they cater only to or prioritize certain religious groups (Christians for the former and Muslims for the latter). Conversely, however, providing services for out-of-group communities does not necessarily mean that the strategy is disinterested, especially in the age of sectarian-based welfarism. Nevertheless, what is relevant here is their institutional and constitutional frameworks (specifically, their medical staffs and managing boards), which are configured along sectarian lines. In addition, the religious signifiers in the names of these two hospitals in a country steeped in sectarianism and ghettoized neighborhoods cannot but reinforce the sectarian character of these two institutions.

The paradox of ʿAṣfūriyyeh is that though a Quaker missionary founded it, nonsectarianism was the word of the day. It is true that the Hospital was not disinterested, but neither was this stance merely a matter of public relations. In time, nonsectarianism, which was inscribed in the Hospital's constitution, became a core principle and ideology. The Beirut and London committees enrolled trustees from other faiths (especially Muslims), culminating with the appointment of Shukayr as chairman of the BEC—which became the de facto governing body of the Hospital once the LGC relinquished its power.

The sectarianization of health care that was exposed by the dissolution of ʿAṣfūriyyeh when it closed its doors in 1982 was possible because of a weak central state and a confessional system that enabled different political parties to use the provision of welfare and health care as a political card to enroll adherents and partisans in their various causes and agendas. But above all the sectarianization was possible because of the path that postindependence politicians took to sanctify the sectarian system in Lebanon, rather than secularize it. As this chapter has shown, the 1951 law marks the sectarianization of charity in modern Lebanon. If the Protestant church today reclaims ʿAṣfūriyyeh as a Protestant waqf, it is precisely because this law naturalized and sanctified the sectarianization of the waqf institution.

Epilogue

> And I will remember the land.
>
> —Leviticus 26:42

The history of ʿAṣfūriyyeh reflects in many ways the history of modern Lebanon, with its entanglement of macro- and micropolitics. As we have seen throughout this book, although ʿAṣfūriyyeh was frequently on the verge of ruin amid various geopolitical upheavals and economic uncertainties, it managed to survive for many years. Founded in 1896 more than three decades after the civil strife that had engulfed the Near East (and opened the door for foreign penetration), ʿAṣfūriyyeh continued to flourish and function unscathed until the civil war.

The two world wars and their respective aftermaths were, precarious times for patients and staff alike. The Hospital narrowly averted closure on two key occasions. During the First World War, its legal status as a charitable endowment (waqf) spared the Hospital from being confiscated for Ottoman military purposes. In the aftermath of the Second World War, the Hospital secured a major government grant from the nascent Republic of Lebanon and implemented a vigorous fund-raising campaign that managed to raise substantial amounts of money both locally and from abroad (including for the first time the emerging petrodollar economies), all in the hope of saving what was now widely perceived to be a national institution that was worth preserving. Indeed, in 1983, Adnan Mroueh, who was then minister of health and not yet the Hospital's mutawallī, referred to the "national interest" as he called for saving the Hospital from bankruptcy.[1]

As we have seen in chapters 5 and 6, it was the Lebanese civil war that delivered the most painful blow to ʿAṣfūriyyeh. Besides the violence and trauma inflicted on both bodies and stones, it was the inflation and dramatic drop in the numbers of private patients from wealthy neighboring countries (worsened by a weak and bankrupt state that was unable to meet its financial obligations) that led to a financial collapse in the late 1970s and the ultimate closure of the Hospital in 1982. Moreover, the rehabilitation of the new Hospital in ʿAramūn, which was also heavily damaged during the civil war, looked even bleaker when the Protestant religious court that now claimed to be the legal owner of ʿAṣfūriyyeh aborted the project to rebuild the Hospital. As I argued in chapter 6, although the Hospital was founded by a Quaker missionary, it was never officially considered a Protestant or missionary hospital—not in the waqfiyyah, the Hospital's constitution, or even in its publicity material. Rather, it is what I call the sectarianization of health care in postwar Lebanon that put a hold on the possibility of giving the Hospital a new life.

War and Medicine

One aspect that stands out in the long history of ʿAṣfūriyyeh is the violence that was inflicted on its patients, staff, and infrastructure during the civil war. Alas, such violence against medical personnel and patients is not specific to the story of ʿAṣfūriyyeh. It is a natural consequence of the changing nature of armed conflict, the development of modern warfare, and the aerial bombardment of urban areas—which has become not only inevitable but often strategic for punishment and deterrence purposes.

The Geneva conventions and protocols form the core of international humanitarian law, which regulates the conduct of armed conflict and seeks to limit its effects. The original Geneva Convention of 1864 included provisions for military but not civilian hospitals. While the 1907 Hague Conventions contained some provisions on the protection of civilian hospitals, strikingly it is only in the fourth Geneva Convention, signed in 1949, that they were first mentioned explicitly.[2] Since the Second World War, the struggles for decolonization, and especially the surge in civil wars in the 1960s and 1970s, transgressions against the neutrality and sanctity of shelters for the sick and wounded have continued to occur—which resulted in the signing in 1977 of two additional protocols that are specifically concerned with the treatment of the victims of war.[3]

However, what is flagrant and perhaps distinctive of our era is the ways in which hospitals have been used as tools of war. In earlier centuries, it was rather diseases (like smallpox or the plague) that served the purpose of military strategies—for example, to decimate populations.[4] It was during the Second World War—with the development of all-metal monoplanes equipped for the first time with bombs—that hospitals, including civilian ones, became targets. Although an inventory of hospitals still needs to be made, it will suffice to mention a few examples. In 1939, the Luftwaffe bombarded Polish hospitals, and in 1943 the Allies bombarded the Hôtel-Dieu in Nantes, France (the major civilian hospital in the city), though in both cases the targeted buildings were clearly marked as hospitals.[5]

More recently, Médecins Sans Frontières, the international medical community, the WHO, and other nongovernmental and humanitarian organizations as well as numerous journalists and independent witnesses have emphasized the radical shift toward deliberately and repeatedly targeting hospitals—and the scale of such targeting—to demoralize and terrorize civilians in contemporary armed conflicts.[6] Not only are hospital facilities no longer neutral zones (as defined by the Geneva conventions), but they have also become weaponized for strategic military purposes, and—perhaps more pertinently—their ruins are used as a warning against committing any act of resistance to or defiance of the status quo (astonishingly, most of these deliberate actions have been carried out by state actors).[7] Indeed, the repetitive targeting of physicians, medical convoys, and above all hospitals (as in Syria, Yemen, Gaza, and Afghanistan)[8] makes us think about how and when we moved from a time when the rules of conducting wars were respected to some extent to an era in which they are entirely dismissed. The story of ʿAṣfūriyyeh invites us to think about the latest transformations of modern hospitals from sacred spaces to tools and targets of war, as well as from spaces of hope and cure to places of death, misery, oblivion, and ruin.

Medical Ruins

War is not the only force behind the emergence or visibility of what we might call "modern medical ruins." There are at least three other forces.

First, there are sociopolitical and economic factors, as was the case with the wave of so-called deinstitutionalization in Europe and North America in the 1960s and 1970s.[9] Recently, artists have started to provide a more nostalgic look at these abandoned Victorian institutions with their magnificent facades and picturesque landscapes. Photographers have brought to life traces of these desolate and dilapidated monuments, with their crumbling interiors and rotting artifacts that once belonged to patients.[10]

Another force is the process of decolonization. Medical anthropologists have started to chronicle the history and examine the debris of Africa's medical and scientific colonial institutions.[11] They are meticulously laying out the traces of such remains not as an exercise in curious peregrinations across postmodern and postcolonial landscapes but as a way to upset the hegemonic, if simplistic, formulaic "vertical" or top-down prescriptions of global health actors.[12] In contrast, the horizontal excavations of medical and scientific sites invite a problematization of power relations: traces of imagined and embodied pasts, presents, and futures.

The third—and perhaps most obvious—factor is poor governance, be it on the micro (hospital or institutional) level or the macro (national) level. The case of Venezuela and its crumbling health care infrastructure, especially its mental health facilities, is a case in point.[13] Another striking example is the psychiatric hospital at Blida, in Algeria, where the Martinique psychiatrist Frantz Fanon taught and worked in the mid-1950s and where a generation of French-Algerian psychiatrists was trained under his leadership.[14] The Hôpital Psychiatrique de Blida-Joinville was once the pride of the colonial Algerian school of psychiatry and viewed as avant-garde, innovative, progressive, and experimental (though also profoundly racist).[15] Today it is underfunded and neglected. Its wards look more like prison cells, and the visitor can hear patients behind bars screaming or begging for money and cigarettes.[16] An additional striking example is the currently crumbling psychiatric infrastructure in France. The situation is so dire—there is a shortage of psychiatrists, the nursing personnel are overworked, the infrastructure is dilapidated, and patients feel abandoned—that journalists and psychiatrists are speaking of a national crisis.[17]

ʿAṣfūriyyeh today stands desolate, derelict, and overtaken by weeds (figure 7.1) in an erratically urbanized and gentrified city, waiting to be destroyed and converted into another commodity in a laissez-faire economy that dreads the past and secures the interests of wealthy stakeholders in times of war as in times of peace.[18] As a microcosm of Lebanon, ʿAṣfūriyyeh is a victim of both modernity (including modern warfare) and a mercantile mentality.[19] It is this heavy sense of ruin and desolation, of lost opportunity and crumbling institutions, and of bereavement that weighs on ʿAṣfūriyyeh today.[20] But there is more to this sense of loss and mourning.

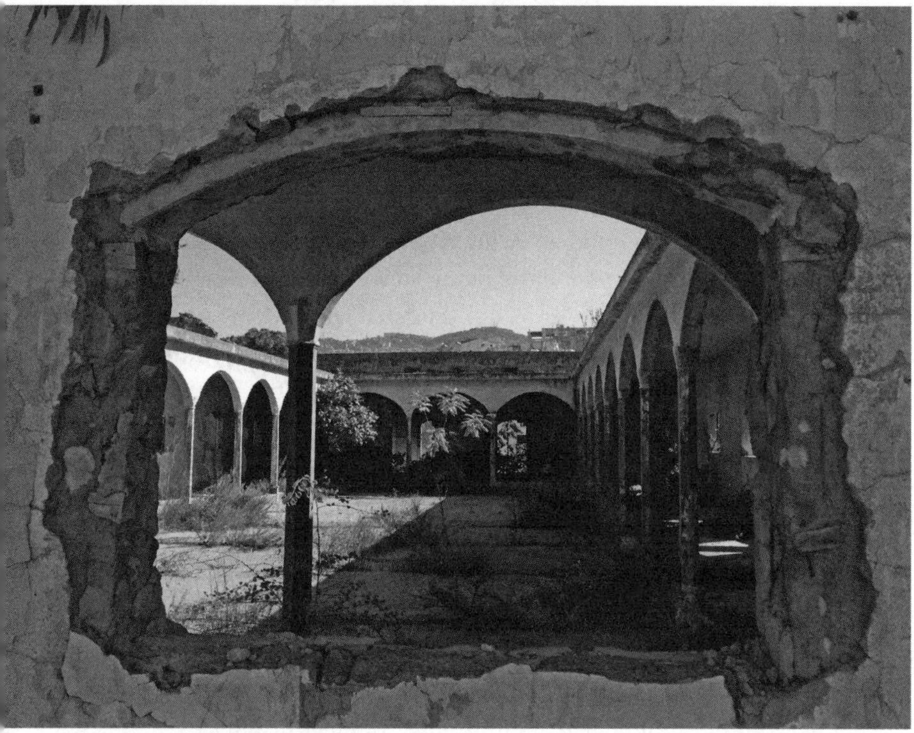

Figure 7.1
The remains of Webster House, ʿAṣfūriyyeh, October 2013.
Source: Courtesy of Delphine Darmency.

A New Psychiatric Landscape

Some may argue that the collapse of ʿAṣfūriyyeh and its ultimate closure was perhaps for the best, since after all these large psychiatric hospitals often turned out to be places of abuse, coercion, and neglect. But today there is increasing and widespread criticism of the movement that led to the deinstitutionalization of the mentally ill. The authors of a 2015 article in the *Journal of the American Medical Association* even call for reinstitutionalization.[21] They provocatively argue that the asylum should be brought back as a way to cope with the many consequences of deinstitutionalization, including the displacement of the patient populations of mental hospitals to the streets, emergency departments, and (perhaps most disturbingly) jails and prisons—which in recent years have become the largest mental health care facilities in the United States.[22] That is precisely why rather than romanticizing, reminiscing about, or fetishizing the landscape of abandoned asylums and psychiatric facilities, we should see that landscape as an opportunity to critique and call into question the current politics of life, which reinforces precarity rather than treats every life equally.

In fact, what the ruins of 'Aṣfūriyyeh reveal is a new psychiatric landscape that has two features: the recriminalization of substance abuse and the repopulation of prisons with people afflicted with mental health issues.[23] These two outcomes have resulted from a lack of specialized facilities to treat disorders related to substance use, as well as a lack of mental health specialists and the infrastructure necessary to provide such services in prisons.[24] Between the 1960s and its closure in 1982, 'Aṣfūriyyeh had a forensic unit that provided treatment for substance-related disorders and for convicted criminals who suffered from a range of mental illnesses. Nonetheless, 'Aṣfūriyyeh cannot be said to have been the main site of incarceration in the country, since the number of these patients was not significant in the long history of the Hospital. Today, however, like in the United States (or in France as Didier Fassin has shown)[25]—but of course on a less impressive scale—prisons are populated with a large number of inmates who suffer from various mental health issues and the prison seems to have displaced the lunatic asylum as the main site of incarceration.[26] Unlike in the United States, the reason is not deinstitutionalization—which did not occur in the modern Middle East, as mentioned below—but a lack of expertise and specialized facilities that could provide an alternative place of confinement and care.[27]

There are two additional departures from the demise of large psychiatric hospitals in the United States and Europe. First, in the context of modern Lebanon is the sectarian framework of public goods that has emerged from the collapse of national and nonsectarian institutions during the civil war (explored in chapter 6). In this new configuration, life and health have become mere commodities that are traded by different political and sectarian groups. Second, in the broader context of the Middle East and North African region is the emergence of large psychiatric institutions as places of last resort in the postcolonial or postindependence period, to which I now turn.

Failed Modernity

The ruins of ʿAṣfūriyyeh belie alternative paths and historical trajectories. As the anthropologist Shannon Lee Dawdy rightly puts it, modern ruins are paradoxical: if they are "contemplated for too long, they can reveal the contradictions of progress."[28] ʿAṣfūriyyeh's ruins—its decaying and abandoned buildings in both the old and new sites, one overtaken by weeds and the other destroyed by war—fit very well into the creative process of ruins facilitated by "capitalism's fast-moving frontiers and built-in obsolescence, as well as political hubris and social conflicts."[29]

More significantly, the ruins are also a reflection of a failed project of modernity. The remains of ʿAṣfūriyyeh exemplify national as well as sociopolitical failure. The downfall of ʿAṣfūriyyeh is part of a story of decline, inefficiency, and the breakdown of both society and the state that have failed to meaningfully support a generation's dream of renewed modernity. Indeed, Antranig Manugian's grand vision of a revamped, state-of-the-art, hypermodern psychiatric institute never materialized and is now buried under the rubble of war.

However, modernity is not only about technology, faith in the possibility of progress, and the rupture with tradition. It is also, and perhaps more so, about the "reflexive appropriation of knowledge," as Anthony Giddens puts it, and more specifically about the ability for "reflexivity" and "self-analysis," which Pierre Bourdieu sees as the essential features of scientific knowledge and practice.[30] Yet in blatant contrast to the Nahḍa intellectuals (see chapter 1), the generation of psychiatrists that had dominated the field of psychiatry and influenced much of the mental health policies in the region until the 1980s failed to be self-reflexive and critical of its own discourse. More specifically, those psychiatrists failed to question and problematize their faith in unabated progress; their assumptions about a triumphalist version of psychiatry; and the ways in which normality and pathology are articulated, defined, produced, and reproduced. More generally, they failed to see how the Western discourse that they so cherished was fallible and vulnerable to criticism.

No leading voice à la Thomas Szasz, R. D. Laing, or Franco Basaglia can be said to have emerged from either Lebanon or the broader Middle East in that crucial period of the 1960s-1970s. There were no voices that had an impact like that of the antipsychiatry movement of the 1960s, which had consequential implications for the ways in which psychiatry is practiced and conceptualized today.[31] Although the Algerian revolutionaries adopted Fanon (he was even buried in Algeria) as one of their brothers in arms, in fact Fanon embraced psychiatry and used it to critique and denounce colonialism as dehumanizing, traumatic, and alienating.[32] And even if we put aside the case of antipsychiatry as an outlying critique and look at how psychoanalysis took hold in the Arab world—for instance, among the Egyptian intelligentsia in the 1950s—what we see is a reluctant embrace of psychoanalysis. Yet the reluctance is not related to a critique of psychoanalysis but rather to a deep suspicion of the Western psychoanalytic project.[33]

Of course, it is not enough to simply mimic the critics of the psychiatric discourse and practice in the West, which would defeat the purpose of self-reflexivity. In his influential *Al-Naqd al-Dhātī Baʿd al-Hazīma* (*Self-Criticism after the Defeat)* originally published in 1968, the Syrian philosopher Sadik Jalal al-Azm diagnosed a lack of self-critique (*naqd dhātī*) in the general mind-set of Arab intellectuals (including the progressive intellectuals of his time) during that momentous period in the history of the region—a lack he blamed on the ossified yet hegemonic authoritarian regimes.[34] This was said in the context of the Six-Day War with Israel in 1968, which the Arab (more specifically, Egyptian) armies spectacularly lost.

A year later, al-Azm published yet another provocative book that led to his trial and imprisonment for "inciting confessional strife in Lebanon" and for daring to challenge religious authorities.[35] In *Naqd al-Fikr ad-Dīnī* (*Critique of Religious Thought*), originally published in 1969, al-Azm undertakes a critique of "religious mentality," which he denounces as being pervasive in the Arab world to their detriment since the religious and political elites have been using religion as an "ideological weapon" to pacify the people and stifle their social and revolutionary struggles.[36] As Hisham Sharabi has shown, al-Azm was part of a coterie of Arab intellectuals (many of whom were very much influenced by the 1960s's revolutionary and emancipatory ethos) who had become vocally critical of neopatriarchal structures and especially of the sacrosanct nature of religion in such societies, which they believe was an impediment to tangible progress, intellectual renewal, and true emancipation.[37]

More than a decade later, al-Azm applied this same critique astonishingly to Edward Said's influential *Orientalism,* which critically appraised the Western's denigrating, phantasmagoric, and essentialist representations of the Orient (and by extension—though anachronistic—contemporary Arab societies).[38] Although Albert Hourani was the first to identify one of the key weaknesses in Said's work—namely, his construction of an ideal type of the Orientalist—al-Azm and other Marxist thinkers expanded the critique to include several more flaws, including the use of a unilinear, ahistoric, immutable, and omnipotent conception of Orientalism rather than a more pragmatic approach to both human nature and politics.[39] But more relevant to our discussion of self-critique, al-Azm identified what he called "Orientalism in reverse" by which he meant the use of those same orientalist assumptions, techniques, and pronouncements by intellectuals, scholars, and other researchers from the Arab and Islamic world who ironically were inspired by Said's work not only to make essentialist pronouncements about Islam and the Orient (as being superior or antithetic to the West) but also to promulgate the idea that the only salvation of the Orient is through a return to political Islam.[40] Interestingly, al-Azm's critique was made as an exercise in self-critique in the aftermath of Iran's 1979 Islamic Revolution.

Along the same line, one can argue that a similar kind of self-critique of the conditions of possibility of psychiatric power is precisely what is missing in the genealogy of medical and psychiatric practice in the Middle East of the 1960s and 1970s and to some extent until today. It would go beyond the scope of this book to try to account for the reasons behind the widespread lack of self-critique and reflexivity. Suffice it to mention sociocultural and political reasons that have to do with the brain drain of physicians, especially since the 1960s; religious power and its monopoly on truth; authoritarianism; and opportunism or simply self-preservation on the part of the medical elite.[41]

Ironically, there is no need to bring the asylum back to the Middle East since it never left in the first place. The difference is that in contrast to Europe and North America, lunatic asylums as well as psychiatric hospitals were originally on a much smaller scale. Despite the fact that today psychiatric needs in the Middle East are immense, especially given the scale and impact of war, terrorism, and socioeconomic distress in Iraq, Syria, or Yemen, there is a lack of mental health care facilities and resources.[42] Yet the largest numbers of psychiatric beds in the Arab world are overwhelmingly in mental hospitals rather than in community-based residential settings or other alternative hospital-based settings.[43] And although Israel has by far the largest number of psychiatric beds per 100,000 population in the region, its largest psychiatric facility, the Sha'ar Menashe Mental Health Center, contains only 420 beds.[44]

In contrast, some of the largest psychiatric hospitals in the world today are in the Middle East. Dayr al-Ṣalīb, in Mount Lebanon, has at least 1,100 beds and an average of 2,200 patients per year; Egypt has two large mental hospitals, namely ʿAbbasiyya (mentioned in the introduction) has around 1,500 beds and a staggering 100,000 annual consultations while El-Khanka mental hospital has around 2,109 beds and 1,500–1,600 monthly consultations; and Al-Rashad Hospital (colloquially known as *al-Shamāʿiyya*) in Iraq was built with a maximum capacity of 1,200 beds though it currently has 1,356 inpatients.[45] Most of these beds are for people with chronic conditions, and given the latest exposés regarding the overcrowded and neglected conditions in several of these institutions,[46] they have conspicuously become places of last resort—or, to borrow Andrew Scull's words, "convenient places for inconvenient people."[47]

A Vanishing Plural World

Medical ruins are arguably part of a broader set of modern ruins—or "ruins of modernity"[48]—that include postindustrial wasteland cities with their abandoned shops and businesses, deserted facilities, and crumbling infrastructures. But what should we make of hybrid institutions like ʿAṣfūriyyeh that cut through different temporalities and do not fit into one typology of modern medical ruins? Although ʿAṣfūriyyeh was a casualty of war and was used as a tool of war, it was also a casualty of poor management and a changing moral economy (from missionary to petrodollar). And what should we make of institutions whose hybrid nature makes them more than just "imperial debris"?[49] They owe much to local and global agencies in terms of their success and failure, or their rise and fall. They are the result not only of the benevolence of both ruler and ruled but also of imperial ambitions and neocolonial intrusions (as well as of national pride), and of hopes of a better world (as well as of despair, suffering, and violence).

In the Middle East specifically, violence is used not only to knock out protesters and dissidents (from Istanbul's Gezi Park to Cairo's Tahrir Square). It is also deployed to destroy ideals and narratives of pluralism and common humanity. The destruction of cultural and architectural sites of world heritage by the so-called Islamic State of Iraq and Syria (ISIS) is not just cultural cleansing, but is part of a more insidious "necropolitics"[50]—that is, those forms and politics of violence that are perpetrated against bodies and lands. The destruction is driven by hubris as well as a profound dislike of both life and the cross-fertilization of cultures and civilizations.[51] What is worse, a similar necropolitics is carried out by other, more banal postcolonial subjects who are driven by the desire for capitalist gains and who are indifferent to the vital importance of spaces of cosmopolitanism, coexistence, and pluralism in the "age of extremes," renewed nationalism, and protofascism.[52]

Such a landscape of ruins naturally evokes a feeling of sadness and melancholy.[53] But this is not simply an affect of pensive sadness over ancient ruins. The most poignant and recurrent image that people mentioned when asked about what they remembered about ʿAṣfūriyyeh was that of a desolate and abandoned site full of memories, both good and bad.[54] More striking was the sense of loss and precariousness that the imagery conjured up. Someone suggested that ʿAṣfūriyyeh was an endangered place that needs to be placed on a heritage list for protection. Another person said that she was not even sure if ʿAṣfūriyyeh had ever really existed.

This sense of a shattered and vanishing world and the urge to preserve it (even in relation to a place of suffering and illness) is arguably quite symptomatic of our time. Waste accumulation and "wasted lives"[55] have been disposed of at the margins of growing and global capitals, and dying cities have become a normal sight in our rapidly changing urban landscapes.[56] Yet this sense of loss is perhaps more acutely felt in the Middle East, where new forms of authoritarianism, repression, and violence are resurging while the region's once-cherished and celebrated pluralism and openness are vanishing before our eyes.[57]

Why would people want to preserve the old buildings of ʿAṣfūriyyeh? What kind of museum, memorial, or living archive do they want these buildings to turn into, and for what purpose? As the anthropologist William Cunningham Bissell has suggested, "the past provides precisely an imaginative resource—a realm rich in invention, critical in possibility—for people struggling with the present, hoping to secure what can no longer be found in the future."[58] The key term here is "the present." Today many people across the Middle East, as well as around the world, are thinking of their failed states and dashed hopes for a better future. They are reminiscing about a past that looks brighter than the current apocalyptic scenes of endless war, suffering, mass migration, and refugee displacement.[59] There is nostalgia for a lost pluralism and tolerance for differences, even if these involve communitarian arrangements.[60] There is nostalgia for greener landscapes unspoiled by urbanization and neoliberal capitalistic ventures. There is a return to local forms of social and solidary economies and a reappropriation of the common goods by the people.[61] There is even nostalgia for the Ottoman Empire and, paradoxically enough, fallen dictators.[62]

Is this a defeatist attitude, or are we doomed to see the past through rose-colored glasses? In the case of Lebanon, nostalgia has been a pervasive feeling and leitmotif ever since the postwar period of the 1990s.[63] What is mobilizing people and civil society is an urge to save what is left of a common history of diversity and pluralism that is at risk of total obliteration. This is more than mere resistance to the post–Ta'if Accords state-sanctioned amnesia.[64] It is resistance to the homogenization of the very fabric of the Levant. Many grassroots initiatives and nongovernmental organizations have been created in recent years to promote, preserve, and defend historical, cultural, and urban sites that have come under increased threat of destruction through rampant urbanization or simple neglect by an indifferent political class.[65] More intriguingly, there has also been a surge of interest in the Levant's lost (or soon-to-be lost), dispersed, and ancestral communities.[66] This malaise with the sense of loss and being robbed of a past that is the product of diverse layers of civilizations that are often at odds with one another, has also intensified in reaction to ISIS's methodical politics of destruction of historical artifacts that reflect a cross-pollination among diverse civilizations. ISIS's aim has been to systematically turn these artifacts into rubble—a tabula rasa on which the self-proclaimed caliphate can rewrite its own history.[67]

Topo-History

ʿAṣfūriyyeh has become a *lieu de mémoire* (memory space) in the popular imagination.[68] Like Beirut's Martyrs' Square or other public memorials and monuments (which undergo continuous metamorphoses alongside the radically changing sociopolitical landscape),[69] ʿAṣfūriyyeh can be said to have become a monument with a life of its own. While the name ʿAṣfūriyyeh initially denoted the area where the Hospital was situated, over the years it became synonymous with the Hospital itself. Then, just as the meanings associated with the thirteenth-century British asylum "Bedlam" (the Bethlem Royal Hospital) mutated, ʿAṣfūriyyeh became a stigmatizing term: a byword for severe mental illness, madness, deviance, and even mere eccentricity. The metaphor traveled beyond the confines of Ottoman Mount Lebanon, and mental hospitals are now called "ʿAṣfūriyyeh" in Palestine,

Syria, and Jordan. The Lebanese singer Sabah who passed away a few years ago made a popular song in which her lover takes her to ʿAṣfūriyyeh (presumably because she is madly in love with him).[70] ʿAṣfūriyyeh has also come to symbolize both the insanity and political folly of a nation, immortalized in the influential play "Fīlm Amīrkī Ṭawīl" (The American Motion Picture) in which the Lebanese artist and playwright Ziad Rahbani criticizes the sectarian nature of politics in Lebanon in the context of the civil war—specifically, the years 1978–1980. The setting of the play is a "mental hospital," which is widely and popularly presumed to be ʿAṣfūriyyeh (though Rahbani never mentions it explicitly), which becomes the reflection of a torn society at war with itself.[71]

Unlike more celebrated *lieux de mémoire*, however, which are often landmarks that reflect pride in a nation and its accomplishments, ʿAṣfūriyyeh is in many ways also a *non-lieu* (nonspace) whose inhabitants are anonymous, anonymized, or silent. The French Marxist philosopher Louis Althusser even used the term *non-lieu* (a legal term meaning "no grounds" for further prosecution) metaphorically to refer to the state of being a living dead (*un mort-vivant*) in the context of his own psychiatric hospitalization following the murder of his wife—which he committed in a psychotic and delusional state.[72] In contrast to the anthropologist Marc Augé, for whom the *non-lieu* is a space of hypermodernity (an airport is the example par excellence),[73] I use the term to describe a space of bare modernity.

Today remembered with both dread and fascination, ʿAṣfūriyyeh is a space at the margins of a city and history, not worthy to be part of a history that glorifies national achievements, which the *lieux de mémoire* are supposed to represent. And unlike other glorious spaces of memory, this liminal space deals with the forgotten and downtrodden, "the dead which cannot be buried" as the medical missionary Cornelius Van Dyck referred to the poor insane more than a century ago.[74] A non-lieu deals with suffering, pain, and disease, as well as shattered dreams and painful lives. Althusser referred to the psychiatric hospital as the "tombstone of the *non-lieu*, of silence and public death."[75]

Although the concept of a duty to remember (*devoir de mémoire*) has had its supporters and detractors over the years and is itself a contingent invocation, it still provides a way to think more critically about the traces and remains of events and people.[76] The French philosopher Paul Ricoeur advanced three reasons for valuing the duty to remember.[77] Ricoeur was concerned with ways to reach a "just memory" (*une mémoire juste*), not in the sense of justice or equity but in the Aristotelian sense of the golden mean or equipoise (i.e., neither an excessive or abusive kind of memory nor an insufficient one).[78] This just memory was supposed to form the "ethico-political foundation" of memory, which thus invokes the past to better construct the future.

The first reason, according to Ricoeur, is straightforward and consists of rescuing events from natural oblivion and erosion. This is what chroniclers do, they immortalize events (wars, plagues, conquests etc.), heroes, and villains. "Zakhor," a Talmudic injunction, which means "remember," takes, however, a different meaning after the Shoah. Here, Ricoeur draws on Hannah Arendt's *The Human Condition* (published in 1958), in specific on her notion of action as characterizing the human condition in the face of death and the "erosion of traces" to suggest that the second reason for the duty to remember rests in the power of promise and forgiveness for "to forgive is basically to be liberated from the burden of the past, to be untied or unbound, while promising enjoins the capacity to be bound by one's own word."[79] Finally, the third reason is to memorialize the victims of history: the voiceless, abandoned, and forgotten.[80]

But what do we make of spaces or sites at the margins of sociopolitical life that have been destroyed (or are on the brink of destruction) not by the inevitable passage of time and the unfolding of world history but by deliberate acts of amnesia? These acts could be state-sanctioned (as in the case of postwar Lebanon),[81] ideologically driven (as in the case of ISIS), the result of a post-traumatic instinct to forget in the name of life and survival (what the artist and philosopher Jalal Toufic aptly calls "post-traumatic amnesia"),[82] or driven by personal financial gains (such as investment or vandalism).

As mentioned in chapter 5, today Solidere is the proprietor of the original estate of ʿAṣfūriyyeh. This company has been responsible for the destruction of many buildings of historical significance during the reconstruction efforts of postwar Beirut. For instance, Zukak el-Blat, a historical quarter that is contiguous to Solidere's project, is today crumbling and rapidly gentrifying, with many of its historical houses being replaced by high-rise buildings. In the nineteenth century, the neighborhood was the cultural and intellectual center of the Nahḍa movement (as well as where SPC—today, AUB—was first established, before moving to Rass Beirut), and it was a quarter for communal coexistence and national awakening.[83] Zukak el-Blat, nevertheless, represents an intellectual epoch that is not only specific to Lebanon but also to the whole Middle East. The destruction of its historical significance consequently affects not only the memory of that specific quarter or of Beirut but of an entire network of intellectuals and sociopolitical movements across the region.

Like in the case of Zukak el-Blat, the plan is to convert ʿAṣfūriyyeh into an insipid and amnesiac site of consumption. But can the dreary remains of war be so easily forgotten? Are they so easily fungible? And what shall we make of such prosaic sites in a dystopian age that is past both truth and memory? Does it make even sense to speak of a fourth duty: to remember these prosaic and derelict sites, these *non-lieux* that are anticlimactic and at the margins of history?

They are certainly (and paradoxically) less visible than the events and people the philosopher Avishai Margalit invokes us to remember in his *Ethics of Memory*.[84] Yet these sites are equally significant: in fact, they are part and parcel of what makes the memory of people and events meaningful. They provide the context (from the Latin *textere*, to weave) that enables memory in the first place. Attempts to erase and destroy institutions, entire villages (as in the case of Palestine),[85] and other similar debris of *non-lieux* constitute a "war against traces"[86] of worldviews that resist both oblivion and homogenization.

The remains of such mundane and hybrid institutions are hence more than a reflection of postcolonial and postmodern landscapes. As with the remains of the hundred hospitals shelled in war-torn Syria, they are also collectively and individually the debris of shattered lives, dreams, and hopes of better futures. Thus, they present an opportunity to reflect on both local and global agencies and interests. The process of identifying and reconstituting these ruins—perhaps even inventorying them—while situating them in a broader framework of regional and global "memoryscapes" not only denaturalizes them but above all presents an opportunity to question and problematize the memories of these sites and the politics of memory formation.[87] It is in this latter sense that this book is a biography—indeed, a *topo-history* (from the Greek *topos*, for "space") of a modern medical ruin.

Notes

Method

Besides the various archival material and other primary sources cited in the endnotes, I have used a quantitative analysis of patterns and trends in the various psychiatric diagnoses and their underlying socioeconomic and demographic characteristics to get a better sense of the kinds of mental illnesses and individuals who were brought to ʿAṣfūriyyeh for treatment.

The tables and figures are based on data collected from the annual reports (ARs) published by the Lebanon Hospital for Mental and Nervous Disorders (LHMND). Most ARs are available from the American University of Beirut, Saab Medical Library (AUB-SML), digital archives. These cover the years from 1900 through 1976, although reports are missing for 1909–1911, 1963–1968, and 1972–1974. The ARs for the period 1974–1981 may be found at the School of Oriental and African Studies (SOAS) Archives and Special Collections (Lebanon Hospital [LH], boxes 13 and 15); unfortunately, they are devoid of any statistical tables for the relevant categories that I analyzed. Some statistics related to the Hospital were compiled from various other materials at SOAS. Some data in the ARs available from the AUB-SML digital archives are missing for patients' discharges, religious denominations, and regional distributions (1963–1976); professional backgrounds (1947–1976); and diagnoses (1963–1968 and 1972–1974). These gaps have been remedied whenever relevant by the use of representative samples from the individual patient records, which are available at AUB-Jafet Library [JL] archives. The total number of patients admitted (excluding the missing years) was 22,834. One can assume that including the missing years and given the trends over the years, the number was perhaps between 25,000 and 30,000—and given the frequent readmissions, probably closer to the higher number than the lower. The subsample of randomly selected private records includes 17,443 patients, representing almost 60 percent of the likely total.

Of the 206 people who answered the anonymous online survey I conducted in 2014, 95 percent were Lebanese, 52 percent had heard of ʿAṣfūriyyeh in the context of a figure of speech or metaphor for madness or mental illness, roughly 40 percent had heard about it from family members or friends, and about 7 percent used to live near

ʿAṣfūriyyeh. Sixty-three percent thought that ʿAṣfūriyyeh had played an important role in society and 66 percent believed that it was not a sectarian institution (i.e, privileged one sect over another). Seventy-eight percent knew that ʿAṣfūriyyeh referred to a psychiatric hospital, a mental institution, a madhouse, or a lunatic asylum, while 32 percent thought that it was a metaphor or figure of speech for mental illness.

Archival Sources

Australia

Australian War Memorial (digital archives at https://www.awm.gov.au): I consulted eight photographs and a remarkable documentary footage of Australian soldiers being treated at ʿAṣfūriyyeh and of their occupation of the Hospital's premises during the Second World War.

France

Archives des Capucins de France (ACF), Paris: Fond de la province de Lyon; côte: 651.93 Z.46, documents divers relatifs au procès de béatification du R. P. Jacques de Ghazir; côte: 651.93 Z.46, Père Jacques et les soeurs de la croix 1930–1947; côte: 651.93 Z.45, Liban documents pour l'histoire; côte: 685.13 Z54, sous-dossier 3 Liban Père Jacques; côte: 685.13 Z43, sous-dossier 4 Liban Père Jacques photos diverses; côte: 65 193 Z46, Liban rapports officiels, sous-dossier 9; côte: 65 173 Z43, courier trié.

Bibliothèque médicale Henri Ey, Hôpital Sainte Anne, Paris: côte: 08–2143, Khalaf Abdul-Massih (ancien interne des hopitaux psychiatriques de Île-de-France), mémoire pour le Certificat d'Études Spécialisées en psychiatrie, "De l'assistance psychiatrique en Syrie," 1980.

Bibliothèque nationale de France (BnF), Paris: Many nineteenth-century and early twentieth-century manuscripts listed under primary sources, as well as government documents such as the *Bulletin officiel des actes administratifs du haut-commissariat,* were consulted on Gallica, the digital platform of the library. They include the Haut-commissariat de la république française en Syrie et au Liban, *Bulletin officiel des actes administratifs du haut-commissariat 15ème année, no. 6* (April 15, 1936) and *Bulletin officiel des actes administratifs du haut-commissariat 17ème année, no. 23* (December 15, 1938).

Ministère des affaires étrangères (MAE), Archives diplomatiques, Paris (La Courneuve): côte: 175 CPCOM/8, 175CPCOM/9, 175CPCOM/25, 175CPCOM/26, 371QONT/639; 380QONT/282, 380QONT/348; 381QONT/527, 380QONT/354, 371QONT/962. Microfilms: sous-série: Syrie-Liban-Cilicie (côte Mnesys: 50CPCOM): vol. 103–111, vol. 385–387, vol. 603–604. Sous-série Turquie (51CPCOM): vol. 527–528.

Lebanon

American University of Beirut, Jafet Library, Archives and Special Collections (AUB-JL): volume 1 (1908), volume 2 (1910–1930), Minutes of the Faculty of Medicine, AA:

3.9.3 Medical Division Faculty Minutes (1908–1978); file 1, box 4, School of Medicine relation with St. John Hospital (1884–1918); file 1, box 5, School of Medicine, correspondence with French officials re: School of Medicine and School of Dentistry (1920–1923); file 1 (1920–1927), box 8, School of Medicine, Minutes of Meetings (1910–1930); file 6/4 Hospital 1886–1919, the Lebanon Hospital for the Insane, Asfuriyeh, Syria (undated leaflet); files 1–4, box 6, School of Medicine Hospital Development and Laboratory 1886–1927; file 1, box 7, School of Medicine Reports to the Rockefeller Foundation 1924–1939; files 1–7, School of Medicine, Correspondence (1871–1947), second miscellaneous reports; AA: 6 AUBites folder: Harvey Porter and file and AA: 6 AUBites folder: Henry Watson Smith; Annual reports, board of managers, Syrian Protestant College, 1866–1867 through 1901–1902; AUB faculty 1867–1909, George Edward Post Collection; BEC Minutes 1938–1947, 1954–1957, 1959–1970, 1973–1977, LHMND.

American University of Beirut, Saab Medical Library, Archives and Special Collections (AUB-SML): The annual reports of ʿAṣfūriyyeh (1898–1978) referred to as ARs have been digitized (see http://ddc.aub.edu.lb/projects/saab/asfouriyeh/annual-reports /overview.html), although some are missing. The collection for LHMND is divided into seven cabinet files, thirty-two boxes, and large ledger books, including a large patient record and a visitors' book. I consulted the LHMND collection at AUB-SML where it was located originally. The collection was subsequently transferred to AUB-JL where it will likely be reorganized.

Near East School of Theology (NEST), Archives and Special Collections, Beirut: A few manuscripts were consulted, especially those by Cornelius Van Dyck, Butrus al-Bustani, and Amin A. Khairallah. I also consulted "Board letters" for 1900–1909 and 1910–1914.

United Kingdom

Library of the Religious Society of Friends (TLRSF), London: Rufus Jones, *Eli and Sybil Jones: Their Life and Work* (Philadelphia: Porter and Coates, 1889); Harris H. Lyn and Rosina D. Harvey, "Asfuriyeh: The Place of Birds," *Friend* 113 (1955), 445–448; "A Pioneer in Lebanon," *Friends' Quarterly Examiner* 80, no. 319 (1946), 162–163; Annual report of the Friends' Syrian Mission: Friends' Syrian Mission, 1875–1883; Report of the Friends' Lebanon Mission, 1875; Twentieth Report of the Friends' Mission in Syria and Palestine, 1889.

National Archives (TNA), Kew Gardens (previously the Public Records Office): CO 733/155/13, CO 733/225/4, OD 34/224, OD 34/431, FO 371/52911, FO 383/94, FO 1018/67, FO 371/134185, WO 372/23/15605.

School of Oriental and African Studies (SOAS), Archives and Special Collections, London: The collection related to the Lebanon Hospital (LH) is organized in seventeen boxes (box 17 is sealed until 2045); CBMS/01/H/03/07/05, box 125, Conference of British Missionary Societies (CBMS).

University of York, Borthwick Institute for Archives (UY-BIA): RET 8/3, papers related to the Lebanon Hospital for the Insane, Syria.

United States

Rockefeller Foundation Archives, Online Collections and Catalog: Record Group 1.1 Projects, Series 833: Lebanon, 12 boxes, 1920–1967.

Personal Communications

Anonymous inmate of Webster House

Herant Katchadourian

Samar Labban

Adnan Mroueh

Hilda Nassar

John Racy

George Sabra

Periodicals, Journals, and Magazines

Arabic

As sources of medical and popularized medical and psychological knowledge (the years consulted are in parentheses):

al-Jinān (1870–1876)

al-Muqtaṭaf (1876–1956)

ash-Shifā' (1886–1891)

at-Ṭabīb (1874–1914; it was called *Akhbār Ṭibbiyah* in 1874–1882 and was suspended in 1877–1880)

English and French

As sources of medical, psychiatric, and missionary writings:

American Journal of Insanity

Annales d'hygiène publique et de médecine légale

Annales médico-psychologiques

Atlantic Monthly

Boston Medical and Surgical Journal (1828–1928), renamed in 1928 the *New England Journal of Medicine*

British Medical Journal

Bulletin de l'Académie nationale de médecine

Churchman

Contemporary Review

Gazette hebdomadaire de médecine et de chirurgie

Gazette médicale d'Orient

International Journal of Social Psychiatry

Journal médical libanais/Lebanese Medical Journal

Journal of Abnormal Psychology

Journal of Mental Science (1858–1962), renamed in 1963 the *British Journal of Psychiatry*

Journal of the American Medical Association

Journal of the American Oriental Society

Journal of the Royal Naval Medical Service

Lancet

Medical Times and Gazette

Missionary Review of the World

Orient

Our Missions: Friends' Missionary Magazine

Transactions of the American Clinical and Climatological Association

Endnotes

Transliteration, Translation, Terminology, and Monetary Values

1. Legislative decree of September 9, 1983, no. 72, article 20. "Riʿayat wa-ʿilāj wa-ḥimāyat al-marḍa al-ʿaqliyyīn," *al-Jaridat al-Rasmiyya/Journal officiel libanais*, no. 38, September 9, 1983: 912–915.

2. Darrel A. Regier, Emily A. Kuhl, and David J. Kupfer, "The DSM-5: Classification and Criteria Changes," *World Psychiatry* 12, no. 2 (June 2013): 92–98.

3. See Butrus al-Bustani, *Muḥīṭ al-Muḥīṭ: Ay Qāmūs Muṭawwal lil-Lughah al-ʿArabiyyah* (Beirut: n.p., 1867), 1: 1042. For more on the etymology of "Syria" and the misuse of the term "Greater Syria," see Daniel Pipes, *Greater Syria: The History of an Ambition* (New York: Oxford University Press, 1990).

4. See Leila Fawaz, *A Land of Aching Hearts: The Middle East in the Great War* (Cambridge, MA: Harvard University Press, 2014), 17.

5. Vincent Capdepuy, "Proche ou Moyen-Orient? Géohistoire de la notion de Middle East," *L'espace géographique* 37, no. 3 (September 22, 2008): 225–238.

6. "Data Series: Exchange Rates USD/LBP," Banque du Liban, 2020, https://www.bdl.gov.lb/statistics/table.php?name=t5282usd.

7. Lawrence H. Officer and Samuel H. Williamson, "Computing 'Real Value' over Time with a Conversion between U.K. Pounds and U.S. Dollars, 1774 to Present," *MeasuringWorth.com*, 2020, http://www.measuringworth.com/exchange/.

Preface

Epigraph: AUB-SML, LHMND, Annual Report (hereafter, AR), 1914–1915, 4.

1. Alexandre Brièrre de Boismont, "De l'influence de la civilisation sur le développement de la folie," *Annales d'hygiène publique et de médecine légale* 21 (1839): 262.

2. Michel Foucault, *Histoire de la folie à l'âge classique: Folie et déraison* (Paris: Librairie Plon, 1961). The book was originally translated into English in an abridged version as Michel Foucault, *Madness and Civilization: A History of Insanity in the Age of Reason*, trans. Richard Howard (New York: Pantheon Books, 1965). For a complete translation of the French text, see Michel Foucault, *History of Madness*, trans. Jonathan Murphy and Jean Khalfa (London: Routledge, 2006).

3. Friedrich Wilhelm Nietzsche, *On the Genealogy of Morals*, trans. Walter Kaufmann and R. J. Hollingdale (New York: Vintage Books, 1989), 93.

4. Katharine Park and Lorraine J. Daston, "Unnatural Conceptions: The Study of Monsters in Sixteenth- and Seventeenth-Century France and England," *Past and Present*, no. 92 (1981): 20–54.

5. Tarek El-Ariss, "Majnun Strikes Back: Crossings of Madness and Homosexuality in Contemporary Arabic Literature," *International Journal of Middle East Studies* 45, no. 2 (2013): 302. For the definition/etymology of ʿAṣfūriyyeh, see footnote 7 of the Introduction.

6. For insightful papers on the elusive nature of disease, see Charles E. Rosenberg, "Disease in History: Frames and Framers," *Milbank Quarterly* 67, supp. 1 (1989): 1–15, and "The Tyranny of Diagnosis: Specific Entities and Individual Experience," *Milbank Quarterly* 80, no. 2 (2002): 237–260.

7. Nikolas Rose, *The Politics of Life Itself: Biomedicine, Power, and Subjectivity in the Twenty-First Century* (Princeton, NJ: Princeton University Press, 2007), 80–81. Also see Didier Fassin, *La vie: Mode d'emploi critique* (Paris: Seuil), 35–67.

8. Jonathan Metzl, *The Protest Psychosis: How Schizophrenia Became a Black Disease* (Boston: Beacon Press, 2009).

9. Jacques Derrida, *Archive Fever: A Freudian Impression*, trans. Eric Prenowitz (Chicago: University of Chicago Press, 1996), 1–4.

10. Laurence Naish to C. M. Dalley, April 20, 1983, LH/08/22, box 14, LH, SOAS.

Introduction

1. "Lebanon Hospital for the Insane," *British Medical Journal* 2, no. 2534 (July 24, 1909): 229.

2. M. A. Partridge, "Psychiatry in the Levant," *Journal of the Royal Naval Medical Service* 32 (April 1946): 115–126.

3. Jens Hanssen, *Fin de Siècle Beirut: The Making of an Ottoman Provincial Capital* (Oxford: Clarendon Press of Oxford University Press, 2005), especially 115–137; Leila Fawaz, "The Changing Balance of Forces between Beirut and Damascus in the

Nineteenth and Twentieth Centuries," *Revue du monde musulman et de la méditerranée* 55, no. 1 (1990): 208–214.

4. Several plague and cholera outbreaks affected the main cities of the Near East in the period 1840–1890, including Damascus, Beirut, and Aleppo. See Charles Philip Issawi, *The Fertile Crescent, 1800–1914: A Documentary Economic History* (New York: Oxford University Press, 1988), especially 15–23.

5. Theophilus Waldmeier, *The Autobiography of Theophilus Waldmeier, Missionary: Being an Account of Ten Years' Life in Abyssinia; and Sixteen Years in Syria* (London: S. W. Partridge and Co., 1886), especially 171–175 (hereafter, *The Autobiography of Theophilus Waldmeier, Missionary)*; Henry Harris Jessup, *Fifty-Three Years in Syria* (New York: Fleming H. Revell, 1910), especially 1:157–214. For more on the 1840s and 1860s massacres in Damascus and Mount Lebanon, see Kamal S. Salibi, *The Modern History of Lebanon* (London: Weidenfeld and Nicolson, 1965), especially 40–52; Leila Fawaz, *An Occasion for War: Civil Conflict in Lebanon and Damascus in 1860* (Berkeley: University of California Press, 1994); Jonathan Frankel, *The Damascus Affair: "Ritual Murder," Politics, and the Jews in 1840* (Cambridge: Cambridge University Press, 1997); Caesar E. Farah, *The Politics of Interventionism in Ottoman Lebanon, 1830–1861* (Oxford: Centre for Lebanese Studies, 2000); Carol Hakim, *The Origins of the Lebanese National Idea 1840–1920* (Berkeley: University of California Press, 2013), especially 65–98.

6. Theophilus Waldmeier, *Appeal for the First Home for the Insane in Bible Lands* (London: Headly Brothers, 1896), 8, LHMND, AUB-SML (hereafter, Waldmeier, *Appeal*).

7. ʿAṣfūriyyeh—today part of Ḥazmiyyeh—was an area in Mount Lebanon known for its golden finches. See Shahin Salibi, *Tisʿūn Taḥkī* (Beirut: Lebanese University, 1987), 90. There are several other possible explanations for the name—one being that the name is related to the family name of the landowner (ʿAṣfūr). However, this is not convincing because the land belonged to the Jumblatt family. Yet another fancy but undocumented explanation is that the Ottoman pasha who governed Mount Lebanon at the time had a golden cage full of birds. Curiously, birds have long been used as symbols of freedom and peace, and encaging them has been a symbol of confinement and oppression. The connotation between madness and birds has been popularized by Ken Kesey's 1962 novel, *One Flew Over the Cuckoo's Nest* (New York: Viking Press). In the case of ʿAṣfūriyyeh, the connotation should be considered purely coincidental until proven otherwise.

8. Clipping from July 1957, *Le Soir*, LHMND, AUB-SML.

9. Charles E. Rosenberg, "What Is an Epidemic? AIDS in Historical Perspective," *Daedalus* 118, no. 2 (April 1, 1989): 2.

10. One major exception is a recent book whose author uses the history of a Cuban madhouse as a window into the history of Cuba. See Jennifer L. Lambe, *Madhouse:*

Psychiatry and Politics in Cuban History (Chapel Hill: University of North Carolina Press, 2017), 233.

11. Gregory Zilboorg, *A History of Medical Psychology* (New York: Norton, 1941); Albert Deutsch, *The Mentally Ill in America: A History of Their Care and Treatment from Colonial Times* (New York: Columbia University Press, 1946); Gerald N. Grob, "The History of the Asylum Revisited: Personal Reflections," in *Discovering the History of Psychiatry*, ed. Mark S. Micale and Roy Porter (New York: Oxford University Press, 1994), especially 260–261.

12. Jan Goldstein, *Console and Classify: The French Psychiatric Profession in the Nineteenth Century* (Chicago: University of Chicago Press, 1981), 80–104; Roy Porter, *Madness: A Brief History* (Oxford: Oxford University Press, 2002), 129–132.

13. Pinel and Tuke adopted moral treatment on different motivational bases: the former on a secular and republican basis, and the latter on Quaker principles. See Anne Digby, *Madness, Morality, and Medicine: A Study of the York Retreat, 1796–1914* (Cambridge: Cambridge University Press, 1985); Goldstein, *Console and Classify*. Interestingly, Foucault omits to mention in *Madness and Civilization* Hegel's praise of Pinel, whose services "deserve the highest acknowledgement," see Laure Murat, *L'homme qui se prenait pour Napoléon: Pour une histoire politique de la folie* (Paris: Gallimard, 2011), 80.

14. Ottomans interchangeably used *darüşşifa*, a Turkish term based on the Arabic *dār ash-shifāʾ* (literally, "house of healing"); *şifahane* ("house of recovery"); *darüssıha*, from the Arabic *dār as-suḥa* ("house of health"); and *bimarhane* ("house of the sick") to refer to the *bīmāristān*.

15. Michael W. Dols, "The Origins of the Islamic Hospital: Myth and Reality," *Bulletin of the History of Medicine* 61, no. 3 (1987): 379.

16. Aḥmad ʿĪsá, *Histoire des bimaristans (hôpitaux) à l'époque islamique. Discours prononcé au Congrès médical tenu au Caire à l'occasion du centenaire de l'École de médecine et de l'Hôpital Kasr-el-Aïni en Décembre 1928* (Cairo: Imprimerie Paul Barbey, 1928); D. M. Dunlop, G. S. Colin, and Bedi N. Şehsuvaroğlu, "Bīmāristān," in *Encyclopaedia of Islam*, 2nd ed., ed. P. Bearman, Th. Bianquis, C. E. Bosworth, E. van Donzel, W. P. Heinrichs, accessed March 6, 2020, http://dx.doi.org/10.1163/1573-3912_islam_COM_0123; Ahmed Ragab, *The Medieval Islamic Hospital: Medicine, Religion, and Charity* (New York: Cambridge University Press, 2015), especially 12–40; Emiliano Fiori, "Jundīshāpūr," in *Encyclopaedia of Islam*, 3rd ed., ed. Kate Fleet, Gudrun Krämer, Denis Matringe, John Nawas, Everett Rowson, accessed March 6, 2020, http://dx.doi.org/10.1163/1573-3912_ei3_COM_27563.

17. Michael W. Dols, "Insanity in Byzantine and Islamic Medicine," *Dumbarton Oaks Papers* 38 (January 1, 1984): 135–148, and "Insanity and Its Treatment in Islamic Society," *Medical History* 31, no. 1 (January 1987): 1.

18. Michel Foucault, *Histoire de la folie à l'âge classique : Folie et déraison* (Paris: Librairie Plon, 1961), 15–19.

19. "Treatment of the Insane in the East," *Lancet* 156, no. 4023 (October 6, 1900): 1025.

20. "Lunacy in Syria," *Lancet* 149, no. 3838 (March 1897): 825–826; "The Lebanon Hospital for the Insane," *Lancet* 153, no. 3935 (January 28, 1899): 248; "Insanity in Palestine," *British Medical Journal* 2, no. 2435 (August 31, 1907): 542–543; "Lebanon Hospital for the Insane," *British Medical Journal* 2, no. 2534 (July 24, 1909): 229; "Bethlem Royal Hospital," *British Medical Journal* 2, no. 1438 (1888): 134; "Insanity in Palestine," *British Medical Journal* 2, no. 2435 (August 31, 1907): 542–543; "Hospital and Dispensary Management: Lebanon Hospital for the Insane," *British Medical Journal* 2, no. 2429 (July 20, 1907): 183; "Lebanon Hospital for the Insane," *British Medical Journal* 2, no. 2534 (July 24, 1909): 229; "An International Mental Hospital in Syria," *British Medical Journal* 2, no. 4166 (November 9, 1940): 637; "Lebanon Hospital for Mental Diseases," *British Medical Journal* 2, no. 4618 (July 9, 1949): 67; "Sir Thomas Smith Clouston, Kt., MD Edin., LlD Edin. and Aberd., formerly Medical Superintendent, Royal Asylum, Edinburgh," *British Medical Journal* 1, no. 2834 (April 24, 1915): 744; "Henry Watson Smith, OBE, MD, Medical Director, Lebanon Hospital for Mental Diseases," *British Medical Journal* 1, no. 3833 (June 23, 1934): 1146–1147; and "Lebanon Hospital for Mental Diseases," *British Medical Journal* 1, no. 3883 (June 8, 1935): 1187.

21. Theophilus Waldmeier, *The Autobiography of Theophilus Waldmeier, Comprising Ten Years in Abyssinia and Forty-Six Years in Syria, with Some Description of the People and Religions of These Countries*, ed. Stephen Hobhouse (London: Friends' Bookshop, 1925), 276–277 (hereafter, *The Autobiography of Theophilus Waldmeier*), 283, 310, and 312.

22. Papers relating to the Lebanon Hospital for the Insane, Syria RET 8/3, UY-BIA.

23. Digby, *Madness, Morality, and Medicine*.

24. For more on Süleymaniye Bimarhanesi, see Fatih Artvinli, *Delilik, siyaset ve toplum: Toptaşı Bimarhanesi (1873–1927)* (Istanbul: Boğaziçi Üniversitesi Yayınevi, 2013) and "Insanity, Belonging and Citizenship: Mentally Ill People Who Went to and/or Returned from Europe in the Late Ottoman Era," *History of Psychiatry* 27, no. 3 (September 1, 2016): 268–277; Cihangir Gündoğdu, "'Are There No Asylums?' The Ottoman State and the Insane, 1856–1908" (PhD diss., University of Chicago, 2014). For more on ʿAbbasiyya, see Marilyn Anne Mayers, "A Century of Psychiatry: The Egyptian Mental Hospitals" (PhD diss. Princeton University, 1984), especially 28–79; Valérie Baqué, "Regards sur l'asile et la folie dans l'Égypte du XIXe siècle," *Annales islamologiques*, no. 26 (1992): 197–206, and "Du bimaristan à l'asile moderne: Mise en place de l'institution et de la médecine psychiatriques en Égypte, 1882/1930" (PhD diss., Université de Provence, 1995); Eugene Rogan, "Madness and Marginality:

The Advent of the Psychiatric Asylum in Egypt and Lebanon," in *Outside In: On the Margins of the Modern Middle East*, ed. Eugene Rogan (London: I. B. Tauris, 2002), especially 110–111.

25. Gündoğdu, "'Are There No Asylums?,'" especially 35–86.

26. By elite—professional, political, economic, or intellectual—I mean the most visible, vocal (i.e., the most engaged), and dominant group of a particular society at a particular time. See John Scott, "Pareto and the Elite,'" in *Vilfredo Pareto: Beyond Disciplinary Boundaries*, ed. Joseph V. Femia and Alasdair J. Marshall (Burlington, VT: Ashgate, 2012), 9–19. To use Bourdieusian terminology, if there is one particular "distinction" that these elites have (as will become clear by the end of this book), it is their involvement in the wider "circulation" (another term borrowed from Vilfredo Pareto) of knowledge and its condition of possibility. See Pierre Bourdieu, *La distinction: Critique sociale du jugement* (Paris: Éditions de Minuit, 1979). On the urban and political notables (in Arabic, *aʿyan*), see Albert H. Hourani, "Ottoman Reform and the Politics of Notables," in *Beginnings of Modernization in the Middle East in the Nineteenth Century*, ed. William R. Polk and Richard L. Chambers (Chicago: University of Chicago Press, 1968), 41–68; Philip S. Khoury, *Urban Notables and Arab Nationalism: The Politics of Damascus, 1860–1920* (Cambridge: Cambridge University Press, 1983), especially 8–23.

27. See Habib Badr, "Mission To 'Nominal Christians': The Policy and Practice of the American Board of Commissioners for Foreign Missions and Its Missionaries Concerning Eastern Churches Which Led to the Organization of a Protestant Church in Beirut (1819–1848)" (PhD diss., Princeton Theological Seminary, 1992), especially 9–11.

28. Louis Mongeri, "Études sur l'aliénation mentale en Orient," *Gazette médicale d'Orient* 4, no. 9 (1860): especially 39–40; Baqué, "Regards sur l'asile," 204.

29. Waldmeier, *The Autobiography of Theophilus Waldmeier*, 310.

30. "Lebanon Hospital for the Insane," *British Medical Journal* 2, no. 2534 (July 24, 1909): 229.

31. For Ottoman Turkey, see Fatih Artvinli, *Delilik, siyaset ve toplum*, "Insanity, Belonging and Citizenship," and "'Pinel of Istanbul': Dr. Luigi Mongeri (1815–82) and the Birth of Modern Psychiatry in the Ottoman Empire," *History of Psychiatry* 29, no. 4 (December 2018): 424–37; Fatih Artvinli and Şeref Etker, "Bimarhaneler ve Mecanin Yönetimi: İki Taslak ve Süregelen. Tartışma," *Osmanlı Bilimi Araştırmaları* 14, no. 2 (2013): 1–40; Gündoğdu, "'Are There No Asylums?'"; Burçak Özlüdil Altın, "Psychiatry, Space, and Time: Case of an Ottoman Asylum," *Journal of the Ottoman and Turkish Studies Association* 5, no. 1 (Spring 2018): 67–89; Yucel Yanikdag, "Ottoman Psychiatry and the Great War," in *The First World War as Remembered in the Countries of the Eastern Mediterranean*, ed. Olaf Farschid, Manfred Kropp, and Stephan Dähne (Beirut: Orient-Institut, 2006), 163–178. For Ottoman Egypt, see Baqué, "Regards

sur l'asile" and "Du bimaristan à l'asile moderne"; Mayers, "A Century of Psychiatry"; Rogan, "Madness and Marginality," 104–125.

32. "Ezrat Nashim Hospital," Central Zionist Archives, accessed April 7, 2020, http://www.zionistarchives.org.il/en/AttheCZA/AdditionalArticles/Pages/EzratNashim.aspx.

33. For Ezrat Nashim and ʿAṣfūriyyeh, see Jacob Margolin and Eliezar Witztum, "Prakim be-Historia Hapsichiatri be-Eretz Yisra'el ve-Besvivatai bei: Beit Ha-holim le-Pagu'ei Nefesh ''asfuria' bi-Levanon," *Harefuah* 140, no. 8 (August 2001): 790–794.

34. For Ezrat Nashim, see Rakefet Zalashik, "Psychiatry, Ethnicity and Migration: The Case of Palestine, 1920–1948," *Dynamis* 25 (2005): 403–422, and *Ad Nefesh: Mehagrim, ʿolim, Peliṭim Ṿeha-Mimsad Ha-Psikhi'aṭri Be-Yisra'el* (Tel Aviv: Ha-Ḳibuts Ha-Me'uḥad, 2008); Margalit Shilo, *Princess or Prisoner? Jewish Women in Jerusalem, 1840–1914* (Hanover, NH: University Press of New England, 2005). For Dayr al-Ṣalīb, see Elias Aboujaoude, "The Psychiatric Hospital of the Cross: A Sane Asylum in the Middle East," *American Journal of Psychiatry* 159, no. 12 (December 2002): 1982; Jean Ducruet, "Les premières décennies de psychiatrie au Liban (1900–1960)," *Travaux et jours*, no. 74 (2004): especially 61–67.

35. See Samir Khalaf, *Protestant Missionaries in the Levant: Ungodly Puritans, 1820–60* (Milton Park, UK: Routledge, 2012), especially 193–213; Ussama S. Makdisi, *The Culture of Sectarianism: Community, History, and Violence in Nineteenth-Century Ottoman Lebanon* (Berkeley: University of California Press, 2000), especially 15–27.

36. David A. Dorman, "The Artillery of Ideology: A Critique of Ussama Makdisi's *The Artillery of Heaven*. A Review Essay," *Theological Review* 30, no. 2 (2009): 235. Also see Biswamoy Pati and Mark Harrison, eds., *Health, Medicine, and Empire: Perspectives on Colonial India* (Hyderabad, India: Orient Longman, 2001); Olivier Faure, "Missions religieuses, missions médicales et 'mission civilisatrice' (XIXe et XXe s.): Un regard décalé," *Histoire, monde et cultures religieuses* 21, no. 1 (March 1, 2012): 5–18.

37. For instance, see Caesar. E. Farah, "A Tale of Two Missions," in *Arabic and Islamic Garland: Historical, Educational and Literary Papers Presented to Abdul-Latif Tibawi* (London: Islamic Cultural Centre, 1977), 81–91.

38. Frantz Fanon, *L'an V de la révolution algérienne* (Paris: La Découverte [1959] 2011), 110. George Antonius had made a similar argument about the role of Western education two decades earlier in his influential *The Arab Awakening: The Story of the Arab National Movement* (London: H. Hamilton, 1939), 93.

39. George Sabra, lecture, "AUB and Religion. Never the Twain Shall Meet … Again?" General lecture series of the Anis Makdisi program in Literature, American University of Beirut, February 2, 2005; Pamela E. Klassen, *Spirits of Protestantism: Medicine, Healing, and Liberal Christianity* (Berkeley: University of California Press, 2011).

40. I borrow the term "anticlerical" from Jan Goldstein, "The Hysteria Diagnosis and the Politics of Anticlericalism in Late Nineteenth-Century France," *Journal of Modern History* 54, no. 2 (June 1982): 209–239.

41. Elizabeth Thompson, *Colonial Citizens: Republican Rights, Paternal Privilege, and Gender in French Syria and Lebanon* (New York: Columbia University Press, 2000), 58. See also Thompson, *Colonial Citizens,* 77; Ronald Edward Robinson and John Gallagher, *Africa and the Victorians: The Official Mind of Imperialism* (London: Macmillan, 1961); Benjamin N. Lawrance, Emily Lynn Osborn, and Richard L. Roberts, eds., *Intermediaries, Interpreters, and Clerks: African Employees in the Making of Colonial Africa* (Madison: University of Wisconsin Press, 2006).

42. On the English consular protection of American missionaries, see Abdul Latif Tibawi, *American Interests in Syria, 1800–1901: A Study of Educational, Literary and Religious Work* (Oxford: Clarendon Press of Oxford University Press, 1966), 19–23. On the French support of Jesuits, see Chantal Verdeil, "L'Université Saint-Joseph et la troisième république," in *Une France en Méditerranée: Écoles, langue et culture françaises, XIXe–XXe siècles,* ed. Patrick Cabanel (Paris: Créaphis, 2006), 235–252, and *La mission jésuite du Mont-Liban et de Syrie, 1830–1864* (Paris: Les Indes Savantes, 2011).

43. R. Hingston Fox, Waldmeier's biographer, wrote, "Waldmeier's long residence in the East has made him almost an oriental." See R. Hingston Fox, *Theophilus Waldmeier* (London: Friends' Foreign Mission Association, 1916), 20, LH/10/01, box 15, LH, SOAS. As for Cornelius Van Dyck (see below in the text), he was known not only for his fluency in Arabic but also for adopting Syrian attire, the traditional *'abāya* (a long sleeveless overblouse) and the fez. See Lutfi M. Sa'di, George Sarton, and W. T. Van Dyck, "Al-Hakîm Cornelius Van Alen Van Dyck (1818–1895)," *Isis* 27, no. 1 (May 1, 1937): 20–45.

44. E. Mittwoch, "Hakim," in *E. J. Brill's First Encyclopaedia of Islam, 1913–1936,* ed. M. T. Houtsma (Leiden, the Netherlands: E. J. Brill, 1987), 3: 224.

45. Theophilus Waldmeier letter to "Friends and other Christians to whom this may come," October 20, 1898, LH/07/04, box 9, LH, SOAS. Waldmeier also mentions "the dead which cannot be buried" and the "half dead" in *Appeal,* 1896, 15, LHMND, AUB-SML and AR, 1904, 18, AUB-SML; Theophilus Waldmeier, *Appeal for the First Home for the Insane in Bible Lands* (London: Headley Brothers, 1897), 11, RET 8/3/1, UY-BIA, and "The Lebanon Hospital for the Insane," *Missionary Review of the World* 21, no. 7 (July 1898): 535.

46. See Philip Sheldrake, *Spaces for the Sacred: Place, Memory, and Identity* (Baltimore, MD: Johns Hopkins University Press, 2001), 29.

47. Waldmeier, *The Autobiography of Theophilus Waldmeier, Missionary,* 58.

48. On the poor being the "necessary and indeed nonnegotiable access point of access to the Kingdom of God," see Gary A. Anderson, *Charity: The Place of the Poor in the Biblical Tradition* (New Haven, CT: Yale University Press, 2013), 3.

49. Waldmeier, *The Autobiography of Theophilus Waldmeier*, 276–277; Patrick Adams, "In Lebanon, Mental Health Is on the Mend," *Lancet* 377, no. 9767 (February 26, 2011): 708.

50. Beverly Ann Tsacoyianis, "Making Healthy Minds and Bodies in Syria and Lebanon, 1899–1961" (PhD diss., Washington University in St. Louis, 2014), 6.

51. N. M. Kronfol, "Health Services to Groups with Special Needs in the Arab World: A Review," *Eastern Mediterranean Health Journal* 18, no. 12 (December 2012): especially 1250–1251.

52. For the pervasiveness of stigmatization in Europe and North America, see US Department of Health and Human Services, "Mental Health: A Report of the Surgeon General" (Rockville, MD: US Department of Health and Human Services, 1999); Regional Committee for Europe, Sixty-Third Session, "The European Mental Health Action Plan" (Çeşme Izmir, Turkey: World Health Organization, September 16, 2013).

53. See, for example, Jürgen Unützer, Ruth Klap, Roland Sturm, Alexander S. Young, Tonya Marmon, Jess Shatkin, and Kenneth B. Wells, "Mental Disorders and the Use of Alternative Medicine: Results from a National Survey," *American Journal of Psychiatry* 157, no. 11 (November 2000): 1851–1857; Ronald C. Kessler, Jane Soukup, Roger B. Davis, David F. Foster, Sonja A. Wilkey, Maria I. Van Rompay, and David M. Eisenberg, "The Use of Complementary and Alternative Therapies to Treat Anxiety and Depression in the United States," *American Journal of Psychiatry* 158, no. 2 (February 2001): 289–294. For medical miracles in the modern world, see Jacalyn Duffin, *Medical Miracles: Doctors, Saints, and Healing in the Modern World* (Oxford: Oxford University Press, 2009).

54. See Nikolas S. Rose, *Governing the Soul: The Shaping of the Private Self* (London: Routledge, 1990), and "Neurochemical Selves," *Society* 41, no. 1 (2003): 46–59.

55. Jack Drescher, "Out of DSM: Depathologizing Homosexuality," *Behavioral Sciences* 5, no. 4 (December 4, 2015): 565–575.

56. See Joseph El-Khoury and Andres Barkil-Oteo, "Letter to the Editor: Lebanese Psychiatrists Take Stand on Homosexuality," *Psychiatric News*, October 9, 2013, https://doi.org/10.1176/appi.pn.2013.L15; Hazem Zohny, "Homosexuality Not a Disease, Says Lebanese Psychiatric Society," *Nature Middle East*, August 21, 2013, http://blogs.nature.com/houseofwisdom/2013/08/homosexuality-not-a-disease-says-lebanese-psychiatric-society.html.

57. Ahmed Okasha, Elie Karam, and Tarek Okasha, "Mental Health Services in the Arab World," *World Psychiatry* 11, no. 1 (February 2012): 52–54.

58. Rogan, "Madness and Marginality," 104.

59. Sigmund Freud, *Psychopathology of Everyday Life*, trans. A. A. Brill (New York: Macmillan Company, 1914).

60. Andrew T. Scull, "The Decarceration of the Mentally Ill: A Critical View," *Politics and Society* 6, no. 2 (1976): 173–212; David Mechanic and David A. Rochefort, "Deinstitutionalization: An Appraisal of Reform," *Annual Review of Sociology* 16 (January 1, 1990): 301–327.

61. David J. Rothman, "New Light on the Origins of the Asylum," *Contemporary Sociology* 19, no. 5 (September 1, 1990): 659, and *The Discovery of the Asylum: Social Order and Disorder in the New Republic* (Boston: Little, Brown, 1971); Robert Castel, *L'ordre psychiatrique: L'âge d'or de l'aliénisme* (Paris: Éditions de Minuit, 1977); Andrew T. Scull, *Museums of Madness: The Social Organization of Insanity in Nineteenth-Century England* (London: Allen Lane, 1979); Marcel Gauchet and Gladys Swain, *La pratique de l'esprit humain: L'institution asilaire et la révolution démocratique* (Paris: Gallimard, 1980).

62. See Moshe Ma'oz, *Ottoman Reform in Syria and Palestine, 1840–1861: The Impact of the Tanzimat on Politics and Society* (Oxford: Clarendon Press of Oxford University Press, 1968); M. Şükrü Hanioğlu, *A Brief History of the Late Ottoman Empire* (Princeton, NJ: Princeton University Press, 2008), especially 72–108.

63. Salibi, *The Modern History of Lebanon*, 47–48; Fawwaz Traboulsi, *A History of Modern Lebanon* (London: Pluto Press, 2007), especially 24–40; Hakim, *The Origins of the Lebanese National Idea*, especially 23–25 and 49–50.

64. The Maronites, a Christian sect, trace their roots to the fifth century. They were persecuted and sought refuge in Mount Lebanon starting in the ninth century. They united with Rome in the twelfth century as a Uniate church, while retaining their liturgy and priesthood. They were influential in establishing the modern state of Lebanon. Today the Maronites are the dominant Christian group in Lebanon. The Druzes follow an esoteric doctrine that is considered an offshoot of Shīʿī Ismāʿīlīsm, which developed during the tenth century. They are named after one of the founders of the sect, Muḥammad Ibn Ismaʿīl al-Darazī. Together with the Maronites, the Druzes have played a key role in the history of modern Lebanon. See Salibi, *The Modern History of Lebanon*, especially xi–xxvii; Kais Firro, *A History of the Druzes* (Leiden, the Netherlands: E. J. Brill, 1992).

65. See Engin Deniz Akarli, *The Long Peace: Ottoman Lebanon, 1861–1920* (Berkeley: University of California Press, 1993), especially 6–33.

66. Jessup, *Fifty-Three Years in Syria*, especially 1: 215–232. Also see J. D. Maitland-Kirwan, *Sunrise in Syria: A Short History of the British Syrian Mission, from 1860–1930* (London: British Syrian Mission, 1930).

67. Hakim, *The Origins of the Lebanese National Idea*, 68.

68. Waldmeier, *The Autobiography of Theophilus Waldmeier, Missionary*, 149. For more on the history of the British Syrian Mission and its founder, Elizabeth Bowen Thompson, see Maitland-Kirwan, *Sunrise in Syria*. For more on American missionaries and the

American Board of Commissioners for Foreign Missions (founded in Boston in 1810), see Tibawi, *American Interests in Syria*; Christine Leigh Heyrman, *American Apostles: When Evangelicals Entered the World of Islam* (New York: Hill and Wang, 2015).

69. See, for example, Davide Rodogno, *Against Massacre: Humanitarian Interventions in the Ottoman Empire, 1815–1914* (Princeton, NJ: Princeton University Press, 2012).

70. See Allan Young, *The Harmony of Illusions: Inventing Post-Traumatic Stress Disorder* (Princeton, NJ: Princeton University Press, 1995); Ben Shephard, *A War of Nerves: Soldiers and Psychiatrists in the Twentieth Century* (Cambridge, MA: Harvard University Press, 2001).

71. Charles Baddoura, "Santé mentale et guerre libanaise," *Bulletin de l'Académie nationale de médecine* 174, no. 5 (May 1990): 583–90; discussion 590–593; E. G. Karam, D. B. Howard, A. N. Karam, A. Ashkar, M. Shaaya, N. Melhem, and N. El-Khoury, "Major Depression and External Stressors: The Lebanon Wars," *European Archives of Psychiatry and Clinical Neuroscience* 248, no. 5 (1998): 225–30; E. G. Karam, J. C. Noujeim, S. E. Saliba, A. H. Chami, and S. Abi Rached, "PTSD: How Frequently Should the Symptoms Occur? The Effect on Epidemiologic Research," *Journal of Traumatic Stress* 9, no. 4 (October 1996): 899–905; U. S. Yatkin and S. Labban, "Traumatic War. Stress & Schizophrenia," *Journal of Psychosocial Nursing and Mental Health Services* 30, no. 6 (June 1992): 29–33; L. K. Zahr, "Effects of War on the Behavior of Lebanese Preschool Children: Influence of Home Environment and Family Functioning," *American Journal of Orthopsychiatry* 66, no. 3 (July 1996): 401–408.

72. For the former, see Rogan, "Madness and Marginality," especially 115. For the latter, see Ussama Makdisi, "Reclaiming the Land of the Bible: Missionaries, Secularism, and Evangelical Modernity," *American Historical Review* 102, no. 3 (June 1, 1997): 691, and *The Culture of Sectarianism*.

73. The term "antipsychiatry" was coined in 1967 by the South African psychiatrist David Cooper, who was part of the movement that questioned the legitimacy of psychiatric practice. See Henry A. Nasrallah, "The Antipsychiatry Movement: Who and Why," *Current Psychiatry* 10, no. 12 (December 2011): 4–53.

74. Edward Hallett Carr, *What Is History?* (New York: Vintage Books, 1961), 179.

75. Quoted in "Lebanon Hospital for Mental Diseases," *British Medical Journal* 2, no. 4618 (July 9, 1949): 67.

76. Erwin H. Ackerknecht, *A Short History of Medicine*, rev. ed. (Baltimore, MD: Johns Hopkins University Press, 1982), 210.

77. In one such exposé in *Life* magazine, the author (who had gone as an undercover reporter to two state asylums, in Cleveland and Philadelphia) compared state asylums to Nazi concentration camps. See Albert Maisel, "Bedlam 1946," *Life*, May 6, 1946, 102–118.

78. See Thomas Stephen Szasz, *The Myth of Mental Illness: Foundations of a Theory of Personal Conduct* (New York: Hoeber-Harper, 1961); R. D. Laing, *The Divided Self: A Study of Sanity and Madness* (Chicago: Quadrangle Books, 1960), and *The Self and Others: Further Studies in Sanity and Madness* (London: Tavistock Publications, 1961); Foucault, *Histoire de la folie à l'âge classique*; Erving Goffman, *Asylums: Essays on the Social Situation of Mental Patients and Other Inmates* (Garden City, NY: Anchor Books, 1961).

79. Goffman, *Asylums*, 12.

80. Rothman, *The Discovery of the Asylum*; Castel, *L'ordre psychiatrique*; Scull, *Museums of Madness.*

81. See Jacques Derrida, "Cogito et histoire de la folie," *Revue de métaphysique et de morale* 68, no. 4 (1963): 460–494; Jürgen Habermas, *The Philosophical Discourse of Modernity: Twelve Lectures* (Cambridge, MA: MIT Press, 1987), especially 238–293; Andrew Scull, "Michel Foucault's History of Madness," *History of the Human Sciences* 3, no. 1 (February 1, 1990): 57–67. For a broader overview of the critique of Foucault's work and approach, see Allan Megill, "The Reception of Foucault by Historians," *Journal of the History of Ideas* 48, no. 1 (1987): 117–141.

82. Foucault, *Histoire de la folie à l'âge classique*, especially chapter 4, "Naissance de l'asile," 576–632. Also see Gladys Swain, *Le sujet de la folie: Naissance de la psychiatrie* (Paris: Calmann-Lévy, 1997); Dora B. Weiner, "'Le Geste de Pinel': The History of a Psychiatric Myth," in *Discovering the History of Psychiatry*, ed. Mark S. Micale and Roy Porter (New York: Oxford University Press, 1994), 232–247.

83. Michael W. Dols, *Majnūn: The Madman in Medieval Islamic Society*, ed. Diana E. Immisch (Oxford: Clarendon Press of Oxford University Press, 1992), especially 128–129. For an analysis of Dols's take on the history of madness, see Boaz Shoshan, "The State and Madness in Medieval Islam," *International Journal of Middle East Studies* 35, no. 2 (May 1, 2003): 329–340.

84. See Grob, "The History of the Asylum Revisited."

85. See, for instance, Goldstein, *Console and Classify*; Nancy Tomes, *A Generous Confidence: Thomas Story Kirkbride and the Art of Asylum-Keeping, 1840–1883* (Cambridge: Cambridge University Press, 1984); Digby, *Madness, Morality, and Medicine*; Ellen Dwyer, *Homes for the Mad: Life inside Two Nineteenth-Century Asylums* (New Brunswick, NJ: Rutgers University Press, 1987).

86. See Joseph Melling, "Accommodating Madness: New Research in the Social History of Insanity and Institutions," in *Insanity, Institutions, and Society, 1800–1914: A Social History of Madness in Comparative Perspective*, ed. Joseph Melling and Bill Forsythe (London: Routledge, 1999), 21.

87. See, for example, John McCulloch, *Colonial Psychiatry and "the African Mind"* (Cambridge: Cambridge University Press, 1995); Jonathan Hal Sadowsky, *Imperial*

Bedlam: Institutions of Madness in Colonial Southwest Nigeria (Berkeley: University of California Press, 1999); Megan Vaughan, "Idioms of Madness: Zomba Lunatic Asylum, Nyasaland, in the Colonial Period," *Journal of Southern African Studies* 9, no. 2 (April 1, 1983): 218–238; Richard Keller, "Madness and Colonization: Psychiatry in the British and French Empires, 1800–1962," *Journal of Social History* 35, no. 2 (December 1, 2001): 295–326; Sloan Mahone and Megan Vaughan, eds., *Psychiatry and Empire* (Basingstoke, UK: Palgrave Macmillan, 2007).

88. Perhaps the most original critiques to date have been by those social critics who have emphasized the psychological damage perpetrated by the colonial enterprise itself on colonized populations. See Aimé Césaire, *Discours sur le colonialisme* (Paris: Présence Africaine, 1955); Frantz Fanon, *Les damnés de la terre* (Paris: Éditions la Découverte, 1961) and *Peau noire, masques blancs* (Paris: Éditions du Seuil, 1952); Albert Memmi, *Portrait du colonisé: Précédé du portrait du colonisateur* (Paris: Éditions Corrêa, 1957).

89. Foucault, *Histoire de la folie à l'âge classique*, especially chapter 2, "Le grand renfermement," 68–109.

90. For the African context, see Megan Vaughan, *Curing Their Ills: Colonial Power and African Illness* (Cambridge: Polity, 1991). For a broader critique of the great confinement thesis, see H. C. Erik Midelfort, "Madness and Civilization in Early Modern Europe: A Reappraisal of Michel Foucault," in *After the Reformation: Essays in Honor of J. H. Hexter*, ed. Barbara Malament (Philadelphia: University of Pennsylvania Press, 1980), 247–265.

91. Daniel R. Headrick, *The Tools of Empire: Technology and European Imperialism in the Nineteenth Century* (New York: Oxford University Press, 1981).

92. Waltraud Ernst, *Colonialism and Transnational Psychiatry: The Case of the Ranchi Indian Mental Hospital in British India, c. 1920–1940* (London: Anthem, 2012). Also see Waltraud Ernst, "Crossing the Boundaries of 'Colonial Psychiatry.' Reflections on the Development of Psychiatry in British India, c. 1870–1940," *Culture, Medicine, and Psychiatry* 35, no. 4 (December 1, 2011): 536.

93. Keller, "Madness and Colonization."

94. See Marc Lagana, *Le parti colonial français: Éléments d'histoire* (Sillery, QC: Presses de l'Université du Québec, 1990), especially "Le projet Sarraut," 82–86; Alice L. Conklin, *A Mission to Civilize: The Republican Idea of Empire in France and West Africa, 1895–1930* (Stanford, CA: Stanford University Press, 1997); Richard C. Keller, *Colonial Madness: Psychiatry in French North Africa* (Chicago: University of Chicago Press, 2007).

95 Ernst, *Colonialism and Transnational Psychiatry: The Case of the Ranchi Indian Mental Hospital in British India, c. 1920–1940*, 3–5.

96. Eugene Rogan, ed., *Outside In: On the Margins of the Modern Middle East* (London: I. B. Tauris, 2002); Keller, *Colonial Madness*; Rakefet Zalashik, *Ad Nefesh*, "The

Psychiatric Asylum in Bnei-Brak and 'The Society for the Help of the Insane,' 1929–1939," *Korot* 17 (2003–2004): 47–69 and x, and "Psychiatry, Ethnicity and Migration"; Sara Scalenghe, *Disability in the Ottoman Arab World, 1500–1800* (New York: Cambridge University Press, 2014); Marianna Scarfone, "La psychiatrie italienne au front: L'expérience fondatrice de la guerre de Libye, 1911–1912," *Le mouvement social* 257, no. 4 (2016): 109–126, and "Italian Colonial Psychiatry: Outlines of a Discipline, and Practical Achievements in Libya and the Horn of Africa," *History of Psychiatry* 27, no. 4 (December 1, 2016): 389–405; Christopher Wilson, "Petitions and Pathways to the Asylum in British Mandate Palestine, 1920–1948," *Historical Journal* 62, no. 2 (2019): 451–471. There are also new anthropologic and ethnographic approaches to psychiatry and mental illness. For example, see Orkideh Behrouzan, *Prozak Diaries: Psychiatry and Generational Memory in Iran* (Stanford, CA: Stanford University Press, 2016).

97. Herant A. Katchadourian, "The Historical Background of Psychiatry in Lebanon," *Bulletin of the History of Medicine* 54, no. 4 (1980): 544–553; Ducruet, "Les premières décennies de psychiatrie au Liban," 39–74; Sami Richa, *La psychiatrie au Liban: Une histoire et un regard* (Beirut: Dergham, 2015).

98. Rogan, "Madness and Marginality," 104; Hanssen, *Fin de Siècle Beirut*, 135.

99. Tsacoyianis, "Making Healthy Minds and Bodies in Syria and Lebanon."

100. Fernand Braudel never really defined the duration of the *longue durée*. His initial motivation was to oppose "event-history" (*histoire événementielle*), which relied on a much shorter time scale and focused on political events. See Fernand Braudel, "Histoire et sciences sociales: La longue durée," *Annales. Économies, sociétés, civilisations* 13, no. 4 (1958): 725–753, and *Leçon inaugurale: Faite le Vendredi 1er Décembre 1950* (Paris: Collège de France, 1951). See also Deborah Cohen and Peter Mandler, "The History Manifesto: A Critique," *American Historical Review* 120, no. 2 (2015): 530.

101. Sebastien Conrad, *What Is Global History* (Princeton, NJ: Princeton University Press, 2016). Also see, Lynn Hunt, *Writing History in the Global Era* (New York: W. W. Norton and Company, 2014); Patrick Boucheron, "L'entretien du monde," in *Pour une histoire-monde*, ed. Patrick Boucheron and Nicolas Delalande (Paris: Presses universitaires de France, 2013), 5–23; Sanjay Subrahamanyam, *Leçons inaugurales du Collège de France: Aux origines de l'histoire globale* (Paris: Collège de France, 2014).

102. See, for example, Carla Yanni, *The Architecture of Madness: Insane Asylums in the United States* (Minneapolis: University of Minnesota Press, 2007).

103. See Jean Baudrillard's critique of Foucault's style of writing, which mirrors the power it condemns and rejects (*Oublier Foucault* [Paris: Éditions Galilée, 1977]). For the "medical gaze," see Michel Foucault, *The Birth of the Clinic: An Archaeology of Medical Perception*, trans. A. M. Sheridan Smith (New York: Pantheon Books, 1973).

104. Antranig Manugian, "The Medical Director's Report for the Year 1966," AR, p. 1, LHMND, AUB-SML.

105. Michel de Certeau, *L'écriture de l'histoire* (Paris: Gallimard, 1975), 286.

1 Oriental Madness and Civilization

1. See H. A. Hajar Albinali, "Arab or Islamic Medicine?," *Heart Views* 14, no. 1 (2013): 41–42. An added complication is a recent call to reclaim part of that history as Ottoman medicine. See Miri Shefer Mossensohn, "A Tale of Two Discourses: The Historiography of Ottoman-Muslim Medicine," *Social History of Medicine* 21, no. 1 (2008): 1–12.

2. In the same way, Africa has been defined in terms of absence, nonbeing, and lack—what Achille Mbembe calls "la pensée du negatif" (*De la postcolonie: Essai sur l'imagination politique dans l'Afrique contemporaine* [Paris: Karthala, 2000], 13 and 21).

3. I am inspired by the way in which Megan Vaughan analyzes the colonial psychiatric discourse in the African context as predicated on two kinds of pathological "others": the "abnormal" and "normal" African mind. The main difference here is that in the African context, ethnicity—rather than religion—precedes the psychiatric category and hence is what marks the colonial encounter. See Megan Vaughan, *Curing Their Ills: Colonial Power and African Illness* (Cambridge: Polity, 1991).

4 Robert Walsh, *A Residence at Constantinople: During a Period Including the Commencement, Progress, and Termination of the Greek and Turkish Revolutions* (London: F. Westley & A. H. Davis, 1836), 1:256.

5. Karl Baedeker, ed., *Palestine and Syria: Handbook for Travellers* (London: K. Baedeker, 1876), 135, 277, and 520.

6. Catharine Arnold, *Bedlam: London and Its Mad* (London: Simon and Schuster, 2008), 45 and 93.

7. See Robert Walsh, *A Residence at Constantinople* 1:256.

8. Walsh, *A Residence at Constantinople*, 1:256.

9. R. R. Madden, "The Lunatic Asylum at Cairo Described," *Boston Medical and Surgical Journal* 3, no. 12 (1830): 722. Also see Valérie Baqué, "Regards sur l'asile et la folie dans l'Égypte du XIXe siècle," *Annales islamologiques*, no. 26 (1992): 200.

10. Gustave Flaubert, *Flaubert in Egypt*, trans. Francis Steegmuller (New York: Penguin, 1996), 67. See also *Voyage en Orient (1849–1851): Égypte, Liban-Palestine, Rhodes, Asie Mineure, Constantinople, Grèce, Italie* (Paris: Gallimard, 2006), 106.

11. "Treatment of Lunatics in Syria," *Boston Medical and Surgical Journal* 45 (October 29, 1851): 264–265.

12. Henry M. Wetherill, "The Insane in Some Remote Lands," in *Ninth Report of the Committee on Lunacy of the Board of Public Charities of the Commonwealth of Pennsylvania* (Harrisburg, PA: Edwin K. Meyers, 1891), 167.

13. Wetherill, "The Insane in Some Remote Lands," 167.

14. Labib B. Jureidini, "The Medical Needs of Syria," *Journal of the American Medical Association* 28, no. 18 (May 1, 1897): 817.

15. Post, quoted in Wetherill, "The Insane in Some Remote Lands," 167. See also Jureidini, "The Medical Needs of Syria," 817.

16. Quoted in "Egypt," *Lancet* 159, no. 4111 (June 14, 1902): 1732. Also see Michael W. Dols, *Majnūn: The Madman in Medieval Islamic Society*, ed. Diana E. Immisch (Oxford: Clarendon Press of Oxford University Press, 1992), especially 132–133; Anne-Marie Moulin, "Conscience et représentation de la folie et de la déraison: Une approche historique égyptienne," in *Conscience et représentation de la santé mentale et neurologique*, ed. Christian Mésenge and Jérôme Palazzolo (Paris: Éditions Publibook, 2012), especially 35–40.

17. AR, 1901, 7 and 1905, 17, AUB-SML, LHMND. See also Henry Harris Jessup, *Fifty-Three Years in Syria* (New York: Fleming H. Revell, 1910), 2:524. It is worth noting that cauterization—which was inspired by Galenic medicine and was much in use in the Middle Ages—was still practiced in nineteenth-century Europe. See Michel Foucault, *Psychiatric Power: Lectures at the Collège de France, 1973–1974*, ed. Jacques Lagrange, trans. Graham Burchell (New York: Picador, 2008), 195, note 15.

18. Louis Mongeri, "Études sur l'aliénation mentale en Orient," *Gazette médicale d'Orient*, 4, no.9 (1860): 147–149.

19. "The Lebanon Hospital for the Insane," *Lancet* 153, no. 3935 (January 28, 1899): 248.

20. For a partial but useful list of the different words for madness in Arabic and their definitions, see Karim Hussam el-Din, "Alfāẓ al-Junūn wal-Humq wa-Mafāhīmuhumā fī al-ʿArabiyya," *Alif* 14 (1994): 6–19.

21. The thirteen kinds of mental illness are epilepsy, despair, madness, delirium, damages to the imagination and intelligence, forgetfulness, brutality in the open countryside with wild animals, insomnia, lethargy, roaring in the head, vertigo, swelling, and headache. See Dols, *Majnūn*, 115.

22. Entry entitled "Junūn, Aliénation mentale, Insanity," in Butrus al-Bustani's *Kitāb Dā'irat al-Maʿārif: Wa-Huwa Qāmūs ʿĀmm li-Kull Fann wa-Maṭlab* (Beirut: al-Maʿārif Press, 1882), 6:563–567 and Cornelius Van Dyck, *Uṣūl al-Bathulūjia al-Dākhiliyya al-Kkhāṣa ayy Mabādi' at-Ṭibb al-Basharī al-Naẓarī wal-ʿIlmī* (Beirut: n.p. 1878), 671–700 and 747–751, NEST.

23. For instance, see "The Lebanon Hospital for the Insane," 248.

24. "The Lebanon Hospital for the Insane," 248.

25. Frederick Sessions, "Some Syrian Folklore Notes Gathered on Mount Lebanon," *Folklore* 9, no. 1 (March 1, 1898): 12–13.

26. C. V. A. Van Dyck, "On the Present Condition of the Medical Profession in Syria," *Journal of the American Oriental Society* 1, no. 4 (January 1, 1849): 580.

27. A. H. De Forest, "Insanity in Syria," *American Journal of Insanity* 6 (1850): 351–354. On De Forest, see Jessup, *Fifty-Three Years in Syria*, 2: 95 and 802.

28. De Forest, "Insanity in Syria," 352.

29. De Forest, "Insanity in Syria," 352–353.

30. De Forest, "Insanity in Syria," 353.

31. De Forest, "Insanity in Syria," 354. Also see Wetherill, "The Insane in Some Remote Lands," 166; "Medical News: Lebanon Hospital for the Insane," *Lancet*, 168, no. 4347 (December 22, 1906): 1761; "Treatment of Lunatics in Syria."

32. Wetherill, "The Insane in Some Remote Lands," 166.

33. "Treatment of Lunatics in Syria," 264–265.

34. Wetherill, "The Insane in Some Remote Lands," 166.

35. Sessions, "Some Syrian Folklore Notes Gathered on Mount Lebanon," 12.

36. Jureidini, "The Medical Needs of Syria," 817.

37. J. Rutter Williamson, *The Healing of the Nations: A Treatise on Medical Missions, Statement and Appeal* (New York: Student Volunteer Movement for Foreign Missions, 1899), 28.

38. Theophilus Waldmeier, "The Lebanon Hospital for the Insane," *Missionary Review of the World* 21, no. 7 (July 1898): 535.

39. Theophilus Waldmeier, *Appeal for the First Home of the Insane on Mount Lebanon* (London: Headley Brothers, 1897), 12, LHMND, AUB-SML.

40. Williamson, *The Healing of the Nations*, 28.

41. Williamson, *The Healing of the Nations*, 28.

42. Wetherill, "The Insane in Some Remote Lands," 166.

43. Quoted in Wetherill, "The Insane in Some Remote Lands," 166.

44. Jacques-Joseph Moreau (de Tours), *Recherches sur les aliénés, en Orient: Notes sur les établissements qui leur sont consacrés à Malte (île de), au Caire (Égypte), à Smyrne*

(Asie-Mineure), à Constantinople, (Turquie) (Paris: Imprimerie de Bourgogne et Martinet, 1843), especially 13–14. For epilepsy, see Dols, *Majnūn*, 8.

45. Salvator Furnari, *Voyage médical dans l'Afrique septentrionale ou de l'ophthalmologie considérée dans ses rapports avec les différentes races* (Paris: Chez J.-B. Baillière, 1845), 330. For more on Furnari, see "Medical News," *Medical Times and Gazette* (July 14, 1886): 47.

46. Furnari, *Voyage médical dans l'Afrique septentrionale*, 332.

47. J. G. Paulding, "Diseases and the Practice of Medicine in Damascus," *Boston Medical and Surgical Journal* 46, no. 6 (1852): 91.

48. Paulding, "Diseases and the Practice of Medicine in Damascus," 90–91.

49. Moreau, *Recherches sur les aliénés*, 14.

50. Taylor published with the pseudonym Laorty-Hadji, *La Syrie, la Palestine et la Judée: Pèlerinage à Jérusalem et aux lieux saints* (Paris: Chez Bolle-Lasalle, 1855), 76.

51. Lady Isabel Burton, *The Inner Life of Syria, Palestine, and the Holy Land: From My Private Journal* (London: H. S. King and Co., 1875), 1:64.

52. Quoted in Wetherill, "The Insane in Some Remote Lands," 166.

53. Quoted in Wetherill, "The Insane in Some Remote Lands," 166. Also see al-Bustani, *Muḥīṭ al-Muḥīṭ*, 1:303. The same definition can be found in Ibn Manzur's thirteenth-century dictionary, *Lisān al-ʿArab*, accessed April 11, 2020, http://www.baheth.info/index.jsp.

54. Wetherill, "The Insane in Some Remote Lands," especially 164–166. Jinn or evil spirit possession as a cause of mental illness is still a common belief, not only in the Middle East or Muslim societies but also in countries such as Ethiopia and India. And the body of literature is considerable. See, for instance, Gerda Sengers, *Women and Demons: Cult Healing in Islamic Egypt* (Leiden, the Netherlands: Brill, 2003); Najat Khalifa and Tim Hardie, "Possession and Jinn," *Journal of the Royal Society of Medicine* 98, no. 8 (August 2005): 351; Najat Khalifa, Tim Hardie, Shahid Latif, Imran Jamil, and Dawn-Marie Walker, "Beliefs about Jinn, Black Magic and the Evil Eye among Muslims: Age, Gender and First Language Influences," *International Journal of Culture and Mental Health* 4, no. 1 (2011): 68–77.

55. "Editorials and Medical Intelligence—Palestine," *Boston Medical and Surgical Journal* 44, no. 14 (1851): 281–288, especially 282–283.

56. Jureidini, "The Medical Needs of Syria," 816.

57. Jureidini, "The Medical Needs of Syria," 815.

58. Post, quoted in Wetherill, "The Insane in Some Remote Lands," 168.

59. Post, quoted in Wetherill, "The Insane in Some Remote Lands," 167–168. Van Dyck and Post were among those who founded the SPC in 1866 and were professors

at the faculty of medicine, founded a year later. For more biographical information of Van Dyck, Post, and other founding members of SPC see, Ghada Y. Khoury, *The Founding Fathers of the American University of Beirut: Biographies* (Beirut: American University of Beirut, 1992).

60. Jureidini, "The Medical Needs of Syria," 816.

61. See Rainer Diriwächter, "Völkerpsychologie," in *The Oxford Handbook of Culture and Psychology*, ed. Jaan Valsiner (Oxford: Oxford University Press, 2012), 43–57.

62. Daniel Pick, *Faces of Degeneration: A European Disorder, c. 1848–c. 1918* (Cambridge: Cambridge University Press, 1989); Charles E. Rosenberg, "Pathologies of Progress: The Idea of Civilization as Risk," *Bulletin of the History of Medicine* 72, no. 4 (1998): 714–730.

63. De Forest, "Insanity in Syria," 354.

64. Benoît Boyer, *Conditions hygiéniques actuelles de Beyrouth (Syrie), et de ses environs immédiats* (Lyon, France: Rey, 1897), 131.

65. Boyer, *Conditions hygiéniques actuelles de Beyrouth*, 130.

66. François Emmanuel Foderé, *Traité du délire appliqué à la médecine, à la morale et à la législation* (Paris: Croullebois, 1817), 2:3.

67. "The Lebanon Hospital for the Insane," *Lancet* 162, no. 4174 (August 29, 1903): 624.

68. Quoted in Wetherill, "The Insane in Some Remote Lands," 167.

69. Ussama Makdisi claims the contrary, see "Reclaiming the Land of the Bible: Missionaries, Secularism, and Evangelical Modernity," *American Historical Review* 102, no. 3 (June 1, 1997): 691. Also see, Ussama Makdisi *Artillery of Heaven: American Missionaries and the Failed Conversion of the Middle East* (Ithaca, NY: Cornell University Press, 2008).

70. Quoted in Daniel H. Tuke, "Does Civilization Favour the Generation of Mental Disease?," *Journal of Mental Science* 4 (1858): 106.

71. Tuke, "Does Civilization Favour the Generation of Mental Disease?," 105–106. The logic behind the reasoning is of course tempting: does it mean that most Syrian soldiers did not feel any sense of belonging to their homeland? For a cultural and intellectual history of nostalgia—a term coined in 1688 as a disease of being cut off of one's homeland—see Helmut Illbruck, *Nostalgia: Origins and Ends of an Unenlightened Disease* (Evanston, IL: Northwestern University Press, 2012).

72. Moreau, *Recherches sur les aliénés*.

73. Moreau, *Recherches sur les aliénés*, 20 and 24.

74. Moreau, *Recherches sur les aliénés*, 19.

75. Richard C. Keller, *Colonial Madness: Psychiatry in French North Africa* (Chicago: University of Chicago Press, 2007), 1–2.

76. Burton, *The Inner Life of Syria, Palestine, and the Holy Land*, 1:289.

77. Didier Fassin, "L'ethnopsychiatrie et ses réseaux. L'influence qui grandit," *Genèses* 35, no. 1 (1999): 146–171, and "Ethnopsychiatry and the Postcolonial Encounter: A French Psychopolitics of Otherness," in *Unconscious Dominions: Psychoanalysis, Colonial Trauma, and Global Sovereignties*, ed. Anderson Warwick, Deborah Jenson, and Richard C. Keller (Durham, NC: Duke University Press, 2011), 223–246.

78. See Jan Goldstein, *Console and Classify: The French Psychiatric Profession in the Nineteenth Century* (Chicago: University of Chicago Press, 1981), 319–321.

79. Fodéré, *Traité du délire appliqué à la médecine*, 2:3.

80. Adolphe Kocher, *De la criminalité chez les Arabes au point de vue de la pratique médico-judiciaire en Algérie* (Paris: J.-B. Baillière et Fils, 1884), 36.

81. Wetherill, "The Insane in Some Remote Lands," 167.

82. See Tuke, "Does Civilization Favour the Generation of Mental Disease?"

83. Post, quoted in Wetherill, "The Insane in Some Remote Lands," 167–168. On the abuses of civilization, see Furnari, *Voyage médical dans l'Afrique septentrionale*, 332.

84. Étienne Esquirol, *Des maladies mentales: Considérées sous les rapports médical, hygiénique, et médico-légal* (Paris: Chez J.-B. Baillière, 1838), 2:25.

85. See Luc Huffschmitt, "Folie et civilisation au XIXe siècle," *L'information psychiatrique*, no. 10 (December 1993): 941–948.

86. Alexandre Brièrre de Boismont, "De l'influence de la civilisation sur le développement de la folie," *Annales d'hygiène publique et de médecine légale* 21 (1839): 263–265.

87. Boismont, "De l'influence de la civilization," 262 and 263.

88. Boismont, "De l'influence de la civilization," 263; see also 272–273.

89. Boismont, "De l'influence de la civilization," 284.

90. Boismont, "De l'influence de la civilization," 284

91. Boismont, "De l'influence de la civilization," 273.

92. John Charles Bucknill and Daniel Hack Tuke, *A Manual of Psychological Medicine: Containing the History, Nosology, Description, Statistics, Diagnosis, Pathology, and Treatment of Insanity, with an Appendix of Cases* (Philadelphia: Blanchard and Lea, 1858). Daniel Tuke's great-grandfather was William Tuke, the founder of the York Retreat.

93. Bucknill and Tuke, *A Manual of Psychological Medicine*, 43.

94. Bucknill and Tuke, *A Manual of Psychological Medicine*, 43.

95. See "Feuilleton," *Gazette hebdomadaire de médecine et de chirurgie* 4, no. 47 (November 20, 1857): 822; "Variétés," *Gazette médicale d'Orient* 1, no. 8 (November 1857): 152. For hashish in Egypt, see G. G. Nahas, "Hashish and Drug Abuse in Egypt during the 19th and 20th Centuries," *Bulletin of the New York Academy of Medicine* 61, no. 5 (June 1985): 428–444.

96. Bucknill and Tuke, *A Manual of Psychological Medicine*, 43.

97. Tuke, "Does Civilization Favour the Generation of Mental Disease?," 109.

98. Tuke, "Does Civilization Favour the Generation of Mental Disease?," 105.

99. Williamson, *The Healing of the Nations*, 28.

100. Gabriel Charmes, *Voyage en Syrie: Impressions et souvenirs* (Paris: C. Lévy, 1891).

101. See Edward W. Said, *Orientalism* (New York: Pantheon Books, 1978).

102. In a rare moment of genuine concern for the future of the Orient, Joseph-François Michaud and Jean-Joseph-François Poujoulat convey their hopelessness and helplessness at seeing all the institutions (mosques, hospitals, and schools) that had once been the pride of the Orient in utter ruin and desolation (*Correspondance d'Orient, 1830–31* [Paris: Ducollet, 1835], 14–16).

103. Boismont, "De l'influence de la civilization," 256.

104. Boismont, "De l'influence de la civilization," 257. On the Victorian obsession with time, decadence, and progress, see Jerome Hamilton Buckley, *The Triumph of Time: A Study of the Victorian Concepts of Time, History, Progress, and Decadence* (Cambridge, MA: Belknap Press of Harvard University Press, 1966).

105. Mongeri, "Études sur l'alienation mentale en Orient," 204–205.

106. The history is documented in the massive and meticulous posthumously published Dols, *Majnūn*. Also see Françoise Cloarec, *Bîmâristâns, lieux de folie et de sagesse: La folie et ses traitements dans les hôpitaux médiévaux au Moyen-Orient* (Paris: L'Harmattan, 1998); Aḥmad ʿĪsā, *Histoire des bimaristans (hôpitaux) à l'époque islamique. Discours prononcé au Congrès médical tenu au Caire à l'occasion du centenaire de l'École de médecine et de l'Hôpital Kasr-el-Aïni en Décembre 1928* (Cairo: Imprimerie Paul Barbey, 1928). On the broader topic of charitable care during the rise of Islam, see Michael David Bonner, Mine Ener, and Amy Singer, eds., *Poverty and Charity in Middle Eastern Contexts* (Albany: State University of New York Press, 2003).

107. Boismont, "De l'influence de la civilization," 256.

108. Paulding, "Diseases and the Practice of Medicine in Damascus," 91.

109. Wetherill, "The Insane in Some Remote Lands," 167. The hospital Nūr al-Dīn was converted to the Museum for Science and Medicine in 1975.

110. Henri Gûys, *Voyage en Syrie: Peinture des moeurs musulmanes, chrétiennes et israélites* (Paris: J. Rouvier, 1855), 105.

111. Ekmeleddin İhsanoğlu, *Al-Mu'assasāt al-Ṣiḥḥīyah al-ʿUthmānīyah al-Ḥadīthah Fī Sūrīyah: Al-Mustashfayāt wa-Kullīyat Ṭibb al-Shām* (Amman, Jordan: Lajnat Tārīkh Bilād al-Shām, 2002), 13; ʿĀmir Mubayyiḍ, *Bīmāristānāt Ḥalab, Mafkharat al-ʿImārah al-Islāmīyah: Fī Dimashq Buniya Awwal Bīmāristān Fī al-Tārīkh* (Aleppo: Syria, Dār al-Qalam al-ʿArabī, 2006), 115.

112. In 2012, activists started to post online videos of the damage to the bīmāristān. Further damage due to the ongoing conflict in Syria was reported in 2015. See Michael D. Danti, Richard L. Zettler, Cheikhmous Ali, Abdalrazzaq Moaz, Tate Paulette, Kathryn Franklin, Allison Cuneo, and David Elitzer, "Planning for Safeguarding Heritage Sites in Syria and Iraq," American School of Oriental Research's Cultural Heritage Initiatives, Weekly Report 31, March, 2015, 28–29.

113. Gûys, *Voyage en Syrie*, 105.

114. Gûys, *Voyage en Syrie*, 105.

115. Christopher de Bellaigue, "Turkey's Hidden Past," *New York Review of Books*, March 8, note 1, https://www.nybooks.com/articles/2001/03/08/turkeys-hidden-past/. Notwithstanding the historians who have contested the "decline thesis" or the "decline paradigm," (namely, the thesis that the Ottoman Empire declined politically, economically, and culturally from the death of Suleiman I in 1566 to the late eighteenth century), this is what Nicholas I is reported to have said to the British envoy to St. Petersburg in 1853, two years before he died. For a review of the literature on the decline thesis, see Dana Sajdi, "Decline, Its Discontents and Ottoman Cultural History: By Way of Introduction," in *Ottoman Tulips, Ottoman Coffee: Leisure and Lifestyle in the Eighteenth Century*, ed. Dana Sajdi (London: I. B.Tauris, 2007), 1–40.

116. See Yasser Tabbaa, "The Functional Aspects of Medieval Islamic Hospitals," in *Poverty and Charity in Middle Eastern Contexts*, 112–113; Gary Leiser and Michael Dols, "Evliyā Chelebi's Description of Medicine in Seventeenth-Century Egypt: Part II: Text," *Sudhoffs Archiv* 72, no. 1 (January 1, 1988): 49; Dols, *Majnūn*, especially 122–128; Bahaeddin Yediyıldız, *Institution du vaqf au XVIIIè siècle en Turquie: Étude socio-historique* (Ankara: Imprimerie de la société d'histoire turque, 1985), 160–162.

117. Quoted in Wetherill, "The Insane in Some Remote Lands," 167.

118. AR, 1902, 12, LHMND, AUB-SML.

119. ʿĪsā suggests very broadly the end of the "Islamic era" (*Histoire des bimaristans (hôpitaux) à l'époque islamique*, 2). Dols suggests an even broader period, "the Middle Ages" (*Majnūn*, 112–113). According to Peter E. Pormann, "by the eleventh century,

the term *bīmarīstān* (hospital) acquired the more specific and restricted meaning of mental asylum" (*Rufus of Ephesus, On Melancholy*, ed. Pormann [Tubingen, Germany: Mohr Siebeck, 2008], 194). And according to Anne-Marie Moulin, such a shift occurred between the "eleventh and the eighteenth centuries" ("Conscience et représentation de la folie et de la déraison," 35). If we consult both Ismāʿīl ibn Ḥammād al-Jawharī's dictionary, *as-Ṣiḥāḥ*, which was compiled in the tenth century, and Ibn Manzur's, *Lisān al-ʿArab*, it is the term *marastān* (not *māristān*, as it is usually transliterated in the literature), that is used in the sense of bīmarīstān. In other words, the meaning was a hospital *(dār al-marḍa)*, not a lunatic asylum. In any case, it is clear that by the seventeenth century when Ibn Jubayr (1145–1217) traveled to the region, *māristān* had taken on the meaning of a lunatic asylum. See Ibn Jubayr, *Riḥla (Travels)*, ed. William Wright and M. J. de Goeje (Leiden, the Netherlands: Brill, 1907). The same linguistic shift is noted in Ottoman Turkish, in which *darüşşifas* (mentioned in the introduction) evolved into mental asylums (vulgarized as *tımarhanes*). See Gábor Ágoston and Bruce Alan Masters, *Encyclopedia of the Ottoman Empire* (New York: Facts on File, 2009), 358.

120. Gaston Bachelard, *La formation de l'esprit scientifique: Contribution à une psychanalyse de la connaissance objective* (Paris: J. Vrin, 1938), 19.

121. Al-Bustani has an entry for bīmarīstān in which he mentions *dār al-marḍa*, but remarkably he does not mention *mustashfa* in his entry on *shafiya* (to heal) (*Muḥīṭ al-Muḥīṭ*, 2:1967 and 1:1103–1104). For the emergence of *mustashfa* at the end of the nineteenth century in the Arab East, see Peter Behnstedt and Manfred Woidich, eds., *Wortatlas der arabischen Dialekte* (Leiden, the Netherlands: Brill, 2012), 2:186.

122. I tend to disagree with those who think that "renaissance" is a problematic translation because it could refer to the Italian Renaissance. It is not a mere coincidence that *al-Muqtaṭaf* published several articles on archaeology in an attempt to revive the ancient roots of Arab intellectual thought and achievements (Greco-Roman, Phoenician, Semitic, and Arab-Islamic) in an age marked by decadence and degeneration. See Nadia Farag, "Al-Muqtataf, 1876–1900: A Study of the Influence of Victorian Thought on Modern Arabic Thought" (PhD diss., University of Oxford, 1969), especially chapter 6. For more on the Nahḍa, see Leyla Dakhli, *Une génération d'intellectuels Arabes: Syrie et Liban, 1908–1940* (Paris: Karthala, 2009).

123. Gerges Effendi El-Khoury, "Fil-Junūn," *al-Jinān* 17 (September 1, 1873): 590–593.

124. See Farag, "Al-Muqtataf."

125. "Al-Duktūr Kurnīliūs Fān-Dayk," *al-Muqtaṭaf* 19, no. 12 (December 1, 1895): 883–884.

126. See Farag, "Al-Muqtataf."

127. See Farag, "Al-Muqtataf," especially chapter 5.

128. For more information, see Farag, "Al-Muqtataf," 72–76; Nadia Farag, "The Lewis Affair and the Fortunes of Al-Muqtataf," *Middle Eastern Studies* 8, no. 1 (January 1, 1972): 73–83; Shafiq Juha, *Darwin and the Crisis of 1882 in the Medical Department and the First Student Protest in the Arab World in the Syrian Protestant College (Now the American University of Beirut)*, trans. Sally Kaya (Beirut: American University of Beirut Press, 2004); Marwa Elshakry, *Reading Darwin in Arabic, 1860–1950* (Chicago: University of Chicago Press, 2013).

129. For instance, Charcot is mentioned in a discussion of how the French neurologist practiced hypnosis at the Pitié Hospital in Paris. See "Al-Seḥer al-Ḥadīth," *al-Muqtaṭaf* 24, no. 7 (April 1, 1893): 425–430.

130. Sigmund Freud, *The Interpretation of Dreams*, trans. Abraham Arden Brill (New York: The Macmillan Company, 1913).

131. Interestingly, in one of his famous books *Kitāb ash-Shifā'* (The book of healing), Avicenna did not speak of a "science of the soul" per se, but he classified the study of the soul under physics (*'ilm ṭabī'ī*), he wrote a "treatise" on the soul (*Risāla Fī-n-Nafs*) and a "classification of the rational sciences" (*aqsām al-'ulūm al-'aqliyya*). See Dimitri Gutas, "Avicenna's Eastern ('Oriental') Philosophy: Nature, Contents, Transmission," *Arabic Sciences and Philosophy* 10, no. 2 (September 2000): 159–180; Jon McGinnis, *Avicenna* (Oxford: Oxford University Press, 2010), especially the bibliographical references.

132. "Al-'Ulūm al-'Aqliyya," *al-Muqtaṭaf* 11, no. 4 (January 1, 1887): 211. For the use of the term *bsīkhūlūjīā* in Ottoman Turkish, see, for example, "Maktūb," *Hazine-yi evrak* (1881): 517. *Hazine-yi evrak* was an Ottoman periodical that was published from 1881 to 1886.

133. For the nineteenth-century Ottoman context, see Robert Ian Blecher, "The Medicalization of Sovereignty: Medicine, Public Health, and Political Authority in Syria, 1861–1936" (PhD diss., Stanford University, 2002); Sylvia Chiffoleau, *Genèse de la santé publique internationale: De la peste d'Orient à l'OMS* (Rennes; France: Presses Universitaires de Rennes, 2012); Birsen Bulmuş, *Plague, Quarantines, and Geopolitics in the Ottoman Empire* (Edinburgh: Edinburgh University Press, 2012).

134. "Al-Majanīn Fī Rūsiā," *al-Muqtaṭaf* 5, no. 1 (1880): 100.

135. "Qiyās al-'Uqūl," *al-Muqtaṭaf* 20, no. 2 (December 1, 1896): 884.

136. Michel Foucault, *Security, Territory, Population: Lectures at the Collège de France, 1977–78*, ed. Arnold Davidson (Basingstoke, UK: Palgrave Macmillan, 2009), 87–114. *Al-Muqtaṭaf* published a lecture by the English physiologist Michael Foster, a portion of which touches on the question of science and politics. See Michael Foster, "Al-'Ilm Fī Mi'at 'Ām," *al-Muqtaṭaf* 23, no. 11 (November 1899): 809–820. Also see "Al-Ḥukūma wal-Ṣiḥḥa," *al-Muqtaṭaf* 19, no. 6 (June 1, 1895): 401–404.

137. See "Al-wiqaya Min al-Amraḍ," *al-Muqtaṭaf* 15, no. 2 (September 1, 1891): 809–812.

138. "Junūn al-Malek Lūwiys al-Thānī Malek Bavāryā," *al-Muqtaṭaf* 11, no. 9 (June 1, 1886): 527.

139. "At-Tamaddun wal-Intiḥār," *al-Muqtaṭaf* 15 (June 1, 1891): 648–654.

140. Émile Durkheim, *Le suicide: Étude de sociologie* (Paris: F. Alcan, 1897).

141. "Al-wiqaya Min al-Amraḍ," 809–812.

142. "At-Tamaddun wal-Intiḥār," 644–654.

143. "Al-Junūn," *al-Muqtaṭaf* 28 (July 1, 1903): 601–602. Also see "Jihād al-'Ulamā': al-Nabtha al-Ūla Fī al-Junūn wal-Majānīn," *al-Muqtaṭaf* 15, no. 5 (February 1, 1891): 281–286.

144. "Masā'il wa-Ajwibatuhā," *al-Muqtaṭaf* 12 (December 1, 1887): 184.

145. "Al-Junūn," *al-Muqtaṭaf* 29, no. 12 (December 1, 1904): 1096.

146. "Masā'il wa-Ajwibatuhā," 184.

147. "Masā'il wa-Ajwibatuhā," *al-Muqtaṭaf* 17 (August 1, 1893): 778.

148. "Intishār al-Junūn," *al-Muqtaṭaf* 30, no. 6 (June 1, 1905): 498–499. On the microbial nature of madness, see "Ilāj al-Junūn bet-Talqīḥ," *al-Muqtaṭaf* 19, no. 4 (April 1, 1895): 312; "'Ilāj al-Junūn," *al-Muqtaṭaf* 20, no. 9 (August 1, 1896): 630–631.

149. "Awhām Urūppā," *al-Muqtaṭaf* 13, no. 7 (April 1, 1889): 494–495; "Jihād al-'Ulamā': al-Nabtha al-Rābi'a Fī-s-Ṣir' wal-Histīriā wal-Khūria," *al-Muqtaṭaf* 15, no. 8 (May 1, 1891): 497–502.

150. The unnamed author mistakenly wrote 1868 instead of 1838. See "Awhām Urūppā." In fact, as Goldstein has shown, this law was pivotal in the history of psychiatry in France because it reorganized the psychiatric profession as an appendage of the state (see *Console and Classify*, especially 276–321).

151. A. Motet, "Rapport sur un projet de loi sur les aliénés en Turquie par M. Mongeri," *Annales médico-psychologique* 17 (1877): 86–88.

152. See Farag, "Al-Muqtataf."

153. "Jihād al-'Ulamā': Al-Nabtha al-Ūla Fī-l-Junūn wal-Majānīn."

154. "Al-Junūn."

155. "Jihād al-'Ulamā': Al-Nabtha al-Ūla Fī-l-Junūn wal-Majānīn," 286; "Jihād al-'Ulamā': al-Nabtha al-Rābi'a Fī-s-Ṣir' wal-Histīriā wal-Khūria," 502.

156. Farag, "Al-Muqtataf," especially 232–243.

157. See Pick, *Faces of Degeneration*; John Van Wyhe, *Phrenology and the Origins of Victorian Scientific Naturalism, Science, Technology, and Culture, 1700–1945* (Aldershot, UK: Ashgate, 2004); Stephen Tomlinson, *Head Masters: Phrenology, Secular Education, and Nineteenth-Century Social Thought* (Tuscaloosa: University of Alabama Press, 2005).

158. "Ṭiba' al-Mujrimīn," *al-Muqtaṭaf* 14, no. 10 (July 1, 1890): 760–761.

159. "Admighat al-Majānīn," *al-Muqtaṭaf* 6, no. 5 (1881): 313; "'Ilāj al-Mujrimīn wal-Ma'tūhīn," *al-Muqtaṭaf* 13, no. 11 (August 1, 1889): 731–735; "Ṭiba' al-Mujrimīn."

160. "Fasād al-Frenūlūjiā," *al-Muqtaṭaf* 13, no. 3 (December 1, 1888): 149–150. In another article on phrenology, the journal added a disclaimer that the opinions expressed in the article were the author's and did not express the views of the journal. See "Al-Frenūlūjiā," *al-Muqtaṭaf* 13, no. 3 (November 1, 1888): 119–125. Of course, it might be said that the original phrenological theory was much more sophisticated, but one should remember that *al-Muqtaṭaf*'s purpose was precisely to popularize and therefore simplify science.

161. Of course, there were exceptions, and a striking example is the enthusiastic reception of al-Bustani's encyclopedia by Western intellectuals. See Albert Hourani, "Bustani's Encyclopedia," *Journal of Islamic Studies* 1 (1990): 111–119. Also see E. H. Palmer, "History and Literature of the East," *Contemporary Review* 36 (1879): 359.

162. For more on the life of Shibli Shumayyil, see Susan Laila Ziadeh, "A Radical in His Time: The Thought of Shibli Shumayyil and Arab Intellectual Discourse (1882–1917)" (PhD diss., University of Michigan, 1991).

163. "At-Ṭabīb," *al-Jinān*, no. 11 (June 1, 1875): 364.

164. "At-Ṭabīb," *al-Muqtaṭaf* 6, no. 5 (1881): 640.

165. "I'lān," *at-Ṭabīb*, no. 5 (May 1, 1874): 16; Shibli Shumayyil, "Ḥājātina," *ash-Shifā'* 1, no. 1 (February 15, 1886): 1–5.

166. "Al-Junūn Funūn," *al-Muqtaṭaf* 1, no. 8 (November 1, 1884): 341.

167. "'Ilāj Fī-s-Ṣir'," *at-Ṭabīb*, no. 52 (April 1882): 96; "As-Ṣir' wal-Jirāḥa," *at-Ṭabīb* (1897):170–173; "Shifā' Ba'ḍ Anwā' al-Junūn bel-Estehwā'," *ash-Shifā'* 1, no. 4 (May 15, 1886): 97–101; "Jur'a Musakkana Ḍodd al-Histīriā," *ash-Shifā'* 4 (March 1891): 77.

168. Léon Thivet, "Murāsalāt *ash-Shifā'* al-Khuṣūṣiyya: Kalām 'Ām Fī Ikhṭilāt al-'Aql ayy al-Junūn," *ash-Shifā'* 4 (July 1890): 270–274.

169. "Al-Musakkanāt Fī-l-Junūn," *ash-Shifā'* 2 (May 5, 1887): 128–130; "Gharība Min Gharā'eb al-Ṣir' al-Histīrī," *ash-Shifā'* 2 (October 1, 1887): 344; "Shifā' Baḥḥa Hysteriyya bel-Estehwā' al-Hipnotīssmī," *ash-Shifā'* 3 (February 15, 1888): 30–31; "Al-Junūn al-Iẓṭihādī," *ash-Shifā'* 4 (November 1, 1890): 405–408; "Al-Junūn al-Iẓṭihādī," *ash-Shifā'* 5 (July 1, 1891): 254–256; "Amrāḍ al-Jihāz al-'Aṣabī," *at-Ṭabīb* (1897): 299–300.

170. For the introduction of case-based reasoning in the nineteenth century in medical teaching, see John Forrester, "If P, Then What? Thinking in Cases," *History of the Human Sciences* 9, no. 3 (1996): especially 15–16.

171. "Muqaddima al-Sana al-Sābiʿa," *al-Muqtaṭaf* 7, no. 1 (June 1, 1882): 1.

172. There are many articles on this topic. See, for example, "Taqaddum al-Gharb wa-Āmāl al-Sharq," *al-Muqtaṭaf* 12, no. 3 (November 1, 1888): 121–122; "Ta'akhurnā al-ʿIlmī wa-Asbabahu," *al-Muqtaṭaf* 15, no. 4 (January 1, 1891): 241–247, 15, no. 5 (February 1, 1891): 297–301, 15, no. 6 (March 1, 1891): 388–392, and 15, no. 7 (April 1, 1891): 441. Also see Farag, "Al-Muqtataf," especially chapter 6.

173. Yaʿqūb Ṣarrūf, quoted in Dagmar Glass, "Popularizing Sciences through Arabic Journals in the Late 19th Century: How Al-Muqtaṭaf Transformed Western Patterns," in *Changing Identities: The Transformation of Asian and African Societies under Colonialism: Papers of a Symposium Held at the Centre for Modern Oriental Studies, Berlin, 21–22 October 1993*, ed. Joachim Heidrich (Berlin: Verlag Das Arabische Buch, 1994), 325.

174. Shumayyil, "Ḥājātinā."

175. "At-Ṭabīb," *al-Muqtaṭaf*, no. 7 (January 1881): 192.

176. "Asās at-Taqaddum al-Ḥaqīqī wa-Ḥufẓuhu," *al-Muqtaṭaf* 10, no. 2 (September 1, 1885): especially 719.

177. Farag, "Al-Muqtataf," 165.

178. "Naṣīḥa Ṭubiyya," *at-Tabīb* (1905): 231–232.

179. Shibli Shumayyil, "Inḥiṭāṭ al-Sharq al-Adabī wal-ʿAqlī," *al-Muqtaṭaf* 23, no. 1 (January 1, 1899): 4. Also see L. M. Kenny, "East versus West in Al-Muqtataf, 1875–1900: Image and Self-Image," in *Essays on Islamic Civilization: Presented to Niyazi Berkes*, ed. Donald Presgrave Little (Leiden, the Netherlands: Brill, 1976), especially 149–150.

180. Shumayyil, "Inḥiṭāṭ al-Sharq al-Adabī wal-ʿAqlī," 7.

181. Albert Habib Hourani, *Arabic Thought in the Liberal Age, 1798–1939* (Cambridge: Cambridge University Press, 1983); Elizabeth Suzanne Kassab, *Contemporary Arab Thought: Cultural Critique in Comparative Perspective* (New York: Columbia University Press, 2010), especially 17–47.

182. "Al-Nahḍa al-ʿIlmiyya," *al-Muqtaṭaf* 21, no. 6 (June 1, 1897): 425–431, 21, no. 7 (July 1, 1897): 516–519, and 21, no. 12 (December 1, 1897): 934–935.

183. For instance, see Salim al-Bustani, "Limādhā Naḥnū Fī Ta'akhur," *al-Jinān*, no. 6 (March 1870): 162–164; "Siḥḥat al-'Umma wa-ʿAmaluha," *al-Muqtaṭaf* 9 (October 1884): 58–59.

184. "Al-Bīmāristān al-Lubnānī," *at-Ṭabīb* 8 (1896): 91–92.

185. See Yūsuf As'ad Dāghir, *Maṣādir al-Dirāsāt al-Adabiyyah, Wufqan li-Manāhij at-Ta'līm al-Rasmiyyah. Lubnān, Sūriyā, al-'Irāq, Miṣr* (Saida, Lebanon: Maṭba'at Dayr al-Mukhliṣ, 1950), especially 540–542, 790, and 807–809.

2 The Struggle for Influence and the Birth of Psychiatry

1. Quoted in George E. Post, "Missionary and College Work in the Holy Land," *Churchman* 88, no. 7 (August 15, 1903): 203.

2. Louis Roché (French ambassador in Beirut), "Relations culturelles—Établissements d'enseignement étrangers," confidential letter to the minister of foreign affairs, February 27, 1956, 371, QONT/639, MAE.

3. John P. Spagnolo, "French Influence in Syria prior to World War I: The Functional Weakness of Imperialism," *Middle East Journal* 23, no. 1 (January 1, 1969): 47 and 55, and "Franco-British Rivalry in the Middle East and Its Operation in the Lebanese Problem," in *Lebanon: A History of Conflict and Consensus*, ed. Nadim Shehadi and Dana Haffar Mills (London: Centre for Lebanese Studies, 1988), 101–123; James Barr, *A Line in the Sand: The Anglo-French Struggle for the Middle East, 1914–1948* (New York: W. W. Norton, 2012).

4. Vincent Cloarec, *La France et la question de Syrie: 1914–1918* (Paris: CNRS Éditions, 1998), especially 3–4.

5. Jean-Pierre Filiu, *Les Arabes, leur destin et le nôtre: Histoire d'une libération* (Paris: La Découverte, 2015), 14.

6. Robert M. Khouri, *La médecine au Liban: De la Phénicie jusqu'à nos jours* (Beirut: Éditions ABCD, 1986), and "Histoire de la médecine au Liban," *Journal médical libanais* 58, no. 1 (2010): 28–44; Nada Sehnaoui, *L'occidentalisation de la vie quotidienne à Beyrouth, 1860–1914* (Beirut: Éditions Dar An-Nahar, 2002), especially 57–58.

7. William Osler, *The Evolution of Modern Medicine: A Series of Lectures Delivered at Yale University on the Silliman Foundation, in April, 1913* (New Haven, CT: Yale University Press, 1921), especially 183–217; Charles E. Rosenberg, "The Therapeutic Revolution: Medicine, Meaning, and Social Change in Nineteenth-Century America," in *The Therapeutic Revolution: Essays in the Social History of American Medicine*, ed. Morris J. Vogel and Charles E. Rosenberg (Philadelphia: University of Pennsylvania Press, 1979), 3–25. In the context of the Middle East, see C. V. A. Van Dyck, "On the Present Condition of the Medical Profession in Syria," *Journal of the American Oriental Society* 1, no. 4 (January 1, 1849): 559–591; Alexander Russell, *The Natural History of Aleppo, and Parts Adjacent. Containing a Description of the City, and the Principal Natural Productions in Its Neighbourhood; Together with an Account of the Climate, Inhabitants, and Diseases; Particularly of the Plague, with the Methods Used by the Europeans for Their Preservation* (London: A. Millar, 1756); Miri Shefer-Mossensohn, *Ottoman Medicine:*

Healing and Medical Institutions, 1500–1700 (Albany: State University of New York Press, 2010).

8. Serge Jagailloux, *La médicalisation de l'Égypte au XIXe siècle (1798–1918)* (Paris: Éditions Recherche sur les Civilisations, 1986); Amira el-Azhary Sonbol, *The Creation of a Medical Profession in Egypt, 1800–1922* (Syracuse, NY: Syracuse University Press, 1991); Sylvia Chiffoleau, *Médecines et médecins en Égypte: Construction d'une identité professionnelle et projet médical* (Paris: L'Harmattan, 1997).

9. Sonbol, *The Creation of a Medical Profession in Egypt*, 39–40. For more on the rule of Muhammad Ali, see Afaf Lutfi Sayyid-Marsot, *Egypt in the Reign of Muhammad Ali* (Cambridge: Cambridge University Press, 1984).

10. Sonbol, *The Creation of a Medical Profession in Egypt*, 59 and 62.

11. See Sehnaoui, *L'occidentalisation de la vie quotidienne à Beyrouth*, 76–77, note 1; Khouri, "Histoire de la médecine au Liban," 30. Also see E. M. Gédéon, "L'enseignement médical à l'époque des premiers médecins libanais diplômés," *Bulletin de la Société libanaise d'histoire de la médecine*, no. 3 (1992): 69–72.

12. R. Sarell, "Turkey," in *Dr. Dobell's Reports on the Progress of Practical and Scientific Medicine in Different Parts of the World*, ed. H. Dobell (London: Longmans, Green, Reader and Dyer, 1871), 2:535; Bernard Lewis, *The Emergence of Modern Turkey* (London: Oxford University Press, 1968), 84. Also see Nuran Yıldırım, "Le rôle des médecins turcs dans la transmission du savoir," in *Médecins et ingénieurs ottomans à l'âge des nationalismes*, ed. Méropi Anastassiadou-Dumont (Paris: Maisonneuve et Larose, 2003), 127–170.

13. Quoted in Lewis, *The Emergence of Modern Turkey*, 85.

14. Sarell, "Turkey," 2:537–538.

15. Yıldırım, "Le rôle des médecins turcs," 127–130; Mérope Anastassiadou, *Les Grecs d'Istanbul au XIXe siècle: Histoire socioculturelle de la communauté de Péra* (Leiden, the Netherlands: Brill, 2012), 183.

16. Procurator-general of the Congregation of the Mission (of Lazarists) to the minister of foreign affairs, June 12, 1883, 75ADP/27, MAE. For Jerusalem and Palestine, see Efraim Lev and Yaron Perry, *Modern Medicine in the Holy Land: Pioneering British Medical Services in Late Ottoman Palestine* (London: I. B. Tauris, 2007).

17. Henry Harris Jessup, *Fifty-Three Years in Syria* (New York: Fleming H. Revell, 1910), 1:230.

18. Charles Henry Churchill, *Mount Lebanon: A Ten Years' Residence, from 1842 to 1852, Describing the Manners, Customs, and Religion of Its Inhabitants with a Full & Correct Account of the Druse Religion, and Containing Historical Records of the Mountain Tribes* (London: Saunders and Otley, 1853), 1:121.

19. Sehnaoui suggests 1840 (*L'occidentalisation de la vie quotidienne à Beyrouth*, 62); Leila Fawaz, 1846 (*Merchants and Migrants in Nineteenth-Century Beirut* [Cambridge, MA: Harvard University Press, 1983], 34); Khouri, 1851 ("Histoire de la médecine au Liban," 38); Samir Kassir, 1853 (*Histoire de Beyrouth* [Paris: Fayard, 2003], 264); Jens Hanssen, 1861 (*Fin de Siècle Beirut: The Making of an Ottoman Provincial Capital* [Oxford: Clarendon Press of Oxford University Press, 2005], 241); and Vital Cuinet, 1870 (*Syrie, Liban et Palestine: Géographie administrative, statistique, descriptive et raisonnée* [Paris: E. Leroux, 1896–1901], 57.

20. Stephen B. L. Penrose, *That They May Have Life: The Story of the American University of Beirut, 1866–1941* (New York: Trustees of the American University of Beirut, 1941); Betty S. Anderson, *The American University of Beirut: Arab Nationalism and Liberal Education* (Austin, TX: University of Texas Press, 2011).

21. Jessup, *Fifty-Three Years in Syria*, 1:317.

22. Abdel-Raouf Sinno, "The Emperor's Visit to the East as Reflected in Contemporary Arabic Journalism," in *Baalbeck: Image and Monument 1898–1998*, ed. Helene Sader, Thomas Schefller, and Angelika Neuwirth (Stuttgart: Steiner), 129.

23. "Note sur le nouvel hôpital français à Beyrouth (Syrie)," May 31, 1882, 75ADP/27, MAE.

24. Prefect of the Lazarists in Syria and Egypt to the minister of foreign affairs, July 9, 1883, 75ADP/27, MAE.

25. Publicity material for the School of Medicine, c. 1950s, second miscellaneous reports files 1–7, School of Medicine correspondence 1871–1947, AUB-JL.

26. See Chantal Verdeil, "L'Université Saint-Joseph et la troisième république," in *Une France en Méditerranée: Écoles, langue et culture françaises, XIXe–XXe siècles*, ed. Patrick Cabanel (Paris: Créaphis, 2006), 238.

27. "Extrait d'une lettre du Dr. Bouvier de Beyrouth," 1883, 75ADP/27, MAE.

28. See "Lettre du P. Benoît Planchet au P. Jean Roothaan," January 7, 1847, in Sami Kuri, *Une histoire du Liban à travers les archives des Jésuites: 1846–1862* (Beirut: Dar el-Machreq Editeurs, 2001), 2:28.

29. "L'Hôpital Français du Sacré-Cœur et la faculté française de médecine-leurs rapports-règlements qui doit fixer ces rapports," July 3, 1909, 68–81, 175CPCOM/8, and "Règlement pour l'hôpital français de Beyrouth," December 10, 1910, 102–109, 175CPCOM/9, both MAE.

30. Verdeil, "L'Université Saint-Joseph et la troisième république."

31. Quoted in "École de médecine de Beyrouth, rapport de M. Sandouzy," March 1888, 75ADP/27, MAE.

32. From R. P. (Révérend Père) Cattin to the French consul, August 10, 1911, 179, 175CPCOM/9, MAE. Attached to the letter was a petition signed by forty-six French professors in support of Cattin's request for 30,000 francs to hire new professors.

33. For the former, see Chantal Verdeil, "L'empire, les communautés, la France: Les réseaux des médecins ottomans à la fin du XIXe siècle," in *Hommes de l'entre-deux: Parcours individuels et portraits de groupes sur la frontière de la Méditerranée, XVIe–XXe siècle,* ed. Bernard Heyberger and Chantal Verdeil (Paris: Les Indes Savantes, 2009), 133–150, and "L'Université Saint-Joseph et la troisième république"; Philippe Bourmaud, "Entre science conquérante, confessionnalisme et souveraineté: Trajectoires et images professionnelles des premiers étudiants de la faculté de médecine de l'Université Saint-Joseph de Beyrouth 1883–1914)," in *Une France en Méditerranée: Écoles, langue et culture françaises, XIXe–XXe siècles,* ed. Patrick Cabane (Paris: Créaphis), 253–264; Jennifer M. Dueck, "Educational Conquest: Schools as a Sphere of Politics in French Mandate Syria, 1936–1946," *French History* 20, no. 4 (December 1, 2006): 442–459.

34. Jules Ferry to the minister of foreign affairs, April 19, 1882, 75ADP/27, MAE.

35. Minister of foreign affairs to Jules Ferry, April 14, 1883, 75ADP/27, MAE.

36. "Extrait d'une lettre du Dr. Bouvier de Beyrouth," c. 1884, 75ADP/27, MAE.

37. "Note," July 20, 1911, 110, 175CPCOM/26, MAE.

38. Chancellor of the Jesuit University to the minister of public instruction, May 1886, 75ADP/27, MAE.

39. "Rapport de M. le Docteur Villejean professeur agrégé à la Faculté de Médecine de Paris, Pharmacien en Chef de l'Hôtel-Dieu sur l'École de Médecine de Beyrouth," June 1887, 175CPCOM/26, MAE.

40. Faculté française de médecine de Beyrouth," published in *Le Journal (Paris, France),* August 10, 1911, 175, newspaper clipping, 175CPCOM/9, MAE.

41. Minister of foreign affairs to the minister of commerce and the minister of public instruction, January 8, 1889, 75ADP/27, MAE.

42. French embassy in Constantinople, letter, October 18, 1898, and "Note pour le ministre" on the subject of the faculty of medicine in Beirut, December 28, 1898, 250–252, 206CPCOM/125, MAE.

43. "Note pour le ministre *a.s.* examens de Beyrouth propositions de distinctions," July 5, 1899, 287–288, 206CPCOM/125, MAE.

44. From the Sublime Porte (Ministry of Foreign Affairs) to the American Consultae General in Constantinople and Cairo and SPC, "Note verbale," March 15, 1871, letter no. 29731; and George E. Post, letter to John Robeson (American consul in Beirut), January 8, 1884, both School of Medicine correspondence 1871–1947, AUB-JL.

45. Jessup, *Fifty-Three Years in Syria*, 2:533.

46. From the Sublime Porte (Ministry of Foreign Affairs) to the SPC, May 17, 1909, letter no. 77755/11, School of Medicine correspondence 1871–1947, AUB-JL.

47. "Rapport adressé à M. le Ministre de l'Instruction Publique," November 18, 1899, 318–323, 206CPCOM/125, MAE.

48. The Treaty of Küçük Kaynarca was a pact signed at the conclusion of the Russo-Ottoman War of 1768–1774 at Küçük Kaynarca, Bulgaria, after the defeat of the Ottomans. The pact contained territorial provisions (most notably the cession of the Crimea to Russia); commercial and diplomatic provisions, which gave Russia the rights to establish consulates and enjoy commercial privileges in the Ottoman Empire; and a religious stipulation, which gave Russia the privilege of representing the Greek Orthodox community in Ottoman lands. See Thomas W. Gallant, *Modern Greece: From the War of Independence to the Present* (London: Bloomsbury Academic, 2016), 19.

49. A. L. Tibawi, "Russian Cultural Penetration of Syria—Palestine in the Nineteenth Century (Part I)," *Journal of the Royal Central Asian Society* 53, no. 2 (1966): 172. Also see Derek Hopwood, *The Russian Presence in Syria and Palestine, 1843–1914: Church and Politics in the Near East* (Oxford, UK: Clarendon Press of Oxford University Press, 1969).

50. Jessup, *Fifty-Three Years in Syria*, 2:660.

51. "Jam'iyyat Musā'adāt Marḍa Fī Bayrūt," *al-Muqtaṭaf* 8, no. 7 (May 1884): 441; Cuinet, *Syrie*, 57.

52. P. W. Dill-Russell (ODM), "Visit to the Lebanon 1st–5th August 1968," August 27, 1968, OD 34/224, TNA.

53. See Abdul-Karim Rafeq, "The Syrian University and the French Mandate (1920–1946)," in *Liberal Thought in the Eastern Mediterranean*, ed. C. Schumann (Leiden, the Netherlands: Brill, 2008), 76.

54. General Henri Gouraud to the minister of foreign affairs, "A.s. École Arabe de Médecine de Damas," August 10, 1921, 61–62, 50CPCOM/108, MAE.

55. Allyre-Julien Chassevant, "Rapport sur la Faculté de Médecine de Damas," December 1921, 227, 50CPCOM/108, MAE.

56. *Stamboul*, June 18, 1911, dispatch to the ministry of foreign affairs, 175CPCOM/9, MAE.

57. Jessup, *Fifty-Three Years in Syria*, 1:302.

58. James S. Dennis, *A Sketch of the Syria Mission* (New York: Mission House, 1872), 21.

59. Quoted in Syrian Protestant College, *Annual Report of the Syrian Protestant College to the Board of Trustees* (Beirut: n.p., 1871), 18.

60. Catalogue of the Syrian Protestant College, 1871, 7, and 1885–1886, 23, AUB-JL. Also see Penrose, *That They May Have Life*, 21.

61. Shahe Sarkis Kazarian, *A History of Academic Psychology at AUB, 1870–2016* (Beirut: American University of Beirut Press, 2016) 26; see also, 29.

62. See the Catalogue of the Syrian Protestant College, 1905–1906, 31, accessed February 11, 2020, http://www.dlir.org/archive/items/show/11092.

63. Catalogue of the Syrian Protestant College, 1905–1906, 39; Herbert W. Schneider, *A History of American Philosophy* (New York: Columbia University Press, 1946), 379; Kazarian, *A History of Academic Psychology at AUB*, 31.

64. John M. Broughton, "The Genetic Psychology of James Mark Baldwin," *American Psychologist* 36, no. 4 (April 1981): 398.

65. Penrose, *That They May Have Life*, 44.

66. Nadia Farag, "The Lewis Affair and the Fortunes of Al-Muqtataf," *Middle Eastern Studies* 8, no. 1 (January 1, 1972): 73–83. See also Donald M. Leavitt, "Darwinism in the Arab World: The Lewis Affair at the Syrian Protestant College," *Muslim World* 71, no. 2 (1981): 85–98; Sehnaoui, *L'occidentalisation de la vie quotidienne à Beyrouth*, especially 53–82; Shafiq Juha, *Darwin and the Crisis of 1882 in the Medical Department and the First Student Protest in the Arab World in the Syrian Protestant College (Now the American University of Beirut)*, trans. Sally Kaya (Beirut: American University of Beirut Press, 2004); George Sabra, lecture, "AUB and Religion. Never the Twain Shall Meet … Again?" General lecture series of the Anis Makdisi program in Literature, American University of Beirut, February 2, 2005; Marwa Elshakry, *Reading Darwin in Arabic, 1860–1950* (Chicago: University of Chicago Press, 2013).

67. Khouri, *La médecine au Liban*, 193.

68. Pierre Mazoyer, "Note remise par le P. Mazoyer," April 16, 1883, 75ADP/27, MAE.

69. Theophilus Waldmeier, *Appeal for the First Home for the Insane in Bibles Lands* (London: Headley Brothers, 1896), 2, RET 8/3/1, UY-BIA (hereafter, *Appeal*). See also Jessup, *Fifty-Three Years in Syria*, 2:521.

70. Waldmeier, *The Autobiography of Theophilus Waldmeier*, 263.

71. R. Hingston Fox, *Theophilus Waldmeier* (London: Friends' Foreign Mission Association, 1916), LH/10/01, box 15, LH, SOAS.

72. Theophilus Waldmeier, *The Autobiography of Theophilus Waldmeier, Comprising Ten Years in Abyssinia and Forty-Six Years in Syria, with Some Description of the People and Religions of These Countries*, ed. Stephen Hobhouse (London: Friends' Bookshop, 1925), 4 (hereafter, *The Autobiography of Theophilus Waldmeier*). On Gobat, see Charlotte van der Leest, "Conversion and Conflict in Palestine: The Missions of the Church Missionary Society and the Protestant Bishop Samuel Gobat" (PhD diss., Leiden University, 2008).

73. Alan Moorehead, *The Blue Nile* (New York: Vintage Books, 1972), 211–281; Paul B. Henze, *Layers of Time: A History of Ethiopia* (London: Hurst and Co., 2000), 119–143. Also see Theophilus Waldmeier, *The Autobiography of Theophilus Waldmeier, Missionary: Being an Account of Ten Years' Life in Abyssinia; and Sixteen Years in Syria* (London: S. W. Partridge and Co., 1886) (hereafter, Waldmeier, *The Autobiography of Theophilus Waldmeier, Missionary*), 78–121.

74. Waldmeier, *The Autobiography of Theophilus Waldmeier, Missionary*, 86 and 150.

75. Quoted in Rufus Jones, *Eli and Sybil Jones: Their Life and Work* (Philadelphia: Porter and Coates, 1889), 193–194, TLRSF.

76. Waldmeier is also remembered as the founder in 1873 of a school in Brummana (in Mount Lebanon) that is still in existence. For more on this, see Waldmeier, *The Autobiography of Theophilus Waldmeier, Missionary*, 256 and 320; Jones, *Eli and Sybil Jones*, 193–198.

77. For his distinction in both "medicine and the letters," Wortabet was awarded the Ottoman Order of the Medjidie (*Mecidiye Nişanı*) as well as the Order of the Knights of St. John. See Jessup, *Fifty-Three Years in Syria*, 1: 48–49. See also Jessup, *Fifty-Three Years in Syria*, 1: 216, 303, 312–313, and 345; "Obituary: John Wortabet," *Lancet* 173, no. 4455 (January 16, 1909): 209.

78. Waldmeier, *Appeal*.

79. Waldmeier, *Appeal*. On Brigstocke, see Daniel Bliss, *Letters from a New Campus: Written to His Wife Abby and Their Four Children during Their Visit to Amherst, Massachusetts, 1873–1874*, ed. Douglas Rugh, Belle Dorman Rugh, and Alfred H. Howell (Beirut: AUB Press, 1994), 275, note 60.

80. See "Sir Thomas Smith Clouston, Kt., MD Edin., LlD Edin. and Aberd., formerly Medical Superintendent, Royal Asylum, Edinburgh," *British Medical Journal* 1, no. 2834 (April 24, 1915): 744; Thomas Bewley, "Thomas Smith Clouston (1840–1915)," in *Madness to Mental Illness: A History of the Royal College of Psychiatrists*, Online Archive 9, n.d., https://www.rcpsych.ac.uk/docs/default-source/about-us/library-archives/archives/thomas-smith-clouston-1840-1915.pdf?sfvrsn=16d796e2_4.

81. "Data re: foundation," Second Volume of Minutes, LH/02/05, box 3, LH, SOAS; Waldmeier, *The Autobiography of Theophilus Waldmeier*, 268–269.

82. T. S. Clouston, "Lunacy Law Reform," *Lancet* 125, no. 3204 (January 24, 1885): 176–178; David Yellowlees, "On the Use of the Restraint in the Care of the Insane," *British Journal of Psychiatry* 35, no. 150 (1889): 286–287.

83. David Yellowlees, "Sir Thomas Smith Clouston," *British Journal of Psychiatry* 61, no. 254 (July 1, 1915): 494–495; "Sir Thomas Smith Clouston," 744.

84. Yellowlees, "On the Use of the Restraint in the Care of the Insane; T. S. Clouston, "Rest and Exercise in the Treatment of Nervous and Mental Diseases," *British Journal of Psychiatry* 41, no. 175 (October 1, 1895): 599–622.

85. Henry R. Rollin, "Psychiatry in Britain One Hundred Years Ago," *British Journal of Psychiatry* 183, no. 4 (October 1, 2003): 292–298.

86. Clouston, "Lunacy Law Reform," 177.

87. See Stephen Trombley, *"All That Summer She Was Mad": Virginia Woolf and Her Doctors* (London: Junction Books, 1981).

88. "Bethlem Royal Hospital," *British Medical Journal* 2, no. 1438 (1888): 134.

89. "Obituary: John Wortabet, M.D. Edinb.," *Lancet* 1, no. 6146 (January 16, 1909): 209–210; reprinted 237, no. 6146 (June 14, 1941): 774.

90. For more on the DPM, see Aubrey Lewis, *The State of Psychiatry: Essays and Addresses* (London: Routledge, 2014), especially 113–124.

91. Minutes of the LGC, October 21, 1897, 5, LH/02/01, box 2, LH, SOAS; Waldmeier, *The Autobiography of Theophilus Waldmeier*, 269.

92. Minutes of the LGC, April 25, 1901, LH/02/01, box 2, LH, SOAS.

93. Theophilus Waldmeier, "Report of Theophilus Waldmeier, Business Superintendent," March 31, 1902, Minutes of the LGC, LH/07/01, box 9, LH, SOAS. See also AR, 1903, 23, LHMND, AUB-SML.

94. "Lebanon Hospital for Mental and Nervous Disorders, Constitution and Regulations, 1965," LH/01/02, box 1, LH, SOAS.

95. Appeal by Antranig Manugian, c. 1974, LH/08/07, box 11, LH, SOAS.

96. Waldmeier, *The Autobiography of Theophilus Waldmeier*, 269.

97. Waldmeier, *The Autobiography of Theophilus Waldmeier*, 287. For more on the history of the Frankford Asylum for the Insane, see Patricia D'Antonio, *Founding Friends: Families, Staff, and Patients at the Friends Asylum in Early Nineteenth-Century Philadelphia* (Bethlehem, PA: Lehigh University Press, 2006).

98. Waldmeier, *The Autobiography of Theophilus Waldmeier*, 284.

99. Waldmeier, *The Autobiography of Theophilus Waldmeier*, 288.

100. Waldmeier, *The Autobiography of Theophilus Waldmeier*, 288.

101. Minutes of the LGC, March 11, 1897, box 2, LH/02/01, LH, SOAS.

102. Minutes of the LGC, March 25 and 21 October 1897, box 2, LH/02/01, LH, SOAS.

103. "Preface to the Constitution and Rules," in *Constitution and Rules* (London: n.p., 1907), LH/01/02, box 1, and First Volume of Minutes, March 26, 1943, LH/02/04, box 3, both LH, SOAS. The donations totaled £4,590 (approximately $660,000 in 2019 US dollars), with £2,879 from the British Isles, £934 from the United States and Canada, £712 from Europe, and £65 from Syria.

104. "Memorandum as to the Property of Asfuriyeh," 1911, LH/01/01, box 1, and First Volume of Minutes, March 26, 1943, LH/02/04, box 3, both LH, SOAS.

105. Waldmeier, *The Autobiography of Theophilus Waldmeier*, 297.

106. For more on the emergence of this French colonial project (which started in 1857), see Leila Fawaz, "The Beirut-Damascus Road: Connecting the Syrian Coast to the Interior in the 19th Century," in *The Syrian Land: Processes of Integration and Fragmentation: Bilad al-Sham from the 18th to the 20th Century*, ed. Thomas Philipp and Birgit Schaebler (Stuttgart: Franz Steiner Verlag Stuttgart, 1998), 19–28. In the early twentieth century, that road would also connect Damascus to the inland part of the Arabian Peninsula via the Hijāz railway.

107. "Literal Translation of the Waqf (Vacouf) Deed Covering All the Properties of the Lebanon Hospital for the Insane," LH/01/01 and "Preface to the Rules," LH/01/02, both box 1, both LH, SOAS.

108. AR, 1898, 10, and 1902, 15, LHMND, AUB-SML; Waldmeier, "Report of Theophilus Waldmeier, Business Superintendent," March 31, 1902, 5–6, LH/07/01, box 9, LH, SOAS. On work therapy as a Quaker principle, see Anne Digby, *Madness, Morality, and Medicine: A Study of the York Retreat, 1796–1914* (Cambridge: Cambridge University Press, 1985).

109. Minutes of the LGC, March 11, 1897, LH/02/01, box 2, LH, SOAS.

110. See John Sibbald, "The Cottage System and Gheel," *Journal of Mental Science* 7, no. 37 (April 1861): 31–60; D. Hack Tuke, "On a Recent Visit to Gheel," *British Journal of Psychiatry* 31, no. 136 (January 1, 1886): 481–497.

111. "Al-Bīmāristān al-Lubnānī," *at-Ṭabīb* 8 (1896): 91–92.

112. Waldmeier, *Appeal,* 15–16.

113. The "Constitution and Bye-Laws of the Executive Committee of the Lebanon Asylum for the Insane" was published in Beirut on April 22, 1896, and was amended in 1907, 1915, and 1965, LH/01/02, box 1, LH, SOAS. See also cabinet no. 4, LHMND, AUB-SML.

114. George Sabra categorizes the period as being of a "classic missionary concern" ("AUB and Religion," 2).

115. Theophilus Waldmeier, "Report for the Year Ending 31st March 1907," 32, AR, LHMND, AUB-SML.

116. "Constitution and Bye-Laws of the Executive Committee of the Lebanon Asylum for the Insane," 4.

117. Theophilus Waldmeier, letter, September 10, 1910, RET 8/3/1, UY-BIA.

118. AR, 1898, 14–15, LHMND, AUB-SML.

119. This is the asylum where the first tricyclic antidepressant would be tested in 1957. See Edward Shorter and David Healy, *Shock Therapy: A History of Electroconvulsive Treatment in Mental Illness* (New Brunswick, NJ: Rutgers University Press, 2007), 172.

120. AR, 1899, 8, LHMND, AUB-SML.

121. Minutes of the LGC, January 1, 1903, 55–56, LH/02/01, box 2, LH, SOAS.

122. Minutes, correspondence, publicity, and other papers from H. H. Jessup (secretary) to the LGC, November 29, 1902, RET 8/3/1, UY-BIA.

123. Minutes, correspondence, publicity, and other papers from O. Wolff to the BEC, November 29, 1902, RET 8/3/1, UY-BIA.

124. Theophilus Waldmeier, October 5, 1900, and "Copy of Parts of a Private Letter to Mr. Brading," May 14, 1903, LH/07/01, box 9, LH, SOAS.

125. Theophilus Waldmeier to Hingston Fox, "Confidential for Committee," October 5, 1900, LH/07/01, LH, SOAS.

126. Fareedy Waldmeier to Francis Brading, c. 1904, LH/07/01, box 9, LH, SOAS.

127. Fareedy Waldmeier to Brading.

128. Minutes of the LGC, March 19, 1904, 72, LH/02/01, box 2, LH, SOAS; "Syria. Lebanon Hospital for the Insane," *Our Missions: Friend's Missionary Magazine*, 1904, 179.

129. Minutes of the LGC, October 26, 1905, 91, LH/02/01, box 2, LH, SOAS. Also see Letter to Dr. Powell (one of the candidates for the post of medical superintendent), August 3, 1908, RET 8/3/1, UY-BIA.

130. Theophilus Waldmeier to the LGC, August 30, 1905, LH/07/01, box 9, LH, SOAS.

131. Theophilus Waldmeier to the LGC.

132. Theophilus Waldmeier to Fortescue Fox (chairman of the LGC), June 1, 1908, LH/07/04, box 9, LH, SOAS.

133. Clipping of the obituary of Henry Watson Smith from the *Lancet* (June 23, 1934): 136 and inserted on p. 177 of the Minutes of London General Committee, LH/02/03, box 2, LH, SOAS. Also see AR, 1933–1934, 1, LHMND, AUB-SML; C. A. Webster, "Doctor Henry Watson Smith," *al-Kulliyyah* 20, no. 6 (July 1, 1934), 171, 6–AUBites folder, AA, AUB-JL; "Henry Watson Smith, OBE, MD, Medical Director, Lebanon Hospital for Mental Diseases," *British Medical Journal* 1, no. 3833 (June 23, 1934): 1146–1147.

134. Waldmeier, *The Autobiography of Theophilus Waldmeier*, 309.

135. Minutes of the LGC, September 3, 1903, 61, and Oscar Darton, "Confidential Report," January 3, 1910, both LH/02/01, box 2, LH, SOAS. According to the report,

"It also appears that Mr. Waldmeier has been in the habit of incurring expenditure out of the ordinary routine without consulting the local Committee and that he acts upon his own initiative on important matters when they should be consulted and their advice obtained."

136. Unsigned letter to Fox, 1913, LH/07/04, box 9, LH, SOAS.

137. Unsigned letter to to Fox. Also see AUB-SML, LHMND, AR, 1933–1934.

138. Unsigned letter to Fox.

139. Franklin Moore to Miss Gooch, February 15, 1914, LH/07/04, box 9, LH, SOAS.

140. Minutes of the LGC, June 15, 1910, 152–154, box 2, LH/02/01, LH, SOAS.

141. Moore to Gooch.

142. Arnold Ruegg to Fox, May 5, 1914, LH/07/04, box 9, LH, SOAS.

143. Lily Waldmeier Tabet to Fox, March 18, 1915, LH/07/04, box 9, LH, SOAS.

144. R. A. Mickelwright, report on his second visit to the Hospital, October 1964–February 1965, "Hospital Buildings," appendix V, miscellaneous items, LH/12/01, box 16, LH, SOAS.

145. Nicholas Z. Ajay, "Mount Lebanon and the Wilayah of Beirut, 1914–1918: The War Years" (PhD diss., Georgetown University, 1973), 385–433; Melanie Tanielian, "The War of Famine: Everyday Life in Wartime Beirut and Mount Lebanon (1914–1918)" (PhD diss., University of California, Berkeley, 2012); John P. Spagnolo, "The Famine of 1915–1918 in Greater Syria," in *Problems of the Modern Middle East in Historical Perspective: Essays in Honour of Albert Hourani*, ed. John P. Spagnolo (Reading, UK: Ithaca Press, 1992), 229–258; Leila Fawaz, *A Land of Aching Hearts: The Middle East in the Great War* (Cambridge, MA: Harvard University Press, 2014).

146. AR, 1914–1915, 7, LHMND, AUB-SML.

147. AR, 1930–1931, 18, LHMND, AUB-SML; "Henry Watson Smith, OBE," 1147. On the abolishment of the capitulations and its consequences, see Cloarec, *La France et la question de Syrie*, especially 79–92.

148. AR, 1915–1916, 5, LHMND, AUB-SML.

149. AR, 1916–1917, 3, and 1917–1918, 4–5, LHMND, AUB-SML.

150. "Subject: Lebanon Hospital for the Insane," consular dispatches to Washington, D.C., December 24, 1914, FO 383/94, TNA. Also see AR, 1933–1934, LHMND, AUB-SML; newspaper clipping, "Lebanon Hospital for Mental Diseases Weathered War through Display of Tact," *Philadelphia Record*, June 18, 1919, LH/07/04, box 9, LH, SOAS.

151. Consular dispatch from Washington, D.C., January 5, 1915, FO 383/94, TNA.

152. AR, 1915–1916, 7–8, and 1917–1918, 3, LHMND, AUB-SML.

153. AR, 1915–1916, 6, LHMND, AUB-SML.

154. AR, 1917–1918, 3–4, LHMND, AUB-SML.

155. AR, 1914–1915, 5, LHMND, AUB-SML.

156. AR, 1918–1919, 3, and 1919–1920, 6, LHMND, AUB-SML.

157. AR, 1918–1919, 3, LHMND, AUB-SML.

158. "Subcommittee Minutes," letter from General Allenby thanking the Hospital, March 26, 1919, LH/02/08, LH, box 3, SOAS; "Henry Watson Smith, OBE," 1147. See also AR, 1915–1916, LHMND, AUB-SML.

159. "Le diplôme d'État français de la faculté de médecine et la nouvelle situation politique dans l'Empire Ottoman," September 13, 1919, 50CPCOM/104, MAE.

160. "Le diplôme d'État français de la faculté de médecine et la nouvelle situation politique dans l'Empire Ottoman."

161. Allied and Associated Powers, *The Treaties of Peace, 1919–1923* (New York: Carnegie Endowment for International Peace, 1924), 2:831.

162. For more on the diverse student body at the FFM, see Bourmaud, "Entre science conquérante, confessionnalisme et souveraineté," 253–264.

163. For more, see Fawwaz Traboulsi, *A History of Modern Lebanon* (London: Pluto Press, 2007), especially 75–87; Nadine Méouchy, ed., *France, Syrie et Liban, 1918–1946: Les ambiguïtés et les dynamiques de la relation mandataire* (Beirut: Presses de l'Ifpo, 2013).

164. "Faculté française de médecine de Beyrouth (Syrie)," January 5, 1921, 223, and "Les facultés de médecine du Levant a/s valeurs respectives de leurs diplômes," 18–20, 50CPCOM/108, both MAE; Robert de Caix, the high commissioner, letter, March 29, 1920, AUB to the high commissioner, April 29, 1920, and General Gouraud, letter, June 5, 1920, file 1, box 5, School of Medicine, correspondence with French officials re: School of Medicine and School of Dentistry (1920–1923), AUB-JL. Of course, since AUB graduates had their diplomas recognized by the state of New York, they could pass the state board examination and practice in the United States. The advantage under Ottoman rule was that their imperial diplomas allowed them to practice all over the Ottoman Empire.

165. A. R. Doble to the minister of foreign affairs, "Monsieur le Ministre il serait bon d'avoir l'oeil sur le Collège Américain de Beyrouth (Syrie) qui est anti-français à tous les points de vue. Il a une mauvaise influence sur les Arabes," June 23, 1921, 49, 50CPCOM/105, MAE.

166. FFM, "La Faculté Américaine, fondée dans un but exclusif de propagande confessionnelle, comme il est dit dans son statut d'établissement, n'a pas depuis l'occupation française, de mode bien déterminé d'existence," 223, 50CPCOM/107, MAE.

167. The French authorities managed to sign off on this discriminatory policy with the newly elected Lebanese government in 1944. The policy was publicly criticized by the American Legation a few decades later, in 1951. See Albion Ross, "US Files Protest on Lebanese Bias," *New York Times*, June 7, 1951, newspaper clipping attached to the diplomatic dispatch of July 11, 1951, 380QONT/354, MAE.

168. Université Saint-Joseph, 2012, 18, accessed February 12, 2020, https://www.usj.edu.lb/actualites/images/livret.pdf.

169. French consul in Beirut to Stephen Pichon (minister of foreign affairs), December 10, 1910, 99, 175CPCOM/9, MAE. See also French consul in Beirut to Stephen Pichon (minister of foreign affairs), December 16, 1910, 114, 175CPCOM/9, MAE.

170. R. P. Cattin to the minister of foreign affairs, letters, September 30 and October 1, 1910, 175CPCOM/9, MAE.

171. Berthelot to Abbot Jalabert, September 16, 1930, 417QO/223, MAE.

172. Berthelot to Jalabert; MAE, A. Demons to the minister of foreign affairs, "Rapport à monsieur le ministre de l'instruction publique sur les examens probatoires subis devant le jury Franco-Ottoman par messieurs les etudiants en médecine et en pharmacie de la faculté française mixte de médecine et de pharmacie de Beyrouth du 2 au 9 Novembre 1909 par A. Demons professeur de clinique chirurgicale à la faculté de médecine de l'université de Bordeaux," 50, 175CPCOM/9, MAE.

173. Stanley E. Kerr (associate professor of biological chemistry), "The Medical Science Laboratories School of Medicine AUB, Syria," report, 1931, file 1, box 7, School of Medicine reports to the Rockefeller Foundation 1924–1939, AUB-JL.

174. The foundation gave support to AUB's Medical School (1920–1967), its Arabic studies program (1948–1953), and its School of Nursing (1927–1941). See "Remarks," Lebanon, 12 boxes, 1920–1967, Series 833, Projects, Record Group 1.1, Rockefeller Foundation Archives.

175. John S. Baick, "Cracks in the Foundation: Frederick T. Gates, the Rockefeller Foundation, and the China Medical Board," *Journal of the Gilded Age and Progressive Era* 3, no. 1 (2004): 59–89; E. Richard Brown, *Rockefeller Medicine Men: Medicine and Capitalism in America* (Berkeley: University of California Press, 1979).

176. Robert Caix to the minister of foreign affairs, followed by a report titled "Assistance publique," July 4, 1922, 13, 50CPCOM/382, MAE.

177. Georges Catroux, "Délégation française de Damas rapport trimestriel 192: Introduction au premier rapport trimestriel de 1921," confidential document, 2–3,

folder 1 (box 4H71), series 4H Levant, "renseignements de la délégation française du haut commissariat de Damas sur la situation politique, militaire et financière," Armée du Levant puis commandement supérieur des troupes du Levant, SHD.

178. Virginie de Luca, *Aux origines de l'état-providence: Les inspecteurs de l'assistance publique et l'aide sociale à l'enfance, 1820–1930* (Paris: Institut national d'études démographiques, 2002).

179. "Some Facts about the Hospital," June 16, 1950, Second Volume of Minutes, LH/02/05, box 3, LH, SOAS; "Rapport sur l'organisation et le fonctionnement des services d'hygiène et de l'assistance publique en Syrie," April 16, 1921, 24–56, 50CPCOM/108, MAE.

180. See Colette Bec, *Assistance et république: La recherche d'un nouveau contrat social sous la IIIe république* (Paris: Éditions de l'Atelier, 1994). For the context of the Mandate, see Sylvia Chiffoleau, "Entre bienfaisance, contrôle des populations et agenda international: La politique sanitaire du mandat français en Syrie et au Liban," *Bulletin Canadien d'histoire de la médecine* 30, no. 2 (2013): 1–30.

181. "Rapport sur l'organisation et le fonctionnement des services d'hygiène et de l'assistance publique en Syrie," 25.

182. "Rapport sur l'organisation et le fonctionnement des services d'hygiène et de l'assistance publique en Syrie," 36.

183. R. P. (Révérend Père) Martimprey (chancellor of the FFM) to M. Leygues (minister of foreign affairs), letter, "Objet: Le nouveau régime d'études de 5 ans et la Faculté Américaine de Beyrouth," November 12, 1920, 50CPCOM/107, MAE.

184. General Henri Gouraud (high commissioner of the French Republic in Syria and Lebanon) to the director of AUB, July 10, 1921, file 1, box 5, School of Medicine, Correspondence with French officials re: School of Medicine and School of Dentistry (1920–1923), AUB-JL.

185. Medical Division Faculty Minutes (1908–1978), 1917, 1:151–156, AA: 3.9.3; interim president of the Syrian Protestant College, letter to General Gouraud, September 7, 1921, file 1, box 5, School of Medicine, Correspondence with French officials re: School of Medicine and School of Dentistry (1920–1923); untitled petitions by third-year medical students, February 28, 1924, and medical faculty, December 17, 1926, file 1 (1920–1927), box 8, School of Medicine, Minutes of Meetings (1910–1930), all AUB-JL.

186. Medical Division Faculty Minutes (1908–1978), August 13, 1918, 1:185, AA: 3.9.3, AUB-JL.

187. Letters to Watson Smith, July 11, 1924, and June 4, 1925, AA: 2.5.0, personal box 1 (1924–25), AUB-JL; Minutes of the LGC, May 20, 1925, 8–9, LH/02/03, box 2, LH, SOAS.

188. Medical subcommittee of the senate, August 4, 1924, file 1 (1920–1927), box 8, School of Medicine, Minutes of Meetings (1910–1930), AUB-JL.

189. "Dr. Henry Watson Smith (1879–1934)," AUBites folder, AA: 6, AUB-JL.

190. Letter, November 25, 1921, file 1, box 5, School of Medicine, correspondence with French officials re: School of Medicine and School of Dentistry (1920–1923), AUB-JL.

191. "Schedule of New Fifth-Year Course," July 17, 1917, 151-156, Minutes of the Faculty of Medicine (1867-1920), AUB-JL.

192. Medical faculty minutes, December 17, 1926, file 1 (1920–1927), box 8, School of Medicine, Minutes of Meetings (1910–1930), AUB-JL.

193. AR, 1927–1928, 21, LHMND, AUB-SML.

194. See Nancy Tomes, *A Generous Confidence: Thomas Story Kirkbride and the Art of Asylum-Keeping, 1840–1883* (Cambridge: Cambridge University Press, 1984).

195. AR, 1933–1934, n.p., LHMND, AUB-SML.

196. AR, 1933–1934, n.p., LHMND, AUB-SML.

197. Minutes of the LGC, September 29, 1920, 159, LH/02/02, box 2, LH, SOAS.

198. Charles Corbin (French ambassador in London) to the minister of foreign affairs, "A.s. de l'Asile d'Aliénés du Liban," June 2, 1933, 161–162, and high commissioner in Syria and Lebanon to the minister of foreign affairs, January 11, 1934, 181–184, both 50CPCOM/603, MAE.

199. État de Damas (direction de l'hygiène et de l'assistance publique), quarterly report, second quarter 1923, 4, file no. 2, series 4H Levant, "renseignements de la délégation française du haut commissariat de Damas sur la situation politique, militaire et financière," Armée du Levant puis commandement supérieur des troupes du Levant, SHD. For more on the Ibn Sina Hospital, see Khalaf Abdul Massih, "De l'assistance psychiatrie en Syrie" (PhD diss., University of Paris René Descartes, 1980), especially 45–71, côte: 08–2143, Bibliothèque médicale Henri Ey; Beverly Ann Tsacoyianis, "Making Healthy Minds and Bodies in Syria and Lebanon, 1899–1961" (PhD diss., Washington University in St. Louis, 2014), especially 186–195.

200. "Service d'hygiène et d'assistance publique," 1921, file no. 1, series 4H Levant, "renseignements de la délégation française du haut commissariat de Damas sur la situation politique, militaire et financière," Armée du Levant puis commandement supérieur des troupes du Levant, SHD; AR, 1920–1921, 2–3, and 1924–1925, 2, LHMND, AUB-SML.

201. AR, 1919–1920, 1, LHMND, AUB-SML.

202. The French military finally requisitioned the Prussian hospital, which was also coveted by the Jesuits, and converted it to a military hospital under a new name, the Hôpital Maurice Rottier. See Frédéric Eccard (senator of the Bas-Rhin and president of the French Protestant Associations), "Re: the Prussian hospital (Hôpital St. Jean) and the military occupation," June 22 and July 3, 1926, 50CPCOM/386, MAE. Also see Khouri, "Histoire de la médecine au Liban," 38.

203. Minister of foreign affairs to Charles Corbin (French ambassador in London), "Asile d'aliénés du Liban," June 19, 1933, 50CPCOM/603, MAE. The association was initially founded in 1925 as *L'Église protestante française au Liban* at the request of the high commissioner. See "Syrie Hôpitaux et Dispensaires," February 3, 1925, 55, and February 4, 1925, 56, 50CPCOM/385, MAE. It was renamed *Oeuvres protestantes françaises de Syrie et du Liban.* See "Extrait du procès-verbal de l'assemblée générale du 21 mars 1929," 134, 50CPCOM/387, MAE.

204. High commissioner in Syria and Lebanon to the minister of foreign affairs, letter, January 11, 1934, 181–184, 50CPCOM/603, MAE.

205. R. P. Stéphane (chargé d'affaires, Lyon) to the minister of foreign affairs, "Objet: (Suite à l'entretien du 23.x.52 avec M. Beyer, Chef de cabinet du précèdent Ministre): Appel des missionnaires Capucins français de la Mission 'Liban-Syrie-Turquie,'" December 21, 1952, 371QONT/639, MAE.

206. Minutes of the LGC, February 28, 1934, 165, LH/02/03, box 2, LH, SOAS; Webster "Doctor Henry Watson Smith Honored," *al-Kulliyyah* 20 (December 15, 1933), 49–50, 6–AUBites folder, AA, AUB-JL.

207. Webster, "Doctor Henry Watson Smith," 171.

208. AR, 1934–1935, 22, LHMND, AUB-SML.

209. For more on the transition from the mandate to an independent republic, see Traboulsi, *A History of Modern Lebanon*, especially 99–108.

210. Quoted in AR, 1943, 4, LHMND, AUB-SML.

211. Khouri, "Histoire de la médecine au Liban," 159.

212. AR, 1945, 2, LHMND, AUB-SML. This state of affairs was reversed when 'Aṣfūriyyeh closed its doors in 1982. Since then AUB medical students have been receiving their training in clinical psychiatry at Dayr al-Ṣalīb.

213. Henri Bersot, "Nécrologie: Dr. Albert Brousseau (1888–1955)," *Schweizer Archiv für Neurologie und Psychiatrie* 77 (1956): 454–455; Khouri, *La médecine au Liban,* 160; Véronique Fau-Vincenti, "Aliénés et rebelles: Quérulence et protestation en milieu asilaire (1910–1959)," *Criminocorpus* (October 6, 2014), note 37. See also AR, 1948, 11, LHMND, AUB-SML.

3 The Rise of ʿAṣfūriyyeh and the Decline of Missions

1. Soeurs Franciscaines de la Croix, ed., *Oeuvres du Révérend Père Jacques missionnaire capucin fondateur de l'ordre des Soeurs Franciscaines de la Croix* (Harisa, Lebanon: Imprimerie St. Paul, 1951), especially 34–36, côte: 651.93 Z.46, ACF; "Bl. Jacques Ghazir Haddad (1875–1954)," Vatican, accessed February 13, 2020, http://www.vatican.va/news_services/liturgy/saints/2008/ns_lit_doc_20080622_haddad_en.html.

2. *Oeuvres du Révérend Père Jacques* and "Liste des oeuvres du P. Jacques El-Haddad de Ghazir Capucin fondateur de la congregation des soeurs franciscaines de la croix du Liban 1925–1954," côte: 685.13 Z54, ACF; Christ-Roi is known for its giant statue of Jesus Christ stretching out his hands and embracing the Mediterranean, much like the Christ the Redeemer statue in Rio de Janeiro—which probably served as a model, since the former was erected in the 1950s and the latter in the 1930s.

3. Théophane de Deir el-Kamar, *L'apôtre de la croix: Père Jacques de Ghazir, capucin, 1875–1954* (Beirut: Imprimerie Catholique, 1961), 185–202 and 223–226.

4. Père Jacques de Ghazir, "A travers le Liban," *Le petit messager de Saint François* (1906): 4, côte: 651.93 Z.45, ACF. On the wave of immigration to the Americas in the nineteenth century, see Albert Hourani and Nadim Shehadi, eds., *The Lebanese in the World: A Century of Emigration* (London: Centre for Lebanese Studies, 1992).

5. Père Jacques de Ghazir, letter, March 29, 1939, letters to Père Ernst, the Provincial Capucin of Lyon by P. Jacques Syria 1925–1946, "Père Jacques et les soeurs de la croix 1930–1947," côte: 651.93 Z.46, ACF. The letter said: "Nous arrachons aux protestants de Asfourieh pour cette année 50 malades atteints de démence tranquille c'est ayant encore assez d'esprit pour pouvoir comprendre le bien qu'on leur fait." In another letter in the same collection, dated May 3, 1939, he wrote: "Le Directeur de Asfourieh est furieux contre moi il a fait marcher quelques fonctionnaires du gouvernement libanais pour faire fermer la croix ou du moins pour m'empêcher de lui arracher sa clientèle. Heureusement la Municipalité de Beyrouth et l'Assistance Publique me protègent comme il faut, vive la Croix." These remarks do not appear in Alexandre Najjar's biography, though the latter does acknowledge Père Jacques's aversion to the growing influence of Protestant missionaries (*L'homme de la providence: Abouna Yaacoub* [Beirut: L'Orient des Livres, 2013], especially 48–49).

6. De Deir el-Kamar, *L'apôtre de la croix,* 215–216.

7. De Deir el-Kamar, *L'apôtre de la croix,* 216 and 223.

8. *Oeuvres du Révérend Père Jacques;* de Deir el-Kamar, *L'apôtre de la croix,* especially 167–202 and 215–228.

9. AR, 1943, 3, LHMND, AUB-SML; Medical Director's Report, "Withdrawal of Patients from Assistance Publique Owing to Shortness of Funds," December 12, 1940, and Minutes of the Executive Committee, December 12, 1949, FO 1018/67,

TNA. Also see "An International Mental Hospital in Syria," *British Medical Journal* 2, no. 4166 (November 9, 1940): 637.

10. Medical Director's Report, December 12, 1949, and Acting Director's Report, January 23, 1950, FO 1018/67, TNA.

11. "Le scandale de l'hospitalization des personnes atteintes de maladies mentales," *L'Orient*, October 18, 1939, LHMND, AUB-SML. See also First Volume of Minutes, October, 21 1938, LH/02/04, box 3, LH, SOAS.

12. "Le scandale de l'hospitalization des personnes atteintes de maladies mentales."

13. "L'oeuvre des anormaux prit la plus large extension. Il n'y avait au Liban qu'un seul Hôpital psychiatrique au Liban [*sic*], tenu par des protestants américains. Le mérite du Père Jacques fut de fonder cet Hôpital psychiatrique Catholique au couvent de la Croix, sans cesse aggrandi" ("Historique," n.d., 2, Liban Documents pour l'Histoire, côte: 651.93 Z.45, ACF).

14. AR, 1943, 3–4 and 7, LHMND, AUB-SML. The occasional medical care was provided by Georges Stéphan, a Lebanese physician, starting from 1929. See R. Chemaly, "History of the Neurosciences in Lebanon," *Lebanese Medical Journal* 53, no. 4 (2005): 243.

15. Minutes of the BEC, June 24, 1950, FO 1018/67, TNA; "Minutes of the Special Meeting held in the Country House of Saeb Beik Salam," October 24, 1950, FO 1018/67, TNA.

16. De Deir el-Kamar, *L'apôtre de la croix,* 170.

17. R. Stewart Miller, "Report of the Medical Director," AR, 1941, 8, LHMND, AUB-SML.

18. First Volume of Minutes, November 1, 1939, LH/02/04, box 3, LH, SOAS; AR, 1948, 8, LHMND, AUB-SML.

19. AR, 1941, 8, LHMND, AUB-SML; "Lebanon Hospital for Mental Diseases," *British Medical Journal* 1, no. 3883 (June 8, 1935): 1187.

20. The 1876 decree forbade the opening of any new lunatic asylums without the explicit approval of the Imperial School of Medicine in Constantinople. See Société de législation comparée and Centre français de droit comparé, *Annuaire de législation étrangère publié par la Société de législation comparée contenant la traduction des principales lois votées dans les pays étrangers en 1876* (Paris: A. Cotillon et Co., 1877), especially 675. Astonishingly, ʿAṣfūriyyeh had no such permission in 1900. The Ottoman governor, Naum Pasha (ruled 1892–1902), approved of the initiative, which seems to have sufficed. See a draft letter addressed "To his Excellency Nahum [Yusuf is barred] Pasha," November 2, 1897, LH/07/04, box 9, LH, SOAS. For the text of the 1876 decree, see George Young, *Corps de droit ottoman*, vol. 6 (Oxford: Clarendon Press of Oxford

University Press, 1905–1906), 304 (articles 944 and 945), 306–309 (chapter II), 377 (articles 1457 and 1458), 389 (article 1541), and 395 (article 1573).

21. Laws were passed on the regulation of medical doctors and midwives (both October 11, 1861), pharmacists (November 17–29, 1862), medical doctors and pharmacists (April 16, 1888), druggists and perfumers (May 7, 1885). See Young, *Corps de droit ottoman*, 3:194–211.

22. Young, *Corps de droit ottoman*, 3:205–207.

23. A. Motet, "Rapport sur un projet de loi sur les aliénés en Turquie par M. Mongeri," *Annales médico-psychologique* 17 (1877): 86–88.

24. See chapter 1, article 3 in Young, *Corps de droit ottoman*, 1:71. For more information, see Yehya Houssam, "La protection sanitaire et sociale au Liban (1860–1963)" (PhD diss., University of Nice Sophia Antipolis, 2015), 72–86; Jens Hanssen, *Fin de Siècle Beirut: The Making of an Ottoman Provincial Capital* (Oxford: Clarendon Press of Oxford University Press, 2005), especially 115–137.

25. Jean Ducruet, "Les premières décennies de psychiatrie au Liban (1900–1960)," *Travaux et jours*, no. 74 (2004): 45. Also see AR, 1938, 10, LHMND, AUB-SML. Watson Smith wrote: "The local authorities make ... no attempt whatsoever ... to offer any history of those patients sent here with the usual *Billet d'Hôpital*" (Report of the Director, AR, 1929–1930, 21, LHMND, AUB-SML).

26. For more on El-Khanka Hospital, see John Racy, *Psychiatry in the Arab East* (Copenhagen: Munksgaard, 1970), 43; Marilyn Anne Mayers, "A Century of Psychiatry: The Egyptian Mental Hospitals" (PhD diss. Princeton University, 1984); Valérie Baqué, "Regards sur l'asile et la folie dans l'Égypte du XIXe siècle," *Annales islamologiques*, no. 26 (1992): 197–206, and "Du Bimarîstan à l'asile moderne: mise en place de l'institution et de la médecine psychiatriques en Egypte (1882–1930)" (PhD diss., Université de Provence, 1995). On Miller, see AR, 1933–1934, 3, LHMND, AUB-SML; Minutes of the LGC, April 1, 1933, 186–187, LH/02/03, box 2, LH, SOAS. Regarding Miller's views on drug addiction, see Mayers, "A Century of Psychiatry," especially 200–201. Also see AR, 1933–1934, n.p. (between pages 2 and 3), LHMND, AUB-SML.

27. The text is available in Arabic. See World Intellectual Property Organization," Legislative Decree No. 340 of March 1, 1943: On the Criminal Code," 2010, http://www.wipo.int/wipolex/en/details.jsp?id=6653.

28. Youssef S. Takla, "Corpus juris du mandat français," in *Les mandats français et anglais dans une perspective comparative/The British and French Mandates in Comparative Perspectives*, ed. Nadine Méouchy and Peter Sluglett (Leiden, the Netherlands: Brill, 2004), 100.

29. C. L. Allen, "Reflections Concerning Neuropsychiatry," *California and Western Medicine* 39, no. 5 (November 1933): 298–300.

30. AR, 1937, 10, LHMND, AUB-SML.

31. AR, 1947, 1 and 8, LHMND, AUB-SML; Second Volume of Minutes, November 26, 1947, LH/02/05, box 3, LH, SOAS.

32. AR, 1946, 16, LHMND, AUB-SML.

33. John P. Spagnolo, "The Definition of a Style of Imperialism: The Internal Politics of the French Educational Investment in Ottoman Beirut," *French Historical Studies* 8, no. 4 (1974): 563–584.

34. AR, 1949, 2, LHMND, AUB-SML.

35. W. M. Ford Robertson, "Some Problems Concerning the Approach to a Middle East Psychiatric Service," *Lebanese Medical Journal* 5, no. 1 (January 1952): 12.

36. AR, 1948, 8, 1949, 18, 1952, 15, and 1960, 27, LHMND, AUB-SML; R. G. Turner, nurse tutor, report on the nursing-training course (1966–1967), September 14 1967, OD 34/224, TNA.

37. AR, 1953, 15, LHMND, AUB-SML.

38. See Sarah G. Shahla, "Nursing in Syria," *American Journal of Nursing* 30, no. 12 (1930): 1516.

39. AR, 1952, 15–16, LHMND, AUB-SML.

40. Medical Director's Report, 1962, AUB-SML; paper on the history of the Hospital signed by the chairman, October 8, 1976, Minutes of the BEC, LH/03/03, box 5, LH, SOAS.

41. Heather Green to Miss Prager, August 29, 1968, LH/08/03, box 10, LH, SOAS.

42. "The Lebanon Hospital for Mental and Nervous Disorders: More Progress for Better Service," in English and Arabic, LH/10/01, box 15, LH, SOAS.

43. Minutes of the BEC, January 19, 1982, LH/08/23, box 14, LH, SOAS. See also on Syria: Minutes of the BEC, March–December 1976 and March 15, 1977, LH/03/03, box 5, LH, SOAS; on Saudi Arabia: Minutes of the BEC, March–December 1976 and March 13, 1979, and BEC Minutes 1961–1963 and November 15 1960, LH/03/04, box 6, LH, SOAS; on Ethiopia: AR, 1961, 4, LHMND, AUB-SML, and BEC Minutes 1961–1963, March 14, 1961, LHMND, AUB-JL; on Iraq: AR, 1951, 8, LHMND, AUB-SML; on collaboration with Arab countries: "The Lebanon Hospital for Mental and Nervous Disorders."

44. Cecil King, "Confidential," December 28, 1967, report from the British embassy in Beirut to the Ministry of Overseas Development, OC 34/224, TNA.

45. Second Volume of Minutes, September 13, 1950, LH/02/05, box 3, LH, SOAS.

46. "Report of the Medical Director," January 7, 1952, Second Volume of Minutes, LH/02/05, box 3, LH, SOAS.

47. "Report of the Medical Director," January 7, 1952.

48. "Report of the Medical Director," January 7, 1952; AR, 1955, 17, LHMND, AUB-SML.

49. AR, 1947, 3, LHMND, AUB-SML.

50. AR, 1913–1914, 6, LHMND, AUB-SML.

51. AR, 1957, 8, LHMND, AUB-SML.

52. Physician Superintendent's Report, 1961, LHMND, AUB-SML.

53. Item 824, March 25, 1947, First Volume of Minutes from 1936–1946, LH/02/04, box 3, LH, SOAS.

54. Bayard Dodge, copy of a letter from Dr. Dodge, President of the American University of Beirut, to the Chairman of the General Committee in London, June 15, 1934, AR, 1933–1934, n.p., LHMND, AUB-SML.

55. See Beverly Ann Tsacoyianis, "Making Healthy Minds and Bodies in Syria and Lebanon, 1899–1961" (PhD diss., Washington University in St. Louis, 2014).

56. The data are compiled from various ARs for 1949–1956.

57. Antranig Manugian, Medical Director's Report, AR, 1954, 11, LHMND, AUB-SML.

58. "Some Problems Concerning the Approach to a Middle East Psychiatric Service," 7.

59. "Report of the Medical Director," January 7, 1952. See also AR, 1950, 1, LHMND, AUB-SML.

60. AR, 1955, 17–18, LHMND, AUB-SML.

61. Quoted in Second Volume of Minutes, September 13, 1950, LH/02/05, box 3, LH, SOAS. On the change of the Hospital name, see Minutes of the BEC, December 20, 1950, LH/03/01, and Minutes of the BEC, March 19, 1974, LH/03/02, both box 5 and LH, SOAS.

62. AR, 1950, 4, LHMND, AUB-SML.

63. Medical Director's Report, July 31, 1950, FO 1018/67, TNA.

64. Minutes of the BEC and Medical Director's Report, May 22, 1950 FO 1018/67, TNA.

65. Minutes of the BEC, April 24, 1950, FO 1018/67, TNA.

66. Minutes of the BEC, April 24, 1950.

67. Minutes of the BEC, April 24, 1950.

68. AR, 1955, 18, LHMND, AUB-SML.

69. AR, 1955, 18.

70. Appeal written by Antranig Manugian c. 1974, Sir Geoffrey Furlonge correspondence, LH/08/07, box 11, LH, SOAS.

71. Louis Roché (French ambassador in Beirut) to the minister of foreign affairs, June 5, 1957, 3, 371QONT/639, MAE.

72. Elizabeth Thompson, *Colonial Citizens: Republican Rights, Paternal Privilege, and Gender in French Syria and Lebanon* (New York: Columbia University Press, 2000), 63.

73. Roché to the minister of foreign affairs, "A/s budget des oeuvres culturelles au Liban," July 25, 1956, 371QONT/639, MAE.

74. See Thomas G. Paterson, "Foreign Aid under Wraps: The Point Four Program," *Wisconsin Magazine of History* 56, no. 2 (December 1, 1972): 119–126.

75. French delegate at the Advisory Commission to the Office of Refugees to the French ambassador in Beirut and the French ambassador in Damascus, "A/s aide fournie à des institutions privées américaines dans le cadre du Point IV," May 21, 1951, 380QONT/354, MAE.

76. French delegate at the Advisory Commission, "A/s aide fournie à des institutions privées américaines dans le cadre du Point IV."

77. Francois Puaux to the minister of foreign affairs, "A/s projets des catholiques américans au Liban," January 17, 1957, 371QONT/639, MAE.

78. *Oeuvres du Révérend Père Jacques*, 28.

79. Ayoub remained chief psychiatrist at Dayr al-Ṣalīb for fifty years and was appointed professor of psychiatry at the FFM in 1965. See Ducruet, "Les premières décennies de psychiatrie au Liban," 63; Sami Richa, *La psychiatrie au Liban: Une histoire et un regard* (Beirut: Dergham, 2015), 88.

80. Richa, *La psychiatrie au Liban*, 88.

81. Second Volume of Minutes, January 20, 1951, LH/02/05, box 3, LH, SOAS.

82. Marwa Elshakry, "The Gospel of Science and American Evangelism in Late Ottoman Beirut," *Past and Present* 196, no. 1 (2007): 173.

83. Roché, telegram to the minister of foreign affairs, May 1, 1958, 371QONT/639, MAE.

84. Robert de Boisseson (French ambassador in Beirut) to the minister of foreign affairs, "A/s réunion à Beyrouth du congrès panarabe de médecine," June 15, 1960, 371QONT/962, MAE.

85. Jacques Emile (French ambassador in Damascus) to the minister of foreign affairs, "A/s status des établissements religieux français en Syrie," December 13, 1954, 381QONT/527, MAE.

86. Roché to the minister of foreign affairs, December 12, 1958, 371QONT/639, MAE.

87. Roché to the minister of foreign affairs, "A/s effectifs des écoles françaises au Liban," March 21, 1957, 7, 371QONT/639, MAE.

88. Roché to the minister of foreign affairs, "Avenir de l'Hôtel-Dieu," April 2, 1959, 371QONT/639, MAE.

89. Roché, telegram flagged as "reservé secret," April 6, 1959, 371QONT/639, MAE.

90. Roché to the minister of foreign affairs, "Avenir de l'Hôtel-Dieu," 13.

91. Roché to the minister of foreign affairs, "Avenir de l'Hôtel-Dieu," 9.

92. Roché to the minister of foreign affairs, "Cérémonie d'anniversaire à la faculté française de médecine de Beyrouth," December 10, 1958, 371QONT/639, MAE.

93. Roché to the minister of foreign affairs, "Cérémonie d'anniversaire à la faculté française de médecine de Beyrouth."

94. Roché, telegram flagged as "reservé secret."

95. Roché to the minister of foreign affairs, September 16, 1965, 371QONT/962, MAE.

96. Nada Raad, "Colleagues Remember Antranig Manugian," *Daily Star,* April 12, 2003, http://www.dailystar.com.lb/News/Lebanon-News/2003/Apr-12/20401-colleagues-remember-antranig-manugian.ashx. For a now-outdated but still very useful overview of the different sectarian communities and their political representation, see Luc-Henri de Bar, *Les communautés confessionnelles du Liban* (Paris: Éditions Recherche sur les Civilisations, 1983). Armenians had settled in Lebanon en masse in the aftermath of the Armenian genocide in 1915. In 1947 the Lebanese parliament reaffirmed the confessional (i.e., faith-based) representation and allocated 3 of the 140 seats to Lebanese-Armenians. Today, six seats are allocated to the Lebanese-Armenian community. (The confessional system is discussed at more length in chapter 6.)

97. Of course, this periodization has become questionable. See, for example, A. R. Norton, "Lebanon after Ta'if: Is the Civil War Over?" *Middle East Journal* 45 (1991): 457–473.

98. "Obituary: Manugian," *Main Gate: American University of Beirut Quarterly Magazine* 1, no. 3 (Spring 2003), http://staff.aub.edu.lb/~webmgate/spring03/memorium.html (site discontinued); "Dr. Antranig S. Manugian (1910–2003)," *AUB Bulletin Today* 4, no. 5 (March–April 2003), https://staff.aub.edu.lb/~webbultn/v4n5/12.html; Raad, "Colleagues Remember Antranig Manugian."

99. First Volume of Minutes, March 28, 1938, LH/02/04, box 3, LH, SOAS.

100. First Volume of Minutes, March 28, 1938, and "Particulars about the Present Staff at Asfuriyeh," LH/02/04, both box 3, LH, SOAS.

101. First Volume of Minutes, June 13, 1945, LH/02/04, box 3, and Minutes of the LGC, April 17, 1970, LH/02/06, box 4, both LH, SOAS.

102. Second Volume of Minutes, November 1947, LH/02/05, box 3, LH, SOAS.

103. Second Volume of Minutes, March 25, 1947, LH/02/05, and First Volume of Minutes, December 13, 1938, LH/02/04, both box 3 and LH, SOAS.

104. AR, 1956, 10, and 1957, 6, LHMND, AUB-SML.

105. Antranig Manugian, "Physician Superintendent's Report, 1956," AR, 1956, 8, LHMND, AUB-SML.

106. A. S. Manugian and G. H. Aivazian, "Mental Health in Lebanon: A Review of the Existing Problems in Lebanon and a Plea for a More Active Interest in Mental Health," *Lebanese Medical Journal* 3, no. 3 (1950): 70–80.

107. For example, see Nikolas S. Rose, *The Psychological Complex: Psychology, Politics and Society in England, 1869–1939* (London: Routledge, 1985), *Governing the Soul: The Shaping of the Private Self* (London: Routledge, 1990), and *Inventing Our Selves: Psychology, Power, and Personhood* (Cambridge: Cambridge University Press, 1996).

108. The founder of the mental hygiene movement was Clifford Whittingham Beers, who authored an influential book about his experiences as an institutionalized patient titled *A Mind That Found Itself* (New York, NY: Longmans, Green, 1908). For more information, see Nick Crossley, *Contesting Psychiatry: Social Movements in Mental Health* (London: Routledge, 2006), especially "Mental Hygiene and Early Protests: 1930–60," 61–87; Parry Manon, "From a Patient's Perspective: Clifford Whittingham Beers' Work to Reform Mental Health Services," *American Journal of Public Health* 100, no. 12 (December 2010): 2356–2357.

109. See Manugian and Aivazian, "Mental Health in Lebanon."

110. AR, 1955, 11, LHMND, AUB-SML.

111. AR, 1956, 6, LHMND, AUB-SML. See also Manugian and Aivazian, "Mental Health in Lebanon."

112. AR, 1958, 7, LHMND, AUB-SML.

113. AR, 1958, 6, LHMND, AUB-SML.

114. AR, 1957, 7, LHMND, AUB-SML.

115. AR, 1958, 6, LHMND, AUB-SML.

116. AR, 1957, 7, LHMND, AUB-SML

117. "Extract of a letter from Dr. Manugian," September 30, 1970, Minutes of the BEC, LH/03/03, box 5, LH, SOAS.

118. Minutes of the LGC, September 9, 1970, LH/02/06, box 4, LH, SOAS.

119. Antranig Manugian to Sir Geoffrey Furlonge, November 1, 1979, Minutes of the BEC, LH/03/04, box 6, LH, SOAS.

120. Minutes of the BEC, March 19, 1974, LH/03/02, box 5, LH, SOAS.

121. "Medical Director's Report," May 18, 1976, Minutes of the BEC, LH/03/03, box 5, LH, SOAS.

122. Sir Furlonge, "Note by the Chairman," Minutes of the BEC, January 15, 1976 , LH/03/03, box 5, LH, SOAS.

123. Kamal S. Salibi, *Cross Roads to Civil War: Lebanon, 1958–1976* (Delmar, NY: Caravan Books, 1976); Fawwaz Traboulsi, *A History of Modern Lebanon* (London: Pluto Press, 2007), especially 156–186.

124. Anne Russell to Dill-Russell, September 7, 1967; Lister to Douglas, July 20, 1967; Dill-Russell, July 20, 1967; Dill-Russell, confidential letter titled "Asfouriyeh Mental hospital. Beirut," April 26, 1967, all OD 34/224, TNA.

125. Dill-Russell to Miss Scurfield, April 25, 1967, OD 34/224, TNA.

126. Dill-Russell, August 17, 1967, and January 16, 1968, OD 34/224, TNA.

127. Anne Russell to Dill-Russell, September 7, 1967, OD 34/224, TNA.

128. Dill-Russell, confidential letter entitled "Asfouriyeh Mental hospital." Beirut April 26, 1967, OD 34/224, TNA.

129. Dill-Russell to Cecil King (British ambassador in Beirut), May 17, 1968, OD 34/224, TNA.

130. Ministry of Overseas Development to the British embassy in Beirut, "Confidential," January 18 or 19, 1968, and H. B. McKenzie Johnston, May 15, 1968, both OD 34/224, TNA.

131. H. B. McKenzie Johnston (ODM) to Cecil King (British ambassador in Beirut), September 9, 1968, OD 34/224, TNA.

132. H. B. McKenzie Johnston (ODM) to Cecil King.

133. Confidential letter to be circulated to the London committee signed "Llewellyn," February 29, 1968, LH/08/03, box 10, LH, SOAS. The idea to sell the land had been raised in the 1950s during a period of economic revival. See BEC minutes, January 22, 1957, and March 17, 1959, AUB-JL.

134. Antranig Manugian, July 2, 1975, Minutes of the LGC, 2, LH/02/07, box 4, LH, SOAS.

135. Subcommittee Minutes, April 10, 1973, LH/02/08, box 4, and paper on the history of the Hospital signed by the chairman of the LGC, October 8, 1976, Minutes of the BEC, LH/03/03, box 5, both LH, SOAS.

136. Subcommittee Minutes, April 10 and 17, 1973, LH/02/08, box 4, LH, SOAS.

137. Subcommittee Minutes, May 29, 1974, LH/02/08, box 4, LH, SOAS.

138. Second Volume of Minutes, January 20, 1951, LH/02/05, box 3, LH, SOAS.

139. "The Medical Director's Report for the Year 1974," July 15, 1975, Minutes of the BEC, LH/03/03, box 5, LH, SOAS.

140. See Salibi, *Cross Roads to Civil War,* especially 90–108; Traboulsi, *A History of Modern Lebanon,* especially 186–189.

141. Antun Salih, a graduate of the SPC, replaced Otto Wolff when the latter was on furlough. Salih was also appointed temporary visiting physician until the appointment of Watson Smith as medical director in 1909. Sami Haddad, another graduate of the SPC, became acting director of the Hospital in the absence of the director in 1919. See AR, 1902, 21, and 1909, 26, report for the year 1919, LHMND, AUB-SML.

142. Richa, *La psychiatrie au Liban,* 175–177.

143. Richa, *La psychiatrie au Liban,* 36–737. More recently, two psychiatrists—John Racy and Herant Katchadourian, who both trained at ʿAṣfūriyyeh in the 1950s as part of their medical training at AUB—are today recognized in the US as distinguished experts in their respective fields. Racy was elected Distinguished Life Fellow of the American Psychiatric Association and is a professor of psychiatry and assistant dean of student affairs at the University of Arizona College of Medicine. Katchadourian has received numerous awards and is a popular mentor and emeritus professor of psychiatry and human biology at Stanford University. For more on Katchadourian, see Angelique Dakkak, "Q&A: Professor Katchadourian Talks Hookup Culture," *Stanford Daily,* March 24, 2014.

4 Patriarchal Power and the Gospel of the Modern Care of Insanity

1. Bayard Dodge, AR, 1933–1934, n.p., LHMND, AUB-SML.

2. However, it is worth remembering that this iconography of the mentally ill is part of the clinical tools and positivist methods used to describe, categorize, and diagnose insanity. The most famous user and creator of such iconography is, of course, Jean-Martin Charcot, chief physician at the Salpêtrière. For more, see Georges Didi-Huberman, *Invention de l'hystérie - Charcot et l'iconographie photographique de la Salpêtrière* (Paris: Macula, 1982).

3. Charles E. Rosenberg, "The Tyranny of Diagnosis: Specific Entities and Individual Experience," *Milbank Quarterly* 80, no. 2 (2002): 237–260.

4. Michel de Certeau, *L'écriture de l'histoire* (Paris: Gallimard, 1975), 284.

5. See Marcel Gauchet and Gladys Swain, *La pratique de l'esprit humain: L'institution asilaire et la révolution démocratique* (Paris: Gallimard, 1980).

6. Theophilus Waldmeier, AR, 1900, 18, LHMND, AUB-SML.

7. Otto Wolff, "Brief Notes of the Cases," AR, 1901, 16, LHMND, AUB-SML.

8. Theophilus Waldmeier, "Report of the Lebanon Hospital for the Insane for the year 1903–4," AR, 1904, 18, LHMND, AUB-SML.

9. Theophilus Waldmeier, *The Autobiography of Theophilus Waldmeier, Comprising Ten Years in Abyssinia and Forty-Six Years in Syria, with Some Description of the People and Religions of These Countries*, edited by Stephen Hobhouse (London: Friends' Bookshop, 1925), 296–297 (hereafter, *The Autobiography of Theophilus Waldmeier*).

10. Case nos. 1–25, 1900, patient records, LHMND, AUB-SML.

11. Case no. 11, 1900, patient records, LHMND, AUB-SML.

12. For an account of the persecution and ultimate death of As'ad al-Shidyaq at the hands of the Maronite church, see Butrus al-Bustani, *Qiṣṣat As'ad Al-Shidyāq* (Beirut: n.p., 1860); Ussama Makdisi, *Artillery of Heaven: American Missionaries and the Failed Conversion of the Middle East* (Ithaca, NY: Cornell University Press, 2008), especially 180–213.

13. Waldmeier, *The Autobiography of Theophilus Waldmeier*, 228–244.

14. Case no. 157, 1903, patient records, LHMND, AUB-SML.

15. Daniel Oliver, "Asfuriyeh," *Friend*, January 8, 1904, RET 8/3/1, UY-BIA.

16. Oliver, "Asfuriyeh," n.p.

17. Quoted in AR 1903, 18, LHMND, AUB-SML.

18. AR, 1901, 14–15, LHMND, AUB-SML.

19. AR, 1901, 7, and 1905, 17, LHMND, AUB-SML.

20. Henry Harris Jessup, *Fifty-Three Years in Syria* (New York: Fleming H. Revell, 1910), 2: 523.

21. Minutes of the LGC, June 14, 1901, 41, LH/02/01, box 2, LH, SOAS.

22. AR, 1938, 8, LHMND, AUB-SML.

23. Data on the percentages of patients who had been working or not upon admission in 1900–1946 were compiled from ARs.

24. Herant A. Katchadourian and John Racy, "The Diagnostic Distribution of Treated Psychiatric Illness in Lebanon," *British Journal of Psychiatry* 115, no. 528 (1969): 1315.

25. Harry Thwaites, "Medical Officer's Report," AR, 1908, 25, LHMND, AUB-SML.

26. Quoted in "The Lebanon Hospital, Asfuriyeh, Syria," *British Journal of Psychiatry* 74, no. 305 (April 1, 1928): 343.

27. AR, 1914–1915, 4, LHMND, AUB-SML.

28. Albert Hourani and Nadim Shehadi, eds., *The Lebanese in the World: A Century of Emigration* (London: Centre for Lebanese Studies, 1992); Akram Fouad Khater, *Inventing Home: Emigration, Gender, and the Middle Class in Lebanon, 1870–1920* (Berkeley: University of California Press, 2001).

29. House of Commons, *Report of the Inter-Departmental Committee on Physical Deterioration* (London: HM Stationery Office, 1904), vol. 1.

30. Quoted in House of Commons, *Report of the Inter-Departmental Committee on Physical Deterioration*, 1:356.

31. Thwaites, "Medical Officer's Report," AR, 1907, 42, LHMND, AUB-SML. See also "Insanity in Palestine," *British Medical Journal* 2, no. 2435 (August 31, 1907): 543.

32. Waldmeier, *The Autobiography of Theophilus Waldmeier*, 314–315.

33. Case nos. 1–25, 1900, patient records, LHMND, AUB-SML; "Insanity in Palestine," 542–543.

34. "Insanity in Palestine," 543.

35. Thwaites, "The Doctor's Report," AR, 1906, 24, LHMND, AUB-SML.

36. AR, 1907, 42–43, LHMND, AUB-SML.

37. "Insanity in Palestine," 543.

38. AR, 1907, 42, LHMND, AUB-SML.

39. AR, 1907, 43, LHMND, AUB-SML.

40. Thwaites, "Medical Officer's Report,"AR, 1908, 23, LHMND, AUB-SML.

41. The history of the emergence of the concept of schizophrenia (a term coined by Eugen Bleuler in 1911) and its displacement of dementia praecox is convoluted. See German E. Berrios, Rogelio Luque, and José M. Villagrán, "Schizophrenia: A Conceptual History," *International Journal of Psychology and Psychological Therapy* 3, no. 2 (2003): 111–140; German E. Berrios, *The History of Mental Symptoms: Descriptive Psychopathology since the Nineteenth Century* (Cambridge: Cambridge University Press, 1996), 189; Edward Shorter, *A Historical Dictionary of Psychiatry* (New York: Oxford University Press, 2005), 267–268.

42. Berrios, *The History of Mental Symptoms*, especially 289–331; Allan V. Horwitz and Jerome C. Wakefield, *The Loss of Sadness: How Psychiatry Transformed Normal Sorrow into Depressive Disorder* (Oxford: Oxford University Press, 2007); David Healy, *Mania: A Short History of Bipolar Disorder* (Baltimore, MD: Johns Hopkins University Press, 2008).

43. Thwaites, "Medical Officer's Report," AR, 1908, 23, LHMND, AUB-SML.

44. John S. Billings, *Report on the Insane, Feeble-Minded, Deaf and Dumb, and Blind in the United States at the Eleventh Census, 1890* (Washington: Government Printing Office, 1895), 21.

45. John Racy, "Psychiatry in the Arab East," in *Psychological Dimensions of Near Eastern Studies*, ed. L. Carl Brown and Norman Itzkowitz (Princeton, NJ: Darwin Press, 1977), 294 and 320.

46. Racy, "Psychiatry in the Arab East," 320.

47. Thwaites, "Medical Officer's Report," AR, 1907, 42, LHMND, AUB-SML.

48. Watson Smith, "Medical Officer's Report," AR, 1908, 31, LHMND, AUB-SML.

49. Elaine Showalter, *The Female Malady: Women, Madness, and English Culture, 1830–1980* (New York: Pantheon Books, 1985).

50. A. Motet, "Rapport sur un projet de loi sur les aliénés en Turquie par M. Mongeri," *Annales médico-psychologique* 17 (1877): 88.

51. Quoted in AR, 1907, 9, LHMND, AUB-SML.

52. AR, 1903, 13, LHMND, AUB-SML.

53. Michel Foucault, *Les anormaux: Cours au Collège de France, 1974–1975* (Paris: Éditions de l'École des Études en Sciences Sociales Gallimard Seuil, 1999).

54. Thwaites, "Medical Officer's Report," AR, 1907, 40, AUB-SML, LHMND.

55. G. H. Aivazian, "Medico-Legal Aspects of Psychiatry in Lebanon; with a Review of Some Justice Cases," *Lebanese Medical Journal* 6, no. 1 (January 1953): 37.

56. Aivazian, "Medico-Legal Aspects of Psychiatry in Lebanon," 39.

57. AR, 1959, 5–6, LHMND, AUB-SML.

58. AR, 1961, 2, LHMND, AUB-SML. Also see "R. A. Mickelwright's Report on his Visit to the Hospital," October 1963–January 1964, LH/12/01, box 16, LH, SOAS; A. S. Manugian, "Physician Superintendent's Report," 1961, 2, LHMND, AUB-SML.

59. AR, 1961, 4, LHMND, AUB-SML.

60. Michel Foucault, *Histoire de la folie à l'âge classique: Folie et déraison* (Paris: Librairie Plon, 1961) and *Surveiller et punir : Naissance de la prison* (Paris: Gallimard, 1975); Thomas Stephen Szasz, *The Myth of Mental Illness: Foundations of a Theory of Personal Conduct* (New York: Hoeber-Harper, 1961); Franco Basaglia, *L'Istituzione Negata* (Torino, Italy: Einaudi, 1968).

61. AR, 1951, 7, LHMND, AUB-SML; George Shéhadé, "Le petit univers d'Asfourieh s'en va," *L'Hebdo Magazine*, February 13, 1958, 30–33. The role of psychiatry in prisons remains problematic, however, and the line between treatment and punishment

is perpetually blurred. See Michel Bertrand and Maurice David, eds., *Soigner et/ou punir: Questionnement sur l'évolution, le sens et les perspectives de la psychiatrie en prison* (Paris: L'Harmattan, 1996).

62. See Najwa al-Qattan, "Safarbarlik: Ottoman Syria and the Great War," in *From the Syrian Land to the States of Syria and Lebanon*, ed. Thomas Philipp and Christoph Schumann (Würzburg, Germany: Ergon, 2004), 163–173.

63. AR, 1917–1918, 3, LHMND, AUB-SML.

64. AR, 1917–1918, 3, LHMND, AUB-SML.

65. AR, 1920–1921, 2–3, LHMND, AUB-SML.

66. Shell shock was a disorder that was initially associated with war, albeit under different names—such as "*vent de boulet*" during the French Revolution and Napoleonic wars, "Da Costa's irritable heart" during the US Civil War, and "*Kriegsneurose*" after the Russo-Japanese War. The diagnosis would eventually widen to include broader cases of psychological and physical trauma that were not related to the battlefield. See Marc-Antoine Crocq and Louis Crocq, "From Shell Shock and War Neurosis to Posttraumatic Stress Disorder: A History of Psychotraumatology," *Dialogues in Clinical Neuroscience* 2, no. 1 (March 2000): 47–55. In 1980, the war neuroses were renamed post-traumatic stress disorder in the third edition of the *DSM*.

67. AR, 1920–1921, 3, LHMND, AUB-SML.

68. AR, 1924–1925, 2, LHMND, AUB-SML.

69. Watson Smith mentions the letter from General Gouraud in "Medical Particulars,"AR, 1919–1920, 1, LHMND, AUB-SML; Letter of thanks from E. Allenby, General Commander in Chief of the Egyptian Expeditionary Force, December 1918, LH/02/02, box 2, LH, SOAS.

70. AR, 1940, 8, and table 6, 12, LHMND, AUB-SML. It must be noted that while the report of the medical superintendent mentions 122 military cases, table 6 refers to 100 such cases.

71. R. Stewart Miller, "Report of the Medical Superintendent," AR, 1940, 8, LHMND, AUB-SML.

72. See Allan M. Brandt, *No Magic Bullet: A Social History of Venereal Disease in the United States since 1880* (New York: Oxford University Press, 1985).

73. Frank Fenner, *Nature, Nurture and Chance: The Lives of Frank and Charles Fenner* (Canberra: ANU Press, 2006).

74. Fenner, *Nature, Nurture and Chance*, 31.

75. Fenner, *Nature, Nurture and Chance*, 29.

76. Fenner, *Nature, Nurture and Chance*, 31.

77. Elias S. Srouji, *Cyclamens from Galilee: Memoirs of a Physician from Nazareth* (Lincoln, NE: iUniverse, Inc., 2003), 106–107.

78. AR, 1941, 7, LHMND, AUB-SML.

79. AR, 1944, 4 and 7, LHMND, AUB-SML.

80. AR, 1946, 7, LHMND, AUB-SML. Also see Minutes of the LGC, April 13, 1921, 182, LH/02/02, box 2, LH, SOAS.

81. Waltraud Ernst, *Mad Tales from the Raj: The European Insane in British India, 1800–1858* (London: Routledge, 1991); Frantz Fanon, *Écrits sur l'aliénation et la liberté*, ed. Jean Khalfa and Robert Young (Paris: La Découverte, 2015), 155.

82. First Volume of Minutes, Item number 281, January 16, 1940, LH/02/04, box 3, LH, SOAS.

83. AR, 1944, 4, LHMND, AUB-SML. The United Nations Relief and Rehabilitation Administration was an international relief agency that was founded in 1943 in a conference that brought together forty-four countries under the aegis of the United States. Its primary responsibility was health work, but it also assisted in the repatriation of millions of refugees and managed hundreds of displaced persons after the Second World War. It was dissolved in 1946, and its functions related to sanitation were transferred to the Interim Commission of the WHO on December 1, 1946.

84. AR, 1944, 7, LHMND, AUB-SML.

85. AR, 1945, 1, LHMND, AUB-SML.

86. Second Volume of Minutes, September 13, 1950, LH/0/05, box 3, LH, SOAS.

87. AR, 1948, 5, and 1960, 9, LHMND, AUB-SML. The refugees' fees were covered by the United Nations Relief and Works Agency for Palestine Refugees in the Near East (UNRWA).

88. For more information, see Adel A. Freiha, *L'armée et l'état au Liban, 1945–1980* (Paris: Librairie Générale de Droit et de Jurisprudence, 1980), 166; Stéphane Malsagne, "L'armée libanaise de 1945 à 1975," *Vingtième siècle. Revue d'histoire* 124, no. 4 (September 7, 2014): 15–31.

89. AR, 1946, 7, LHMND, AUB-SML.

90. AR, 1956, 7, LHMND, AUB-SML.

91. "Implications of the War on Hospitals," minute no. 222, Minutes of the BEC, October 16, 1973, 2, LH/03/02, box 5, LH, SOAS.

92. Antranig Manugian, "Medical Director's Report to the BEC," January 18, 1977, Minutes of the BEC, LH/03/03, box 5, LH, SOAS.

93. "Developments since Our Meeting on 25th May, 1982," Minutes of the BEC, LH/08/23, box 14, LH, SOAS.

94. AR, 1926–1927, 30, LHMND, AUB-SML; "Hospital and Dispensary Management: Lebanon Hospital for the Insane," *British Medical Journal* 2, no. 2429 (July 20, 1907): 183.

95. Waldmeier, *The Autobiography of Theophilus Waldmeier*, 313. See also Henry M. Wetherill, "The Insane in Some Remote Lands," in *Ninth Report of the Committee on Lunacy of the Board of Public Charities of the Commonwealth of Pennsylvania* (Harrisburg, PA: Edwin K. Meyers, 1891), 167. For an exhaustive history of the circulation of such substances and their use in medieval Islam, see Sami Hamarneh, "Pharmacy in Medieval Islam and the History of Drug Addiction," *Medical History* 16 (1972): 226–37.

96. Waldmeier, *The Autobiography of Theophilus Waldmeier*, 314.

97. V. R. Puzantian, "Editorial: Problem of Drug Addiction in Lebanon," *Lebanese Medical Journal* 26, no. 3 (1973): 211–213; Herant A. Katchadourian and Jeffrey V. Sutherland, "Psychiatric Aspects of Drug Addiction in Lebanon," *Substance Use and Misuse* 10, no. 6 (1975): 949–962. See also A. Yazbek, "Le trafic de la drogue et la lutte contre les stupéfiants au Liban," *Annales de la faculté de droit de Beyrouth* 35 (1961): 205–223.

98. "La Suisse du Moyen-Orient: Le Liban prend une importance croissante en Méditerranée Orientale," *Le Monde diplomatique*, November 1957, 7, https://www.monde-diplomatique.fr/1957/11/A/22376.

99. Jonathan Marshall, *The Lebanese Connection: Corruption, Civil War, and the International Drug Traffic* (Stanford, CA: Stanford University Press, 2012), especially 14–58.

100. See Michael C. Hudson, *The Precarious Republic: Political Modernization in Lebanon* (Boulder, CO: Westview Press, 1985).

101. The data on patients in 1952–1960 are based on a representative sample of patient records, see "Notes."

102. Charles Baddoura, "Toxicomanie au Liban," *Bulletin de l'Académie nationale de médecine* 176, no. 9 (1992): 1506. Also see Marshall, *The Lebanese Connection*.

103. Yazbek, "Le trafic de la drogue," 219.

104. Yazbek, "Le trafic de la drogue," 219.

105. AR, 1961, 2 and 4, LHMND, AUB-SML.

106. Katchadourian and Sutherland, "Psychiatric Aspects of Drug Addiction in Lebanon," 960.

107. Anonymous inmate of Webster House, personal communication, November 10, 2016.

108. Katchadourian and Sutherland, "Psychiatric Aspects of Drug Addiction in Lebanon," 959–961.

109. Katchadourian and Sutherland, "Psychiatric Aspects of Drug Addiction in Lebanon," 960.

110. Anonymous inmate of Webster House, personal communication, November 10, 2016. Swedenburg passed away on October 16, 2016.

111. AR, 1959, 11, LHMND, AUB-SML.

112. Katchadourian and Sutherland, "Psychiatric Aspects of Drug Addiction in Lebanon," 949; Marshall, *The Lebanese Connection*, 16; Karine Bennafla, "Le développement au péril de la géopolitique: L'exemple de la plaine de la Békaa (Liban)," *Géocarrefour*, 81, no. 4 (2006), April 1, 2010, https://doi.org/10.4000/geocarrefour.1644.

113. Katchadourian and Sutherland, "Psychiatric Aspects of Drug Addiction in Lebanon," 950.

114. Marshall, *The Lebanese Connection*, especially 14–58.

115. Katchadourian and Sutherland, "Psychiatric Aspects of Drug Addiction in Lebanon," 950–951. Baddoura similarly observed that 23 percent of patients treated in the 1970s and 1980s were from "the lower socioeconomic class" ("Toxicomanie au Liban," 1510).

116. Baddoura, "Toxicomanie au Liban"; Marshall, *The Lebanese Connection*, especially 75–112.

117. Charles Baddoura, "Santé mentale et guerre libanaise," *Bulletin de l'Académie nationale de médecine* 174, no. 5 (May 1990): 587. Also see Didier Bigo and Annie Laurent, "Guerre et drogue au Liban. Entretien avec Antoine Boustany," *Cultures & Conflits*, no. 3 (October 17 1991), https://doi.org/10.4000/conflits.2015.

118. Darina Al-Joundi and Mohamed Kacimi, *Le jour où Nina Simone a cessé de chanter* (Arles, France: Actes Sud, 2008), 112, 121, and 126–127.

119. Baddoura, "Toxicomanie au Liban," 1505–1514, and "Santé mentale et guerre libanaise," 587. See also Bigo and Laurent, "Guerre et drogue au Liban," 4; Adnan Houbballah, *Le virus de la violence: La guerre civile est en chacun de nous* (Paris: Albin Michel, 1996), especially 121–131.

120. Baddoura, "Santé mentale et guerre libanaise," 587; Bigo and Laurent, "Guerre et drogue au Liban," 3. Bernard Lewis's history of the Isma'ili sect has been recently deconstructed by Farhad Daftary. See Bernard Lewis, *The Assassins: A Radical Sect in Islam* (New York: Basic Books, 1967); Farhad Daftary, *The Assassin Legends: Myths of the Isma'ilis* (London: I. B. Tauris, 1994).

121. See Andrew Scull, *Hysteria: The Biography* (Oxford: Oxford University Press, 2009).

122. Benoît Boyer, *Conditions hygiéniques actuelles de Beyrouth (Syrie), et de ses environs immédiats* (Lyon, France: Rey, 1897), 130–131.

123. For the orientalist interpretation of Boyer's medical discourse, see Jens Hanssen, *Fin de Siècle Beirut: The Making of an Ottoman Provincial Capital* (Oxford: Clarendon Press of Oxford University Press, 2005), 132.

124. Wadīʿ Effendi Riz'allah Al-Barbārī, "Muʿālajat al-Junūn fi-l-Nisā' al-ʿAṣabiyyāt wal-Muṣābāt bel-Histīriā," *at-Ṭabīb* (June 1895): 10.

125. Hysteria continued to account for 6 percent of all psychiatric diseases in 1967 at the Hôpital Psychiatrique de la Croix, ʿAṣfūriyyeh's rival institution. See A. Habib, "Aspect de l'hystérie au Liban," *Journal médical libanais* 20, no. 3 (June 1967): 182.

126. Habib, "Aspect de l'hystérie au Liban."

127. Carroll Smith-Rosenberg, *Disorderly Conduct: Visions of Gender in Victorian America* (New York: Oxford University Press, 1986).

128. Carroll Smith-Rosenberg, "The Hysterical Woman: Sex Roles and Role Conflict in 19th Century America," *Social Research* 39, no. 4 (1972): 678.

129. John Racy, personal communication, July 1, 2014; Katchadourian, *The Way It Turned Out* (Singapore: Pan Stanford Publishing, 2012), 122 and 174. They both graduated from AUB Medical School and pursued their psychiatric training at the University of Rochester, in New York.

130. Katchadourian and Racy, "The Diagnostic Distribution of Treated Psychiatric Illness in Lebanon."

131. M. Piccinelli and F. Gomez Homen, *Gender Differences in the Epidemiology of Affective Disorders and Schizophrenia* (Geneva: World Health Organization, 1997), especially 61–110. For a useful summary of the scientific debate, see Steven O. Moldin, "Gender and Schizophrenia: An Overview," in *Gender and Its Effects on Psychopathology*, ed. Ellen Frank (Washington: American Psychiatric Press, 2000), 169–186.

132. Rose Ghorayeb, "May Ziadeh (1886–1941)," *Signs* 5, no. 2 (December 1, 1979): 375–382; Carmen Boustani, "May Ziadé: Vie et écriture," *Les Cahiers du GRIF* 43, no. 1 (1990): 163–169; Antje Ziegler, "Al-Haraka Baraka! The Late Rediscovery of Mayy Ziyādah's Works," *Die Welt des Islams* 39, no. 1 (1999): 103–115; Butheina Khaldi, *Egypt Awakening in the Early Twentieth Century: Mayy Ziyādah's Intellectual Circles* (New York: Palgrave Macmillan, 2012).

133. Salma al-Ḥaffār Al-Kuzbarī, *Mayy Ziyādah aw Ma'sāt al-Nubūgh* (Beirut: Mu'assasat Nawfal, 1987), 2: 161.

134. "Memorandum of Dr. Webster's Informal Address to the General Committee on June 2, 1938 at the Office," 1-5 (hereafter, "Memorandum of Dr. Webster"), October 21, 1938, LH/02/04, box 3, LH, SOAS.

135. Salāmah Mūsa, *Tarbiyat Salāmah Mūsa* (Cairo: Hindawi, 2014). Originally published in Arabic in 1941, an English translation was published under the title *The Education of Salamah Musa*, trans. Lein Oebele Schuman (Leiden: Brill, 1961).

136. Case no. 5397, patient records, LHMND, AUB-SML. Emil Kraepelin considered "involutional melancholia" to be a subset of manic-depressive illness and defined it as a form of "agitated depressions occurring for the first time in life after the age 45–55 in contrast to manic-depressive illness which manifest[s] itself at an early age." See Berrios, *The History of Mental Symptoms*, 311.

137. Al-Kuzbarī, *Mayy Ziyādah aw Ma'sāt al-Nubūgh*; Mūsa, *Tarbiyat Salāmah Mūsa*, 225–230.

138. Mūsa, *Tarbiyat Salāmah Mūsa*, 146 and 227–228.

139. Khālid Muḥammad Ghāzī, *Mayy Ziyādah: Sīrat Ḥayātuhā wa-Adabuhā wa-Awrāq lam Tunshar* (Cairo: Wakālat al-Ṣaḥāfah al-ʿArabiyyah, 2015), 175.

140. "Memorandum of Dr. Webster."

141. "Memorandum of Dr. Webster." See also Mayy Ziyādah, *Mayy Ziyādah Fī Mudhakkirātihā* (Beirut: Dār al-Rīḥānī lil-Ṭibāʿah wa-al-Nashr, 1950), especially 185–92; Al-Kuzbarī, *Mayy Ziyādah aw Ma'sāt al-Nubūgh;* Edmond Melhem, "Saving May: The Story of How Saʿadeh Tried to Save May Ziadeh from the Ghoul," *al-Mashriq: A Quarterly Journal of Middle East Studies* 1, no. 3 (2002).

142. "Memorandum of Dr. Webster."

143. Quoted in "Memorandum of Dr. Webster," 2.

144. Quoted in "Memorandum of Dr. Webster,"2.

145. "A la Chambre, la session extraordinaire a été clôturée hier," *Le Jour*, March 1, 1938, newspaper clipping, LHMND, AUB-SML.

146. "Memorandum of Dr. Webster"; AR, 1938, 10, LHMND, AUB-SML.

147. "Où en est l'enquête sur l'Asile d'Asfourieh?," newspaper clipping, *L'Orient*, March 2, 1938, LHMND, AUB-SML.

148. Subcommittee Minutes, October 1, 1913, LH/02/08, box 3, LH, SOAS.

149. AR, 1922–1923, 2, and 1917–1918, 2, LHMND, AUB-SML.

150. AR, 1938, 11, LHMND, AUB-SML.

151. Visitors' book, LHMND, AUB-SML.

152. One case was still making its way through the Lebanese courts in 2020 (Hilda Nassar, personal communication, March 26, 2020).

153. BEC Minutes, May 5, 1955, LHMND, AUB-SML.

154. At least four attendants were fined and their behavior reported to the Ministry of Social Affairs for "ill treating" patients, "neglect of duty to patients," laziness, drunkenness, violence, lewd language, and failure to report to duty, among other things. See "Re: H. N., Incident Requiring Disciplinary Action," March 19, 1953; "Re: M. H.," 1954; "Re: S. T.," October 21, 1953; and "Re: Y. B.," March 19, 1953. In her report on the infliction of a corporal injury on a female patient in August 1956, the matron concluded that the accuser (the patient) deserved "the benefit of the doubt." See "Statement Regarding the Death of E. N., a Prisoner in R. H. Who Died of Barbiturate Poisoning," May 22, 1959, court cases (only initials are given out of concern for patient confidentiality), LHMND, AUB-SML.

155. Al-Joundi and Kacimi, *Le jour où Nina Simone a cessé de chanter*, 142–158.

156. Al-Joundi, *Le jour où Nina Simone a cessé de chanter*, 151–152.

157. Darina Al-Joundi, *Prisonnière du Levant: La vie méconnue de May Ziadé* (Paris: Grasset, 2017).

158. This was according to the 1932 Lebanese Code of Obligations and Contracts (*Qanūn al-Mūjibāt wal-ʿUqūd*).

159. Habermas rather speaks of second-order "reflexiveness" and "concepts," but I think second-order criticism fits well in his critical theory. See Peter Dews, ed., *Autonomy and Solidarity: Interviews with Jürgen Habermas* (London: Verso, 1992), 254; Jürgen Habermas, *The Philosophical Discourse of Modernity: Twelve Lectures* (Cambridge, MA: MIT Press, 1987), 116.

160. Miriam Cooke, "Telling Their Lives: A Hundred Years of Arab Women's Writings," *World Literature Today* 60, no. 2 (April 1, 1986), 212.

161. Mūsa, *Tarbiyat Salāmah Mūsa*, 229.

162. For example, see Stephen Trombley, *"All That Summer She Was Mad": Virginia Woolf and Her Doctors* (London: Junction Books, 1981).

163. Ghorayeb, "May Ziadeh (1886–1941)."

164. Al-Kuzbarī, *Mayy Ziyādah aw Ma'sāt al-Nubūgh*, 2:230–231.

165. Hisham Sharabi, *Neopatriarchy: Theory of Distorted Change in Arab Society* (Oxford: Oxford University Press, 1988), especially 1–25.

166. Hanssen, *Fin de Siècle Beirut*, 135; see also 133–136.

167. Hanssen, *Fin de Siècle Beirut*, 135.

168. The numbers of patients increased after 1935 on an annual basis, reaching 1,011 patients in 1962 (data compiled from AR, 1900–1962, AUB-SML). For an estimation of the population, see Roger Owen, *The Middle East in the World Economy, 1800–1914* (London: Methuen, 1981), especially 244–272.

169. Data on the regional distribution of the admitted patient population in 1900–1916 were compiled from ARs, AUB-SML.

170. At ʿAṣfūriyyeh, members of the immediate family usually initiated the process of hospitalization—as was the case in many North American mental hospitals. See Gerald N. Grob, *Mental Illness and American Society, 1875–1940* (Princeton, NJ: Princeton University Press, 1983), 9.

171. AR, 1960, 3, LHMND, AUB-SML. For more on Chehab, see Kamal Salibi, "Lebanon under Fuad Chehab 1958–1964," *Middle Eastern Studies* 2, no. 3 (1966): 211–226; Stéphane Malsagne, *Fouad Chéhab, 1902–1973: Une figure oubliée de l'histoire libanaise* (Paris: Karthala, 2011).

172. Manugian, "Physician Superintendent's Report," AR, 1960, 3, LHMND, AUB-SML.

173. See Richard C. Keller, *Colonial Madness: Psychiatry in French North Africa* (Chicago: University of Chicago Press, 2007), especially 19–46.

174. Waldmeier, *The Autobiography of Theophilus Waldmeier*, 309.

175. Waldmeier, *The Autobiography of Theophilus Waldmeier*, 315.

176. Waldmeier, *The Autobiography of Theophilus Waldmeier*, 315.

177. Waldmeier, *The Autobiography of Theophilus Waldmeier*, 310.

178. Theophilus Waldmeier, *Appeal for the First Home of the Insane on Mount Lebanon* (London: Headley Brothers, 1897), 13, LHMND, AUB-SML. For more on Heinroth, see H. Steinberg, "Die Geburt des Wortes, 'Psychosomatisch' in der Medizinischen Weltliteratur durch Johann Christian August Heinroth," *Fortschritte der Neurologie und Psychiatrie* 75, no. 7 (October 2007): 413–417. Antoine Porot—the founder of the Algiers School of Psychiatry—saw himself as the liberator of the Maghreb in the same vein. See Keller, *Colonial Madness*, especially 19–46.

179. AR, 1935–1936, 25, and 1945, 2, LHMND, AUB-SML.

180. AR, 1911–1912, 4, LHMND, AUB-SML.

181. AR, 1915–1916, 4, LHMND, AUB-SML.

182. AR, 1935–1936, 25, LHMND, AUB-SML.

183. AR, 1911–1912, 4, LHMND, AUB-SML.

184. AR, 1906, 23, LHMND, AUB-SML.

185. AR, 1961, 1, LHMND, AUB-SML.

186. AR 1938, verso, LHMND, AUB-SML.

187. "Lebanon Hospital for Mental Diseases, Notes for December 20th, 1948," records, LHMND, AUB-SML.

188. AR, 1924–1925, 2, LHMND, AUB-SML.

189. AR, 1902, 15, and 1906, 16, LHMND, AUB-SML.

190. Theophilus Waldmeier, "The Founder's Report,"AR, 1908, 18, LHMND, AUB-SML.

191. Quoted in AR, 1907, 32, LHMND, AUB-SML.

192. AR, 1936, 2; 1937, 3; and 1938, 3, LHMND, AUB-SML.

193. John Racy, *Psychiatry in the Arab East* (Copenhagen: Munksgaard, 1970), 37.

194. AR, 1908, 26, and 1929–1930, 21, LHMND, AUB-SML. Syphilis is another disease with a long history. Before the discovery of the causative agent in 1905 and antibiotic treatment in 1943, the disease was known as the "general paresis of the insane" or "dementia paralytica." For more on syphilis, see Brandt, *No Magic Bullet*; Claude Quétel, *Le mal de Naples: Histoire de la syphilis* (Paris: Seghers, 1986).

195. Manfred Sakel, the Austrian psychiatrist who popularized the use of the therapy, performed it for the first time in Vienna in 1934. See Edward Shorter and David Healy, *Shock Therapy: A History of Electroconvulsive Treatment in Mental Illness* (New Brunswick, NJ: Rutgers University Press, 2007), especially 9–30.

196. R. Stewart Miller, "Report of the Medical Director,"AR, 1937, 7, LHMND, AUB-SML.

197. R. Stewart Miller, "Report of the Medical Director,"AR, 1938, 9, LHMND, AUB-SML.

198. AR, 1937, 7, and 1945, 2, LHMND, AUB-SML. For Ugo Cerlutti's first use of electroconvulsive therapy on a patient and its globalization, see Shorter and Healy, *Shock Therapy*, especially 31–48.

199. "Lebanon Hospital for Mental Diseases." See also AR, 1948, 7, LHMND, AUB-SML.

200. Nobel Prize official website, "The Nobel Prize in Physiology or Medicine 1949," https://www.nobelprize.org/prizes/medicine/1949/summary/. For the rise and fall of lobotomy, see Jack David Pressman, *Last Resort: Psychosurgery and the Limits of Medicine* (Cambridge: Cambridge University Press, 1998).

201. Rakefet Zalashik and Nadav Davidovitch, "Last Resort? Lobotomy Operations in Israel, 1946–60," *History of Psychiatry* 17, no. 1 (2006): 95.

202. A. S. Manugian and Medical Staff, "Medical Report," AR, 1954, 13, LHMND, AUB-SML.

203. Such is Pressman's argument (*Last Resort*). Also see V. W. Swayze, "Frontal Leukotomy and Related Psychosurgical Procedures in the Era before Antipsychotics (1935–1954): A Historical Overview," *American Journal of Psychiatry* 152, no. 4 (April 1995): 505–515. On the pharmacological revolution, see David Healy, *The*

Antidepressant Era (Cambridge, MA: Harvard University Press, 1997) and *The Creation of Psychopharmacology* (Cambridge, MA: Harvard University Press, 2002).

204. A. S. Manugian, "Clinical Director's Report" AR, 1955, 15, LHMND, AUB-SML.

205. For a discussion of the contested history of chlorpromazine, see Healy, *The Creation of Psychopharmacology*, especially 76–128.

206. Foucault, *Histoire de la folie à l'âge classique*, 56.

207. Manugian, "Physician Superintendent's Report," AR, 1958, 8, LHMND, AUB-SML.

208. AR, 1959, 11, LHMND, AUB-SML.

209. Keller, *Colonial Madness*.

210. W. M. Ford Robertson, "Medical Director's Report," AR, 1954, 11, LHMND, AUB-SML.

211. AR, 1958, 8, LHMND, AUB-SML.

212. Manugian, "Physician Superintendent's Report," AR, 1956, 8, LHMND, AUB-SML.

213. AR, 1957, 6, LHMND, AUB-SML.

214. Manugian, "Physician Superintendent's Report," AR, 1961, 2, LHMND, AUB-SML.

215. AR, 1957, 8–9, LHMND, AUB-SML.

216. AR, 1914–1915, 1, LHMND, AUB-SML.

217. AR, 1935–1936, 23, and 1936, 20–21, LHMND, AUB-SML.

218. The Magistrate Civil Court at Baabda, letter presenting the case, the incident, and the legal statement, February 19, 1957, LHMND, AUB-SML.

219. Admission and discharge rates based on ARs 1900–1962.

220. AR, 1957, 8–9, LHMND, AUB-SML.

221. AR, 1931–1932, 17–18, LHMND, AUB-SML.

222. AR, 1908, 26, and 1909, 34, LHMND, AUB-SML.

5 The Downfall of ʿAṣfūriyyeh and the Breakdown of the State

1. Only a few works have documented and examined the impact of war on psychiatric hospitals or the ways in which patients in such institutions made sense of their psychosomatic ailments and of war itself. These works have tended to focus on the two world wars and their aftermaths. See Isabelle von Bueltzingsloewen, *L'hécatombe des fous: La famine dans les hôpitaux psychiatriques français sous l'occupation* (Paris: Éditions Aubier, 2007); Armand Ajzenberg and André Castelli, *L'abandon à la mort … de*

76 000 fous par le régime de Vichy; suivi de, Un hôpital psychiatrique sous Vichy (Paris: L'Harmattan, 2012); Stéphane Tison, "Loin du front, la folie? Les civils internés à l'asile durant la grande guerre," *Guerres Mondiales et Conflits Contemporains*, 1, no. 257 (March 16, 2015): 13–36. Another exception is Frantz Fanon's analysis of noncombatant patients traumatized by Algeria's war of independence at the Blida psychiatric hospital outside Algiers (*Les damnés de la terre* [Paris: Éditions la Découverte, 1963], especially 200–250).

2. See Human Rights Watch, "Still No Justice for Thousands 'Disappeared' in Lebanon's Civil War," August 30, 2017, https://www.hrw.org/news/2017/08/30/still-no-justice-thousands-disappeared-lebanons-civil-war.

3. See Médecins Sans Frontières USA, "Special Report: In Syria, Medicine as a Weapon of Persecution," February 8, 2012, https://www.msf.org/syria-medicine-used-weapon-persecution; Ellen Francis, "The War on Syria's Doctors," *Foreign Policy*, August 11, 2016, http://foreignpolicy.com/2016/08/11/the-war-on-syrias-doctors-assad-medicine-underground/.

4. Adnan Mroueh, personal communication, November 4, 2014. Mroueh is a professor of gynecology and obstetrics at AUB. He served as Lebanon's minister of health, labor, and social affairs in the period 1982–1984.

5. For instance, see Ussama Makdisi, *The Culture of Sectarianism: Community, History, and Violence in Nineteenth-Century Ottoman Lebanon* (Berkeley: University of California Press, 2000), and *Artillery of Heaven: American Missionaries and the Failed Conversion of the Middle East* (Ithaca, NY: Cornell University Press, 2008).

6. See Eugene Rogan, "Madness and Marginality: The Advent of the Psychiatric Asylum in Egypt and Lebanon," in *Outside In: On the Margins of the Modern Middle East*, ed. Eugene Rogan (London: I. B. Tauris, 2002), 115.

7. Charles Winslow, *Lebanon: War and Politics in a Fragmented Society* (New York: Routledge, 1996), 150; Farid El Khazen, *The Breakdown of the State in Lebanon, 1967–1976* (Cambridge, MA: Harvard University Press, 2000), 135.

8. This was in retaliation for the 1968 hijacking of an El-Al airliner in Athens by the Marxist Popular Front for the Liberation of Palestine. See Michael C. Hudson, "The Palestinian Factor in the Lebanese Civil War," *Middle East Journal* 32, no. 3 (1978): 261–278.

9. El Khazen, *The Breakdown of the State in Lebanon*, 167.

10. The PLO was founded in Cairo in 1964.

11. Theodor Hanf, *Coexistence in Wartime Lebanon: Decline of a State and Rise of a Nation* (London: Centre for Lebanese Studies in association with I. B. Tauris, 2015), 177. See also Hanf, *Coexistence in Wartime Lebanon*, especially 160–175; El Khazen, *The Breakdown of the State in Lebanon*, especially 131–175.

12. It was named after the bloody month in 1970 when King Hussein of Jordan had declared military rule, expelling and killing thousands of Palestinian fedayeen following an attempted coup by the PLO. See Christopher Dobson, *Black September: Its Short, Violent History* (New York: Macmillan, 1974).

13. For more information see Kamal S. Salibi, *Cross Roads to Civil War: Lebanon, 1958–1976* (Delmar, NY: Caravan Books, 1976); Elizabeth Picard, *Liban, état de discorde: Des fondations aux guerres fratricides* (Paris: Flammarion, 1988); El Khazen, *The Breakdown of the State in Lebanon*; Hanf, *Coexistence in Wartime Lebanon*.

14. Antranig Manugian to Sir Geoffrey Furlonge, May 4, 1973, LH/08/06, box 11, LH, SOAS.

15. Manugian to Sir Furlonge, May 4, 1973. Also see Hudson, "The Palestinian Factor in the Lebanese Civil War."

16. See Salibi, *Cross Roads to Civil War*; Fawwaz Traboulsi, *A History of Modern Lebanon* (London: Pluto Press, 2007), especially 187–204; El Khazen, *The Breakdown of the State in Lebanon*, especially 283–358.

17. Picard, *Liban, état de discorde*, especially 171–176.

18. Minutes of the BEC, October 13, 1975, LH/03/03, box 5, LH, SOAS. According to a brief history of the AUB Department of Psychiatry, which was posted online in 2019 and is no longer available, Zeidan "greatly enhanced the teaching of psychiatry whether in the classroom, during the clerkships at 'Asfourieh,' or in the outpatient department (OPD) at AUB."

19. Antranig Manugian, "The Medical Director's Report to the BEC," December 16, 1975, 4, Minutes of the BEC, LH/03/03, box 5, LH, SOAS.

20. Picard, *Liban, état de discorde*, 174; Hanf, *Coexistence in Wartime Lebanon*, especially 540–550.

21. Manugian, "The Medical Director's Report to the BEC," November 18, 1975, 3, Minutes of the BEC, LH/03/03, box 5, LH, SOAS.

22. For instances of violence inflicted on civilians from 1975 until 2008, see International Center for Transitional Justice, "Lebanon's Legacy of Political Violence: A Mapping of Serious Violations of International Human Rights and Humanitarian Law in Lebanon, 1975–2008," September 2013, https://www.ictj.org/sites/default/files/ICTJ-Report-Lebanon-Mapping-2013-EN_0.pdf.

23. Manugian, "The Medical Director's Report to the BEC," January 21, 1976, Minutes of the BEC, LH/03/03, box 5, LH, SOAS.

24. Manugian, "The Medical Director's Report to the BEC on Tuesday February 17, 1976," and minutes for January 23, 1976, 2, Minutes of the BEC, LH/03/03, box 5, LH, SOAS.

25. Manugian, "The Medical Director's Report to the BEC," February 21, 1978, Minutes of the BEC, LH/03/04, box 6, LH, SOAS.

26. Nikolas S. Rose, *Governing the Soul: The Shaping of the Private Self* (London: Routledge, 1990).

27. For example in France, Michel Foucault, Pierre Vidal-Naquet, and Jean-Marie Domenach signed a manifesto in 1971 demanding more transparency on the state of prisons and prisoners. In 1977, Simone Veil, then the French minister of health, proposed the establishment of fifteen *centres médico-psychologiques régionaux* (proper psychiatric units) within prisons, which was generally considered to be a pivotal moment in opening up the closed world of confinement in France. See Jean-Louis Senon and Denis Richard, "Punir ou soigner: Histoire des rapports entre psychiatrie et prison jusqu'à la loi de 1994," *Revue pénitentiaire et de droit pénal*, 123, no. 1 (January–March 1999): 97–110.

28. Manugian, "The Medical Director's Report to the BEC," February 21, 1978.

29. Manugian, "The Medical Director's Report to the BEC," April 20, 1976, Minutes of the BEC, LH/03/03, box 5, LH, SOAS.

30. Manugian, "The Medical Director's Report to the BEC meeting on Tuesday April 20, 1976," and minutes for March 16, 1976, 2, Minutes of the BEC, LH/03/03, box 5, LH, SOAS.

31. Manugian, "The Medical Director's Report to the BEC meeting on Tuesday April 20, 1976," and minutes for March 16, 1976, 2, Minutes of the BEC.

32. Manugian, "The Medical Director's Report to the BEC," April 20, 1976.

33. Manugian, "The Medical Director's Report to the BEC," April 20, 1976.

34. Manugian, "The Medical Director's Report to the BEC," April 20, 1976 and minutes for September 21, 1976, Minutes of the BEC, LH/03/03, box 5, LH, SOAS.

35. Manugian, "The Medical Director's Report to the BEC meeting on Tuesday October 19, 1976" and minutes for October 4, 1976, 2, Minutes of the BEC, LH/03/03, box 5, LH, SOAS.

36. "War's Overlooked Victims," *Economist*, January 13, 2011, https://www.economist.com/international/2011/01/13/wars-overlooked-victims.

37. Note by Sir Geoffrey Furlonge, April 6, 1976, LH/08/03, box 10, LH, SOAS.

38. Manugian, "The Medical Director's Report to the BEC," April 20, 1976.

39. Manugian, "The Medical Director's Report to the BEC," November 16, 1976, Minutes of the BEC, LH/03/03, box 5, LH, SOAS.

40. AR, 1929–1930, n.p., LHMND, AUB-SML.

41. Guy Feuer, "La force arabe de sécurité au Liban," *Annuaire français de droit international* 22, no. 1 (1976): 51–61; Rola el-Husseini, *Pax Syriana: Elite Politics in Postwar Lebanon* (Syracuse, NY: Syracuse University Press, 2012).

42. Manugian, "The Medical Doctor's Report to the BEC," January 18, 1977, Minutes of the BEC, LH/03/03, box 5, LH, SOAS.

43. "Matron's Report to the BEC," February 15, 1977, Minutes of the BEC, LH/03/03, box 5, LH, SOAS.

44. "Matron's Report to the BEC, February 21, 1978, Minutes of the BEC, LH/03/04, box 6, LH, SOAS.

45. Manugian to Sir Furlonge, July 19, 1978, LH/08/09, box 11, LH, SOAS.

46. "Matron's Report to the BEC," February 21, 1978.

47. "Matron's Report to the BEC," July 18, 1978, Minutes of the BEC, LH/03/04, box 6, LH, SOAS.

48. Manugian, "The Medical Doctor's Report to the BEC," April 20, 1976 and minutes for March 30, 1976, 7, Minutes of the BEC, LH/03/03, box 5, LH, SOAS.

49. Manugian, "Medical Director's Report for the year 1976," LHMND, AUB-SML.

50. Manugian to Furlonge, January 1, 1976, LH/03/03, box 5, LH, SOAS.

51. Manugian, "The Medical Doctor's Report to the BEC," May 18, 1976, Minutes of the BEC, LH/03/03, box 5, LH, SOAS.

52. Manugian, "The Medical Doctor's Report to the BEC," April 19, 1977, Minutes of the BEC, LH/03/03, box 5, LH, SOAS.

53. Manugian, "The Medical Doctor's Report to the BEC," September 11, 1978, Minutes of the BEC, LH/03/04, box 6, LH, SOAS.

54. Manugian, "The Medical Doctor's Report to the BEC," July 18, 1978, Minutes of the BEC, LH/03/04, box 6, LH, SOAS.

55. Manugian, "To all staff," October 1, 1975, Minutes of the BEC, LH/03/03, box 5, LH, SOAS. See also Manugian, "To all staff," October 15, 1975, Minutes of the BEC, LH/03/03, box 5, LH, SOAS.

56. Manugian, "The Medical Doctor's Report to the BEC," January 20, 1976, Minutes of the BEC, LH/03/03, box 5, LH, SOAS. Curiously, Ḥazmiyyeh, the name of the city where the Hospital is located today, does not appear in the official annual reports. People may have started to use the name Ḥazmiyyeh instead of ʿAṣfūriyyeh (the name of the area, as mentioned in the introduction) more frequently to avoid the stigmatizing connotations that the latter invoked. (I thank Habib Debs and Ishac Diwan for this suggestion.)

57. Manugian, "The Medical Doctor's Report to the BEC," February 17, 1976, Minutes of the BEC, LH/03/03, box 5, LH, SOAS.

58. Marvine Howe, "Special Report: The American University of Beirut: A Year of Tragedy and Hope," *Washington Report on Middle East Affairs*, December 2005, 42–43.

59. Thomas L. Friedman, "University Head Killed in Beirut; Gunmen Escape," *New York Times*, January 19, 1984, http://www.nytimes.com/1984/01/19/world/university-head-killed-in-beirut-gunmen-escape.html.

60. Manugian, "The Medical Doctor's Report to the BEC," October 21, 1975, Minutes of the BEC, LH/08/03, box 10, LH, SOAS.

61. Manugian, "The Medical Doctor's Report to the BEC," May 18, 1976.

62. "Minutes of the LGC," November 8, 1976, Minute Book (January 20, 1964–November 18, 1982), LH/02/06, box 4, LH, SOAS.

63. Manugian, "The Medical Doctor's Report to the BEC," May 18, 1976.

64. Manugian, "The Medical Director's report to the BEC," May 18, 1976.

65. Manugian, "The Medical Director's report to the BEC," July 20, 1976 and minutes for July 25–26, 1976, 5, Minutes of the BEC, LH/03/03, box 5, LH, SOAS.

66. Marcel Gauchet and Gladys Swain, *Madness and Democracy: The Modern Psychiatric Universe*, trans. Catherine Porter (Princeton, NJ: Princeton University Press, 1999), 113–116.

67. S. Nasr, J. Racy, and J. A. Flaherty, "Psychiatric Effects of the Civil War in Lebanon," *Psychiatric Journal of the University of Ottawa / Revue de psychiatrie de l'Université d'Ottawa* 8, no. 4 (1983): 210; L. L. Hourani, H. Armenian, H. Zurayk, and L. Afifi, "A Population-Based Survey of Loss and Psychological Distress during War," *Social Science & Medicine* 23, no. 3 (1986): 269–275; and P. A. Saigh, "The Validity of the DSM-III Posttraumatic Stress Disorder Classification as Applied to Children," *Journal of Abnormal Psychology* 98, no. 2 (1989): 189–192. A systematic review study of PTSD published in 2013 revealed a prevalence in Lebanon ranging from 8.5 percent to 14.7 percent during the civil war. See Khuzama Hijal Shaar, "Post-Traumatic Stress Disorder in Adolescents in Lebanon as Wars Gained in Ferocity: A Systematic Review," *Journal of Public Health Research* 2, no. 2 (September 2, 2013): e17.

68. On the pathologization of politics during the French Revolution until the Commune, see Laure Murat, *L'homme qui se prenait pour Napoléon: Pour une histoire politique de la folie* (Paris: Gallimard, 2011).

69. "'Disturbed, Calm, Normal' Killers in Beirut," *New York Herald Tribune*, December 10, 1977, LH/08/08, box 11, LH, SOAS.

70. Charles Baddoura, "Santé mentale et guerre libanaise," *Bulletin de l'Académie nationale de médecine* 174, no. 5 (May 1990): 589. See also Baddoura, "Santé mentale et guerre libanaise," 586.

71. For the army as a national institution, see Oren Barak, *The Lebanese Army: A National Institution in a Divided Society* (Albany: State University of New York Press, 2009).

72. Alexander Abdennur, "A Cognitively Induced Collective Psychopathology," *International Journal of Social Psychiatry* 28, no. 4 (December 1, 1982): 274–281.

73. Nasr, Racy, and Flaherty, "Psychiatric Effects of the Civil War in Lebanon," 210–211. See also Elise Knutsen, "Experts Say 'Resilient Lebanese' Have Good Overall Mental Health," *Daily Star*, October 22, 2013, http://www.dailystar.com.lb/News/Lebanon-News/2013/Oct-22/235315-experts-say-resilient-lebanese-have-good-overall-mental-health.ashx.

74. Nasr, Racy, and Flaherty, "Psychiatric Effects of the Civil War in Lebanon," 210.

75. Manugian, "The Medical Director's report to the BEC," June 15, 1976, Minutes of the BEC, LH/03/03, box 5, LH, SOAS.

76. Manugian, "The Medical Director's report to the BEC meeting on Tuesday February 21, 1978," AND minutes for October 17, 1978, Minutes of the BEC, LH/03/04, box 6, LH, SOAS.

77. Theophilus Waldmeier letter to "Friends and other Christians to whom this may come," October 20, 1898, LH/07/04, box 9, LH, SOAS.

78. Bayard Dodge, "A Brief History of the University and the Lands Which It Serves," 32–33, AA: 6.2.16.1.1, file 1, AUB Faculty 1867–1909, box 1, George Edward Post Collection, AUB-JL; Stephen B. L. Penrose, *That They May Have Life: The Story of the American University of Beirut, 1866–1941* (New York: Trustees of the American University of Beirut, 1941), 38.

79. Letter to "Le médecin inspecteur Emily, Inspecteur Général du Service d'Hygiène, Assistance à l'Oeuvre Sociale," November 25, 1921, file 1, box 5, "Correspondence with French officials re: the School of Medicine and School of Dentistry, 1920–1923, School of Medicine," AUB-JL.

80. Letter from the lawyer Georges Abi-Nader to the Lebanon Hospital for Mental and Nervous Disorders, "Re: The case of A. A-H" (initials used instead of full name to respect patient confidentiality), March 16, 1956, LHMND, AUB-SML; BEC minutes, March 20, 1956, LHMND, AUB-JL.

81. In contrast, Beverly Ann Tsacoyianis argues that ʿAṣfūriyyeh's finances "never fully recovered from losses suffered during and immediately after WWII." She further argues that because of those losses, administrators decided to sell the land in

the early 1970s and to relocate to ʿAramūn. See Beverly Ann Tsacoyianis, "Making Healthy Minds and Bodies in Syria and Lebanon, 1899–1961" (PhD diss., Washington University in St. Louis, 2014), 151. In contrast, this book argues that this was not the case and it was the civil war that brought about the greatest and irreversible losses.

82. H. Lyn Harris (LGC chairman) and O. M. Darton (LGC treasurer) to the Peter Coats Trust, January 6, 1944, LH/08/02, box 1, LH, SOAS.

83. "Data re: Foundation," Second Volume of Minutes, LH/02/05, box 3, LH, SOAS.

84. See AR, 1929, 19, and 1930, 13–15, LHMND, AUB-SML. Fadlo Hourani was made vice president of ʿAṣfūriyyeh in 1952.

85. See Abdulaziz A. al-Sudairi, *A Vision of the Middle East: An Intellectual Biography of Albert Hourani* (Oxford: Centre for Lebanese Studies, 1999), 17. See also Cecil Hourani and Zelfa Hourani, *Fadlo Hourani: The quiet merchant of Manchester* (Beirut: Antoine, 2020).

86. "Report of Mr. F. Hourani to the Lebanon Hospital Subcommittee," December 20, 1946, First Volume of Minutes, LH/02/04, box 3, LH, SOAS.

87. First Volume of Minutes, June 7 and September 26, 1944, LH/02/04, box 3, LH, SOAS.

88. "For the Glory of God in Lebanon," introduction by Fadlo Hourani on the fiftieth anniversary of ʿAṣfūriyyeh, followed by many quotes of donors who listened to the BBC broadcast, LH/10/01, box 15, LH, SOAS. For more on the fundraising role of Fadlo Hourani in the history of ʿAṣfūriyyeh see, Hourani and Hourani, *Fadlo Hourani*, especially 197–219.

89. "Talk on Asfuriyeh: Its Work Now and in the Future," 3, LHMND, AUB-SML.

90. First Volume of Minutes, June 7, 1944, LH/02/04, box 3, LH, SOAS.

91. First Volume of Minutes, August 2, 1945, LH/02/04, box 3, LH, SOAS.

92. Béchara El Khoury, *Récit d'un destin national,* trans. Roger Geahchan (Beirut: Les Éditions l'Orient-Le Jour, 2012), 174.

93. AR, 1950, 1, LHMND, AUB-SML.

94. Roger Soltau, "Le Liban. Le pays et ses habitants—L'hôpital d'Asfouriyeh," *Le Globe* 89, no. 1 (1950): 6.

95. Minutes of the LGC, July 29, 1980, LH/02/06, box 4, LH, SOAS.

96. Minutes of the LGC, October 25, 1977, LH/02/06, box 4, LH, SOAS.

97. Antranig Manugian, note on the growth of psychiatry in Saudi Arabia in the minutes for January 22, 1980, Minutes of the BEC, LH/03/04, box 6, LH, SOAS.

98. Sir Geoffrey Furlonge, "Note on the Lebanon Hospital for Mental and Nervous Disorders," May 1, 1969, LH/08/03, box 10, LH, SOAS; extract from the report of Dr. Dill-Russell on his visit to Lebanon, July 11–13, 1969, OD 34/224, TNA.

99. Minutes of the LGC, November 8 and 24, 1977, LH/02/06, box 5, LH, SOAS.

100. Although Great Britain withdrew its troops from the Gulf in 1971, it remained a key strategic and financial partner of the Gulf states. See Jane Kinninmont, "Future Trends in the Gulf" (London: Chatham House, February 2015), 5.

101. From P. H. G. Wright (British ambassador in Beirut) to Sir Geoffrey Furlonge, June 15, 1972, LH/08/06, box 11, LH, SOAS.

102. From Paul P. Howel (Middle East Development Division, MOD) to A. J. A. Douglas (MOD), April 11, 1968, 44, OD 34/224, TNA. See Achol Deng, "Obituary: Paul Philip Howell, D. PHIL, CMG, OBE," *Cambridge Anthropology* 17, no. 1 (1994): 69–71. This division of the British Foreign Office was disbanded by Prime Minister Margaret Thatcher's government in 1981, partly because of budgetary constraints but also because of the decline of developmental interests in a region swamped with oil revenues. See Paul W. T. Kingston, *Britain and the Politics of Modernization in the Middle East, 1945–1958* (Cambridge: Cambridge University Press, 1996), 157.

103. Minutes of the LGC, October 6, 1977, LH/02/06, box 4, LH, SOAS.

104. Architects and planning consultants (Challen, Floyd, Slaski, and Todd) to Sir Furlonge, May 30, 1972, LH/08/06, box 11, LH, SOAS.

105. Minutes of the BEC, September 19, 1978, LH/03/04, box 6, LH, SOAS.

106. The inflation was worldwide and unrelated to the political disturbances that preceded the Lebanese civil war. See El Khazen, *The Breakdown of the State in Lebanon*, especially 255–257.

107. AR, 1970, LH/09/04; AR, 1971, LH/09/05; and AR, 1974, LH/09/06, all box 15, LH, SOAS.

108. AR, 1974, LH/09/04, box 15, LH, SOAS; AR, 1941, LHMND, AUB-SML.

109. The Saudis donated LBP 1 million (worth US$3 million in 2019), which (like the British grant) was also used to cover salaries and indemnities. See "Note by the chairman," December 19, 1977, Minutes of the LGC, LH/02/06, box 4 and Minutes of the BEC, February 12, 1980, LH/03/04, box 6, both LH, SOAS; "Lebanon: Assistance to the Asfuriyeh Hospital for Mental and Nervous Disorders," January 1, 1976 to December 31, 1978, both OD 34/431, TNA.

110. Manugian to Sir Furlonge, May 26 and June 4, 1975, LH/08/03, box 10, LH, SOAS.

111. Manugian to Sir Furlonge, June 4, 1975, LH/08/03, box 10, LH, SOAS.

112. Manugian, "The Medical Director's Report to the BEC," March 16, 1976, LH/03/03, box 5, LH, SOAS.

113. Minute book, November 8, 1976, LH/02/06, box 4, LH, SOAS.

114. "Direct Losses due to the War," LH/08/08, box 11, LH, SOAS.

115. See Roger Owen, "The Economic History of Lebanon 1943–1974: Its Salient Features," in *Toward a Viable Lebanon*, ed. Halim Barakat (London: Croom Helm, 1988), 34.

116. An untitled paper on the history of ʿAṣfūriyyeh signed by the chairman, October 8, 1976, Minutes of the BEC, LH/03/03, box 5; Minutes of the LGC, November 1, 1972, and March 22, 1973, and "Aide-memoire," March 7, 1973, LH/02/07, both box 4, all LH, SOAS.

117. On February 17, 1982, the debt was as follows: LBP 6.5–7.0 million for salaries, indemnities, and bonuses; LBP 7.77 million for new hospital debt; LBP 1.5 million for old hospital debt; LBP 15 million to repay a governmental loan; and LBP 600,000 to repay a governmental advance. See Minutes of the LGC and BEC, February 17, 1982, LH/02/06, box 4, LH, SOAS.

118. Decree no. 1645, January 13, 1979, LH/08/09, box 11, LH, SOAS. The LBP 15 million loan is mentioned in the previous note.

119. Sir Furlonge to Manugian, April 1, 1981, LH/08/09, box 11, LH, SOAS.

120. Manugian to Sir Furlonge, April 27, 1981, LH/08/09, box 11, LH, SOAS.

121. Antranig Manugian to O. M. Darton (chairman of the LGC), July 16, 1982, LH/08/18, box 13; Minutes of the BEC, January 19, 1982, LH/08/23, box 14; "Developments since Our Last Meeting on 25 May 1982," Minutes of the BEC, LH/03/05, box 6, all LH, SOAS.

122. Adnan Mroueh, personal communication, November 6, 2014. For more on the Liberation War, see Traboulsi, *A History of Modern Lebanon*, especially 226–252.

123. Shannon Lee Dawdy, "Clockpunk Anthropology and the Ruins of Modernity," *Current Anthropology* 51, no. 6 (December 1, 2010): 777.

124. Minutes of the LGC, March 31, 1981, LH/02/06, box 4, LH, SOAS.

125. "Report of the London General Committee to the Members for the Year 1982," Minutes of the LGC, LH/02/06, box 4, LH, SOAS.

126. Ministry of Health to the Ministry of Overseas Development, May 2, 1968, OD 34/224, TNA. See also Sir Furlonge to Ambassador Wright, December 6, 1971, LH/08/06, box 11, LH, SOAS; Ambassador Wright to Sir Furlonge, April 5, 1974, LH/08/07, box 11, LH, SOAS.

127. Minutes of the BEC, January 20, 1981, LH/03/0, box 6, LH, SOAS.

128. "Replies to Six Questions Posed by the Syndicate," c. 1978, LH/08/09, box 11, LH, SOAS.

129. "77th Annual Report for the Years 1975 to 1981 Inclusive," December 31, 1981, LH/08/20, box 13, LH, SOAS.

130. Minutes of the LGC, January 25, 1982, LH/02/06, box 4, LH, SOAS.

131. Minutes of the LGC, March 2, 1982, LH/02/06, box 4, LH, SOAS.

132. Minutes of the LGC, March 2, 1982.

133. On corruption, forced evictions, and other accusations related to Solidere, see Habib Battah, "Solidere Assailed by Charges of Corruption," *Daily Star*, June 23, 2004, http://www.dailystar.com.lb//Business/Lebanon/2004/Jun-23/1438-solidere-assailed-by-charges-of-corruption.ashx; Peter Beaumont and Mitchell Prothero, "Why 'Mr. Lebanon' Had Many Enemies," *Guardian*, February 19, 2005, http://www.theguardian.com/world/2005/feb/20/syria.lebanon; Reinoud Leenders, *Spoils of Truce: Corruption and State-Building in Postwar Lebanon* (Ithaca, NY: Cornell University Press, 2012).

134. Nadine Kenaan, "Solīdayr ila-l-ʿAṣfūriyyeh," *Al-Akhbar*, February 17, 2012, https://al-akhbar.com/Archive_Turath/65469.

135. W. M. F. Robertson, "Some Problems Concerning the Approach to a Middle East Psychiatric Service," *Lebanese Medical Journal* 5, no. 1 (January 1952): 7.

6 The Politics of Health, Charity, and Sectarianism

1. Christopher Dalley to Muhammad Shukayr, July 2, 1984 and Dalley to the members of the Lebanon Hospital for Mental and Nervous Disorders, in which Dalley (former chairman of the LGC) confirms the steps taken to appoint Shukayr as mutawallī, both LH/08/03, box 10; telegram that mentions the election of Shukayr as mutawallī, February 1, 1984, LH/08/25, box 14, all LH, SOAS.

2. George Sabra, personal communication, March 1, 2016; "Le conseiller présidentiel Mohammed Choucair abattu à son domicile à Beyrouth-Ouest," *L'Orient-Le Jour*, August 3, 1987, 1 and 12; "Choucair est le martyr de l'unité nationale, déclare Gemayel," *L'Orient-Le Jour*, August 4, 1987, 2.

3. Adnan Mroueh, personal communications, April 18 and 20, 2016. Mroueh also provided the author with a copy of the minutes of the General Committee for March 7, 1991.

4. Mroueh, personal communications, November 6 and 8, 2014, and February 26, 2016; Sabra, personal communication, February 29, 2016.

5. Mroueh, personal communication, November 8, 2014; Sabra, personal communication, September 28, 2015.

6. Sabra, personal communication, September 28, 2015.

7. See Judith P. Harik, *"The Public and Social Services of the Lebanese Militias"* (Oxford: Centre for Lebanese Studies, 1994); Nisreen Salti and Jad Chaaban, "The Role of Sectarianism in the Allocation of Public Expenditure in Postwar Lebanon," *International Journal of Middle East Studies* 42, no. 4 (2010): 637–655; Melani Cammett and Sukriti Issar, "Bricks and Mortar Clientelism: Sectarianism and the Logics of Welfare Allocation in Lebanon," *World Politics* 62, no. 3 (2010): 381–421; Melani Cammett, *Compassionate Communalism* (Ithaca, NY: Cornell University Press, 2014).

8. Signed in the Saudi city of Ta'if, the accords are the result of the process of national reconciliation among the different political factions that ended the civil war (1975–1990). Despite the official ending of the war, violence (in the form of political assassinations, suicide bombings, and terrorism) as well as wars (particularly between the Shiite party, Hezbollah, and Israel) and (since October 17, 2019) popular revolts against precarious socioeconomic conditions continue to sporadically disturb this national agreement. It remains to be seen if the Ta'if Accords will be seriously challenged by these recent popular uprisings.

9. For the Beirut municipality and the reforms' contributions to public health, see Jens Hanssen, *Fin de Siècle Beirut: The Making of an Ottoman Provincial Capital* (Oxford: Clarendon Press of Oxford University Press, 2005), especially 115–137.

10. See Daniel Panzac, "Tanzimat et santé publique: Les débuts du conseil sanitaire de l'empire ottoman," in *150 Yilinda Tanzimat*, ed. H. D. Yildiz (Ankara: Türk Tarih Kurumu, 1992), 325–333; Sylvia Chiffoleau, *Genèse de la santé publique internationale: De la peste d'Orient à l'OMS* (Rennes, France: Presses Universitaires de Rennes, 2012).

11. For Jewish and Catholic hospitals in the United States, see Charles E. Rosenberg, *The Care of Strangers: The Rise of America's Hospital System* (New York: Basic Books, 1987), 112. For the black hospital movement, see Vanessa Northington Gamble, "Roots of the Black Hospital Reform Movement," in *Sickness and Health in America: Readings in the History of Medicine and Public Health*, ed. Judith Walzer Leavitt and Ronald L. Numbers (Madison: University of Wisconsin Press, 1997), 369–391. For the Ottoman minority hospitals, see Nuran Yıldırım, *A History of Healthcare in Istanbul: Health Organizations, Epidemics, Infections and Disease Control, Preventive Health Institutions, Hospitals, Medical Education* (Istanbul: Istanbul University, 2010), especially 177–181.

12. "Once a Missionary in Abyssinia," *Missionary Review of the World* 34, no. 6 (June 1911): 464.

13. Data compiled from ARs, 1900–1961. Data missing for 1909–1910, 1930, and 1942–1943.

14. See Eugene Rogan, "Madness and Marginality: The Advent of the Psychiatric Asylum in Egypt and Lebanon," in *Outside In: On the Margins of the Modern Middle East*, ed. Eugene Rogan (London: I. B. Tauris, 2002), 115.

15. Quoted in AR, 1926–1927, 25, AUB-SML. For Patriarch Huwayek, see AR 1903, 18, AUB-SML.

16. See, for instance, Lady Isabel Burton, *The Inner Life of Syria, Palestine, and the Holy Land: From My Private Journal* (London: H. S. King and Co., 1875), 1:192.

17. "Constitution and Bye-Laws of the Executive Committee of the Lebanon Asylum for the Insane, Beirut, 22 April 1896," LHMND, AUB-SML. This article was retained in the amended constitutions of 1907, 1915, and 1965, with the only modification being the deletion of the priority given to "the natives of the country."

18. See, for instance, Davide Rodogno, *Against Massacre: Humanitarian Interventions in the Ottoman Empire, 1815–1914* (Princeton, NJ: Princeton University Press, 2012).

19. See Jürgen Osterhammel, *The Transformation of the World: A Global History of the Nineteenth Century*, trans. Patrick Camiller (Princeton, NJ: Princeton University Press, 2014); Eric J. Hobsbawm, *The Age of Empire, 1875–1914* (New York: Pantheon Books, 1987).

20. Ussama Makdisi, "Reclaiming the Land of the Bible: Missionaries, Secularism, and Evangelical Modernity," *American Historical Review* 102, no. 3 (June 1, 1997): 691.

21. Ussama S. Makdisi, *The Culture of Sectarianism: Community, History, and Violence in Nineteenth-Century Ottoman Lebanon* (Berkeley: University of California Press, 2000), 15.

22. Theophilus Waldmeier, *The Autobiography of Theophilus Waldmeier, Missionary: Being an Account of Ten Years' Life in Abyssinia; and Sixteen Years in Syria* (London: S. W. Partridge and Co., 1886) (hereafter, Waldmeier, *The Autobiography of Theophilus Waldmeier, Missionary*), 226–227.

23. Theophilus Waldmeier, *Appeal for the First Home of the Insane on Mount Lebanon* (London: Headley Brothers, 1897), 3–4, LHMND, AUB-SML (hereafter, Waldmeier, *Appeal*).

24. Waldmeier, *The Autobiography of Theophilus Waldmeier, Missionary*, 326.

25. For accounts of the risk incurred by Muslims for publicly embracing Protestantism, see Waldmeier, *The Autobiography of Theophilus Waldmeier, Missionary*, 250; Henry Harris Jessup, *The Setting of the Crescent and the Rising of the Cross; Or, Kamil Abdul Messiah, a Syrian Convert from Islam to Christianity* (Philadelphia: Westminster Press, 1898); J. D. Maitland-Kirwan, *Sunrise in Syria: A Short History of the British Syrian Mission, from 1860–1930* (London: British Syrian Mission, 1930), 33–34 and 39.

26. Howard S. Bliss, "The Modern Missionary," *Atlantic Monthly*, May 1920, 673.

27. Quoted in Waldmeier, *Appeal*, 20.

28. Quoted in Waldmeier, *Appeal*, 21.

29. "Constitution and Bye-Laws of the Executive Committee of the Lebanon Asylum for the Insane," 3, LHMND, AUB-SML.

30. Minutes of the LGC, May 17, 1929, LH/02/02, box 2, LH, SOAS.

31. Antranig Manugian, "The Medical Director's Report to the BEC," May 18, 1976, 10, Minutes of the BEC, LH/03/03, box 5, LH, SOAS.

32. Though insignificant, some endowments were also created after the deaths of a few trustee members, such as Henry Jessup or Lady Scott Moncrieff. See "Lady Scott Moncrieff Fund/Peter Coats Endowment," 1919–1953, LH/08/02, list of endowment funds, March 1981, LH/08/04, both box 10, both LH, SOAS.

33. AR, 1902, 19; 1907, 6; and 1911–1912, 5, LHMND, AUB-SML.

34. R. A. Mickelwright, "Report on His Second Visit to the Hospital, October 1964 to February 1965," appendix V, "Hospital Buildings," LH/12/01, box 16, LH, SOAS; "Lebanon Hospital for Mental Diseases, Brief History," LHMND, AUB-SML.

35. First Volume of Minutes, June 7 and September 26, 1944, LH/02/04, box 3, LH, SOAS.

36. Minutes of the LGC, February 16, 1932, 125, LH/02/03, box 2, and "Redevelopment Plans—the New Hospital," LH/08/03, box 10, both LH, SOAS; AR, 1946, 3, LHMND, AUB-SML.

37. Minutes of the LGC, September 13, 1922, 215, LH/02/01, box 2, LH, SOAS.

38. See LH/08/06 ("Sir Geoffrey Furlonge, Correspondence, October 1971–December 1973"), LH/08/07 ("Sir Geoffrey Furlonge, Correspondence, January 1974–December 1975"), LH/08/08 ("Sir Geoffrey Furlonge, Correspondence, January 1976–December 1977"), and LH/08/09 ("Sir Geoffrey Furlonge, Correspondence, January 1978–October 1981"), all box 11, all LH, SOAS.

39. From Frank Judd (minister of state) to the Rt. Hon. Mrs. Judith Hart (member of Parliament), "Aid to Lebanon: Asfouriyeh Mental Hospital," December 6, 1977, OD 34/431, TNA.

40. J. E. Rednall (the Middle East and Mediterranean Department, MOD), "Lebanon—Assistance to Asfuriyeh Mental Hospital," December 30, 1977, OD 34/431, TNA.

41. Peter Wakefield (British ambassador to Lebanon), telegram, February 11, 1977, OD 34/431, TNA.

42. Cecil King (British ambassador to Lebanon), "Confidential," to MOD, December 28, 1967, OD 34/224, TNA.

43. "Thirty Years' Pioneer Work, Being the Story of the Lebanon Hospital for Mental Diseases," box 125, CBMS, SOAS.

44. Sabra, personal communication, August 5, 2014.

45. Nada Raad, "Colleagues Remember Antranig Manugian," *Daily Star*, April 12, 2003, http://www.dailystar.com.lb/News/Lebanon-News/2003/Apr-12/20401-colleagues-remember-antranig-manugian.ashx.

46. "For the Glory of God in Lebanon," with an endorsement by Camille Chamoun, c. 1950, LH/10/01, box 15, LH, SOAS.

47. Data compiled from ARs, 1900–1962, LHMND, AUB-SML."

48. *"Constitution and Rules"* of the Lebanon Hospital for the Insane, 1907, LH/01/02, box 1, LH, SOAS,

49. "Note of Consultation with Mr. R.A.K. Wright on 28.1.8," LH/08/20, box 13, and "Sir Geoffrey Furlonge, Correspondence," LH/08/06–09, box 11, both LH, SOAS.

50. *Millet* (the Turkish rendering of the Arabic *milla*) means religion, religious community, or nation. The millet system enabled the numerous religious communities of the empire to coexist while exercising their religious freedom and managing their own communal affairs. See Bernard Lewis and Benjamin Braude, eds., *Christians and Jews in the Ottoman Empire: The Functioning of a Plural Society* (New York: Holmes and Meier, 1982), vol. 1; Ami Ayalon, *Language and Change in the Arab Middle East: The Evolution of Modern Arabic Political Discourse* (New York: Oxford University Press, 1987), especially 16–28; Avigdor Levy, "Millet," in *Encyclopedia of Jews in the Islamic World*, ed. Norman A. Stillman, accessed April 1, 2020, https://referenceworks.brillonline.com/entries/encyclopedia-of-jews-in-the-islamic-world/millet-COM_0015330?s.num=0&s.f.s2_parent=s.f.book.encyclopedia-of-jews-in-the-islamic-world&s.q=MILLET.

51. Cammett, *Compassionate Communalism*.

52. Kamal Salibi, "Lebanon under Fuad Chehab 1958–1964," *Middle Eastern Studies* 2, no. 3 (1966): 221.

53. Roger Melki, "La protection sociale au Liban: Entre réflexe d'assistance et logique d'assurance," in *Linking Economic Growth and Social Development in Lebanon* (Beirut: United Nations Development Programme, 2000), 187–210.

54. See Carolyn Gates, *The Merchant Republic of Lebanon: Rise of an Open Economy* (London: Centre for Lebanese Studies, 1998), 95–96; Hyam Mallat, "La politique de protection sociale au Liban: Évolution, situation et perspectives," January 2004, https://www.issa.int/html/pdf/initiative/reports/1Liban.pdf; Stéphane Malsagne, *Fouad Chéhab, 1902–1973: Une figure oubliée de l'histoire libanaise* (Paris: Karthala, 2011), 272–273.

55. Robert de Boisséson (French ambassador to Lebanon) to the minister of foreign affairs, "A.s., Promulgation par décret de la loi sur la Sécurité Sociale," September 11, 1963, 371QONT/962, MAE.

56. Ḥassān Ḥallāq, *Dār al-ʿAjaza al-Islāmiyya Fī Bayrūt (1954–2004): Ṣafaḥāt Muḍīat Min Tārīkh al-ʿAmal al-Insānī Fī Lubnān wal-ʿĀlam al-ʿArabī* (Beirut: Dār al-ʿAjaza al-Islāmiyya, 2004), 10.

57. AR, 1953, 5, LHMND, AUB-SML; Samar Labban, personal communication, July 18, 2012.

58. See Dār al-ʿAjaza al-Islāmiyya's official website of the hospital, accessed February 16, 2020, https://daih.org. See also Brigitte Khoury and Sarah Tabbarah, "Lebanon," in *Oxford Handbook of the History of Psychology: Global Perspectives*, ed. David B. Baker (Oxford: Oxford University Press, 2012), especially 368–369.

59. For more on Basaglia, see Mario Colucci and Pierangelo Di Vittorio, *Franco Basaglia : Portrait d'un psychiatre intempestif* (Ramonville-Saint-Agne, France: Erès, 2005); John Foot, *The Man Who Closed the Asylums: Franco Basaglia and the Revolution in Mental Health Care* (London: Verso, 2015).

60. Labban, personal communication, July 18, 2012.

61. Harriet Fitch Little, "Spotlight on Mental Illness," *Now Lebanon*, April 7, 2013, https://now.mmedia.me/lb/en/reportsfeatures/spotlight-on-mental-illness.

62. Labban, personal communication, July 18, 2012.

63. Mohammed Zaatari, "Italian Embassy Pledges Support for Mental Health Care in South," *Daily Star*, October 27, 2009, http://www.dailystar.com.lb/News/Lebanon-News/2009/Oct-27/55822-italian-embassy-pledges-support-for-mental-health-care-in-south.ashx.

64. "The American University of Beirut, Directory of Alumni, 1870–1952," 346, AUB-JL.

65. Manugian, "The Medical Director's Report to the BEC," February 21, 1978, Minutes of the BEC, LH/03/04, box 6, LH, SOAS; matron's reports, December 19, 1978, and January 16 and February 6, 1979, all Minutes of the BEC, all LHMND, AUB-JL.

66. Quoted in "'Tragédie sociale, morale et sanitaire': Jabak ordonne la fermeture d'un hôpital psychiatrique insalubre," *L'Orient-Le Jour*, February 17, 2019, https://www.lorientlejour.com/article/1157758/tragedie-sociale-morale-et-sanitaire-jabak-ordonne-la-fermeture-dun-hopital-psychiatrique-insalubre.html.

67. Amal Khalil, "*'Al-Fanār' Min "Aṣfūriyyeh' Ila Muʿtaqal: Wizārat al-Suḥḥa Mas'ūlūn Aiḍan*," *Al-Akhbar*, February 18, 2019, https://al-akhbar.com/Community/266417; "Scandale sanitaire: La propriétaire de l'hôpital al-Fanar entendue le 2 avril prochain," *L'Orient-Le Jour*, March 13, 2019, https://www.lorientlejour.com/article/1161457/scandale-sanitaire-la-proprietaire-de-lhopital-al-fanar-entendue-le-2-avril-prochain.html.

68. Copy of the original Arabic deed and judgment and literal translation of the waqf deed, April 17, 1912, LH/01/01, box 1, LH, SOAS.

69. For more information, see Randi Deguilhem, "The Waqf in the City," in *The City in the Islamic World*, ed. Salma Khadra Jayyusi and Renata Holod (Leiden, the Netherlands: Brill, 2008), 2:923–950; Gábor Ágoston and Bruce Alan Masters, *Encyclopedia of the Ottoman Empire* (New York: Facts on File, 2009), 590–591.

70. George Young, *Corps de droit ottoman* (Oxford: Clarendon Press of Oxford University Press, 1905–1906), 6:113.

71. See Randi Deguilhem, ed., *Le waqf dans l'espace islamique: Outil de pouvoir socio-politique* (Damascus: Institut Français de Damas, 1995).

72. John Robert Barnes, *An Introduction to Religious Foundations in the Ottoman Empire* (Leiden, the Netherlands: E. J. Brill, 1986), 68–69. Precedents of this type of centralization may be found under the Ummayad, the Abbasid, and the Mamluks. For more on the waqf, see Randi Deguilhem-Schoem, "Ottoman Waqf Administrative Reorganization in the Syrian Provinces: The Case of Damascus," *Arab Historical Review for Ottoman Studies/Al-Majalla al-Tārīkhīya al-ʿArabīya li-l-Dirāsāt al-ʿUthmāniyya* 5-6 (February 1992): 31–38.

73. Amy Singer, "Charity's Legacies: Reconsideration of Ottoman Imperial Endowment-Making," in *Poverty and Charity in Middle Eastern Contexts*, ed. Michael David Bonner, Mine Ener, and Amy Singer (Albany: State University of New York Press, 2003), 295–313.

74. See Randi Deguilhem, "On the Nature of Waqf. Pious Foundations in Contemporary Syria: A Break in the Transition," in *Les fondations pieuses (waqf) en Méditerranée: Enjeux de société, enjeux de pouvoir*, ed. Randi Deguilhem and Hénia Abdelhamid (Safat: Kuwait Awqaf Public Fondation, 2004), 395–430.

75. See Marlène Ghorayeb, *Beyrouth sous mandat français: Construction d'une ville moderne* (Paris: Karthala, 2014), especially 76–77.

76. For very useful information, see Maurus Reinkowski, *Ottoman "Multiculturalism"? The Example of the Confessional System in Lebanon* (Beirut: Orient-Institut der Deutschen Morgenländischen Gesellschaft, 1999).

77. *Lisān al-ʿArab*, s.v. "*ṭā'ifa*," accessed April 12, 2020, http://www.baheth.info/index.jsp.

78. Ayalon, *Language and Change in the Arab Middle East*, 24–25; Levy, "Millet."

79. See Choucri Cardahi, "Conflict of Law," in *Law in the Middle East*, ed. Majid Khadduri and Herbert J. Liebesny (Washington: Middle East Institute, 1955), 334–348; Iliya F. Harik, *Politics and Change in a Traditional Society: Lebanon, 1711–1845* (Princeton, NJ: Princeton University Press, 1968), 20. For a challenge to the claim

of judicial autonomy, see Najwa al-Qattan, "Dhimmis in the Muslim Court: Legal Autonomy and Religious Discrimination," *International Journal of Middle East Studies* 31, no. 3 (1999): 429–444.

80. Will Kymlicka calls this configuration a "federation of theocracies" (*Multicultural Citizenship: A Liberal Theory of Minority Rights* [Oxford: Oxford University Press, 1995], 157). Also see Reinkowski, *Ottoman "Multiculturalism"?*

81. Engin Deniz Akarli, *The Long Peace: Ottoman Lebanon, 1861–1920* (Berkeley: University of California Press, 1993), especially 27–29; Leila Fawaz, *An Occasion for War: Civil Conflict in Lebanon and Damascus in 1860* (Berkeley: University of California Press, 1994), 27–28.

82. Akarli, *The Long Peace*, especially 6–33.

83. See Georges Corm, *Le Liban contemporain: Histoire et société* (Paris: La Découverte, 2003), 90–92; Paul W. T. Kingston, *Reproducing Sectarianism: Advocacy Networks and the Politics of Civil Society in Postwar Lebanon* (Albany: State University of New York Press, 2013), 21–53; Faïza Tobich, *Les statuts personnels dans les pays arabes: De l'éclatement à l'harmonisation* (Aix-en-Provence, France: Presses Universitaires d'Aix-Marseille, 2015), 161–183.

84. See Haut-commissariat de la république française en Syrie et au Liban, *Bulletin officiel des actes administratifs du haut-commissariat 15ème année*, no. 7 (April 15, 1936): 173, BnF. Ten Christian, five Muslim, and three Jewish ("Israelite") communities were recognized in 1936. In 1938, an amendment was made (arrêté 146/LR, Article 28) that added the Protestant community. See also, *Bulletin officiel des actes administratifs du haut-commissariat 17ème année*, no. 23 (December 15, 1938): 282, BnF.

85. They had the right to establish and organize religious courts and formulate their personal status codes and family laws. These codes and laws dealt with matters of adoption, divorce, custody, and abuse. Lebanon does not have a civil code regulating matters of personal status. Instead, the country's different recognized religious communities have their own laws, all of which are administered by separate religious courts.

86. The National Pact was an unwritten agreement between President Bechara el-Khoury and Prime Minister Riad al-Solh. First, they agreed to view Lebanon as a neutral, independent, and sovereign entity with an Arab character. Second, they agreed that Lebanon would not seek unity with Syria or the Arab world, nor would it have special ties with France or the West. Third, they agreed to divide power among Christians and Muslims in a six-to-five ratio throughout the government, with the offices of president, prime minister, and speaker of the house assigned to the Maronites, Sunnis, and Shiites, respectively. See Edmond Rabbat, *La formation historique du Liban politique et constitutionnel: Essai de synthèse* (Beirut: Université Libanaise, 1973); Hassan Krayem, "The Lebanese Civil War and the Taif Agreement,"

in *Conflict Resolution in the Arab World*, ed. Paul Salem (Beirut: American University of Beirut, 1997), 441–435.

87. Maher Mahmassani and Ibtissam Messarra, *Statut personnel: Textes en vigueur au Liban* (Beirut: Faculté de droit et des sciences économiques), 336–351.

88. See Georges Moussa Dib, *"Law and Population in Lebanon"* (Medford, MA: Tufts University, Fletcher School of Law and Diplomacy, Law and Population Monograph Series Number 29, 1975), 11–14.

89. Dib, *"Law and Population in Lebanon,"* 18; Kingston, *Reproducing Sectarianism*, 243.

90. The numbers of books published with titles containing the term *ṭā'ifiyya* peaked in the 1970s.

91. Makdisi, *The Culture of Sectarianism*, 7. See also Ussama Makdisi, "The Modernity of Sectarianism in Lebanon: Reconstructing the Nation-State," *Middle East Report* 26, no. 200 (Fall 1996), https://merip.org/1996/09/the-modernity-of-sectarianism-in-lebanon/.

92. Dib, *"Law and Population in Lebanon,"* 12.

93. Sawsan al-Abṭah, "Maqbarat al-Zawāj al-Madanī," *al-Sharq al-Awsaṭ*, February 4, 2013, http://archive.aawsat.com/leader.asp?section=3&issueno=12487&article=715795#.Vz8MRGbVllo.

94. On Syria, see Deguilhem, "On the Nature of Waqf." On Egypt, see Murat Çizakça, *A History of Philanthropic Foundations: The Islamic World from the Seventh Century to the Present* (Istanbul: Boğaziçi University Press, 2000).

95. Reverend F. Audi, "Judgment Rendered by the Court of First Instance of the Protestant Religious Court of Beirut," March 8, 1972, LH/01/03, box 1, LH, SOAS.

96. Mahmassani and Messarra, *Statut personnel*, 337.

97. Minutes of the BEC, minute no. 105, December 21, 1971, LH/03/06, box 6, LH, SOAS.

98. Habib Badr, "Evangelical Missions and Churches in the Middle East," in *Christianity: A History in the Middle East*, ed. Habib Badr, Suad Abu el-Rouss Slim, and Joseph Abou Nohra (Beirut: Middle East Council of Churches, Studies and Research Program, 2005), 714.

99. "Judgment Confirming the Legality of the Wakf When the Former Owner Attempted to Break the Wakf, F. E. Hoskins vs. C. A. Webster" and "Literal Translation of the Wakf Deed Covering All the Properties of the Lebanon Hospital for the Insane," both April 17, 1912, LH/01/01, box 1, LH, SOAS.

100. "Judgment Confirming the Legality of the Wakf When the Former Owner Attempted to Break the Wakf, F. E. Hoskins vs. C. A. Webster" and "Literal Translation of the Wakf Deed Covering All the Properties of the Lebanon Hospital for the Insane."

101. "Judgment Confirming the Legality of the Wakf When the Former Owner Attempted to Break the Wakf, F. E. Hoskins vs. C. A. Webster" and "Literal Translation of the Wakf Deed Covering All the Properties of the Lebanon Hospital for the Insane."

102. Guy Hinsdale, "Dr. R. Fortescue Fox, FRCP," *Transactions of the American Clinical and Climatological Association* 56 (1940): xlii–xliii.

103. See Henry Harris Jessup, *Fifty-Three Years in Syria* (New York: Fleming H. Revell, 1910), 2:503; "Death of Dr. F. E. Hoskins," *Orient* 7, no. 51 (November 17, 1920): 501; "Obituary: Franklin Evans Hoskins '83," *Princeton Alumni Weekly* 21, no. 8 (November 24, 1920): 182.

104. See, for instance, Ron Shaham, "Christian and Jewish Waqf in Palestine during the Late Ottoman Period," *Bulletin of the School of Oriental and African Studies* 54, no. 3 (October 1991): 460–472.

105. "Judgment Confirming the Legality of the Wakf When the Former Owner Attempted to Break the Wakf, F. E. Hoskins vs. C. A. Webster" and "Literal Translation of the Wakf Deed Covering All the Properties of the Lebanon Hospital for the Insane"; "Preface to the Rules."

106. "Petition," June 10, 1968, LH/01/02, box 1, LH, SOAS.

107. "Petition," June 10, 1968, 1.

108. Minutes for November 13, 1981, Minutes of the LGC, LH/02/06, box 4, LH, SOAS.

Epilogue

1. Adnan Mroueh to Muhammad Shukayr (chairman of the BEC), May 23, 1983, LH/08/03, box 10, LH, SOAS.

2. Elzbieta Mikos-Skuza , "Hospitals," in *The 1949 Geneva Conventions: A Commentary*, ed. Andrew Clapham, Paola Gaeta, Marco Sassòli (Oxford: Oxford University Press, 2015), 209.

3. Protocol I (June 8, 1977) relates to the "Protection of Victims of International Armed Conflicts," accessed April 11, 2020, https://ihl-databases.icrc.org/ihl/INTRO/470. Protocol II (June 8, 1977) relates to the "Protection of Victims of Non-International Armed Conflicts," accessed April 11, 2020, https://ihl-databases.icrc.org/applic/ihl/ihl.nsf/INTRO/475. For more about the history of the Geneva Conventions, see Wade Mansell and Karen Openshaw, "The History and Status of the Geneva Conventions," in *The Geneva Conventions Under Assault*, ed. Sarah Perrigo and Jim Whitman (New York: Pluto Press, 2010), 18–41. For an assessment of armed conflict in the twentieth century, see Nils Petter Gleditsch, Peter Wallensteen, Mikael Eriksson, Margareta Sollenberg, and Havard Strand, "Armed Conflict 1946–2001: A New Dataset," *Journal of Peace Research* 39, no. 5 (September 1, 2002): 615–637.

4. See Alfred W. Crosby, *Ecological Imperialism: The Biological Expansion of Europe, 900–1900* (New York: Cambridge University Press, 1993).

5. Michel Cantal-Dupart, "Un hôpital urbain, idéalement implanté dans la ville," *Les tribunes de la santé* 4, no. 37 (2012): 75–81; Bruno Coppieters and Nick Fotion, eds., *Moral Constraints on War: Principles and Cases* (Lanham, MD: Lexington Books, 2002), 74.

6. See, for example, World Health Organization, "Report on Attacks on Health Care in Emergencies" (Geneva: World Health Organization, 2016).

7. World Health Organization, "Report on Attacks on Health Care in Emergencies," 7.

8. Médecins Sans Frontières USA, "Special Report: In Syria, Medicine as a Weapon of Persecution," February 8, 2012, https://www.msf.org/syria-medicine-used-weapon-persecution; Médecins Sans Frontières, "Airstrike Destroys MSF-Supported Hospital in Aleppo Killing 14," April 28, 2016, http://www.msf.org/en/article/syria-airstrike-destroys-msf-supported-hospital-aleppo-killing-14; Médecins Sans Frontières, "Kunduz Hospital Attack," October 3, 2015, http://www.msf.org/en/topics/kunduz-hospital-airstrike; Ellen Francis, "The War on Syria's Doctors," *Foreign Policy*, August 11, 2016, http://foreignpolicy.com/2016/08/11/the-war-on-syrias-doctors-assad-medicine-underground/; Kareem Shaheen, "Hospitals Are Now Normal Targets of War, Says Médecins Sans Frontières," *Guardian*, June 1, 2016, https://www.theguardian.com/world/2016/jun/01/hospitals-are-now-normal-targets-of-war-says-medecins-sans-frontieres-adviser; Matthieu Aikins, "Doctors with Enemies: Did Afghan Forces Target the M.S.F. Hospital?" *New York Times*, May 17, 2016, http://www.nytimes.com/2016/05/22/magazine/doctors-with-enemies-did-afghan-forces-target-the-msf-hospital.html; Christiaan Triebert, Evan Hill, Malachy Browne, Whitney Hurst, and Dmitriy Khavin, "How Times Reporters Proved Russia Bombed Syrian Hospitals," *New York Times*, October 13, 2019, https://www.nytimes.com/2019/10/13/reader-center/russia-syria-hospitals-investigation.html; Physicians for Human Rights and Mwatana for Human Rights, "'I ripped the IV out of my arm and started running:' Attacks on Health Care in Yemen," March 18, 2020, https://phr.org/wp-content/uploads/2020/03/PHR-Mwatana-March-2020-Report-Attacks-on-Health-Care-in-Yemen-ENGLISH.pdf.

9. Andrew T. Scull, "The Decarceration of the Mentally Ill: A Critical View," *Politics and Society* 6, no. 2 (1976): 173–212.

10. For example, see Christopher Payne and Oliver W. Sacks, *Asylum: Inside the Closed World of State Mental Hospitals* (Cambridge, MA: MIT Press, 2009); Darby Penney, Peter Stastny, and Lisa Rinzler, *The Lives They Left Behind: Suitcases from a State Hospital Attic* (New York: Bellevue Literary Press, 2008); Mark Davis, *Asylum: Inside the Pauper Lunatic Asylums* (Gloucestershire, UK: Amberley Publishing, 2014).

11. Paul Wenzel Geissler, Guillaume Lachenal, John Manton, and Noémi Tousignant, eds., *Traces of the Future: An Archaeology of Medical Science in Twenty-First-Century Africa* (Bristol, UK: Intellect, 2016).

12. Geissler, Lachenal and Tousignant, *Traces of the Future*, 24.

13. Meridith Kohut and Nicholas Casey, "Inside Venezuela's Crumbling Mental Hospitals," *New York Times*, October 1, 2016, http://www.nytimes.com/2016/10/02/world/americas/inside-a-dysfunctional-psychiatric-hospital.html; Nicholas Casey, "Dying Infants and No Medicine: Inside Venezuela's Failing Hospitals," *New York Times*, May 15, 2016https://www.nytimes.com/2016/05/16/world/americas/dying-infants-and-no-medicine-inside-venezuelas-failing-hospitals.html.

14. See Alice Cherki, *Frantz Fanon, portrait* (Paris: Seuil, 2000).

15. Richard C. Keller, *Colonial Madness: Psychiatry in French North Africa* (Chicago: University of Chicago Press, 2007).

16. *Al-Shurūq* (Echorouk TV), an Algerian news channel, conducted investigative reportage in 2012 and criticized the dire state of care at the Blida psychiatric hospital, accusing the staff of abuse, violence, and neglect. See "Voilà ce que Joinville de Blida, Frantz Fanon est devenu," October 22, 2012, https://www.youtube.com/watch?v=ITVyMGf2_vI.

17. François Béguin, "La psychiatrie en grande souffrance," *Le Monde*, January 26, 2018, https://www.lemonde.fr/sciences/article/2018/01/26/le-grand-malaise-des-soignants-en-psychiatrie-on-a-le-sentiment-d-etre-maltraitant_5247248_1650684.html; Eric Favereau, "La psychiatrie publique proche du délabrement," *Libération*, June 7, 2018, http://www.liberation.fr/france/2018/06/07/la-psychiatrie-publique-proche-du-delabrement_1657487; "La psychiatrie, un secteur en état d'urgence," editorial, *Le Monde*, August 18, 2018, https://www.lemonde.fr/idees/article/2018/08/18/la-psychiatrie-un-secteur-en-etat-d-urgence_5343765_3232.html.

18. On the Lebanese neoliberal economy and politics, see Reinoud Leenders, *Spoils of Truce: Corruption and State-Building in Postwar Lebanon* (Ithaca, NY: Cornell University Press, 2012); Toufic K. Gaspard, *A Political Economy of Lebanon, 1948–2002: The Limits of Laissez-Faire* (Leiden, the Netherlands: Brill, 2004).

19. See Carolyn Gates, *The Merchant Republic of Lebanon: Rise of an Open Economy* (London: Centre for Lebanese Studies, 1998). The Lebanese politician Michel Chiha coined the term the "merchant republic" (*république marchande*) in *Politique intérieure* (Paris: Éditions du Trident, 1964), 196.

20. On the notion of bereavement, see Rasha Salti, *Beirut Bereft: The Architecture of the Forsaken and Map of the Derelict*, trans. Mohammed Talaat Khedr (Sharjah, the United Arab Emirates: Sharjah Biennial, 2009).

21. Dominic A. Sisti, Andrea G. Segal, and Ezekiel J. Emanuel, "Improving Long-Term Psychiatric Care: Bring Back the Asylum," *Journal of the American Medical Association* 313, no. 3 (January 20, 2015): 243–244.

22. Sisti, Segal, and Emanuel, "Improving Long-Term Psychiatric Care," 243.

23. See Meris Lutz, "Discrimination Persists in Drug Law Application," *Daily Star*, October 20, 2014, http://www.dailystar.com.lb/News/Lebanon-News/2014/Oct-20/274631-discrimination-persists-in-drug-law-application.ashx; Karim Nammour, "Postponed Treatment: The Ongoing Prosecution of Drug Addicts in Lebanon," *Legal Agenda*, March 13, 2015, https://www.legal-agenda.com/en/article.php?id=3066.

24. L. M. Chahine and Z. Chemali, "Mental Health Care in Lebanon: Policy, Plans and Programmes," *La revue de santé de la méditerranée orientale* 15, no. 6 (2009): 1596–1612; The Research Council of Saint Joseph University, the World Health Organization, the Ministry of Public Health and the Institute of Health Management and Social Protection, "National Health Statistics Report in Lebanon," (Beirut: n.p., 2012), 85, https://www.usj.edu.lb/intranet/annonce/files/pdf/175_pdf_1.pdf; Catharsis, "Mental Health in Lebanese Prisons: Prevalence Study of Severe Mental Illness among Inmates in Roumieh and Baabda Prisons," 2015, http://www.catharsislcdt.org/Prevalence%20study%20Severe%20Mental%20Illness%20LebPrisons_en.pdf.

25. Didier Fassin, "L'asile et la prison," *Esprit*, no. 3 (March–April 2015): 82–95. Also see Didier Fassin, *L'ombre du monde: Une anthropologie de la condition carcérale* (Paris: Éditions du Seuil, 2015).

26. Major depression was the most common mental health condition in a 2009 survey of twenty prisons in Lebanon (which excluded Roumieh, the largest prison in the country, where data could not be gathered.) See "National Health Statistics Report in Lebanon," 88. The statistics remain inadequate, but these numbers do provide a good sense of the scope of the problem.

27. For the US, for instance, see E. Fuller Torrey, "Jails and Prisons—America's New Mental Hospitals," *American Journal of Public Health* 85, no. 12 (December 1995): 1611–1613; Ana Swanson, "A Shocking Number of Mentally Ill Americans End Up in Prison Instead of Treatment," *Washington Post*, April 30, 2015, https://www.washingtonpost.com/news/wonk/wp/2015/04/30/a-shocking-number-of-mentally-ill-americans-end-up-in-prisons-instead-of-psychiatric-hospitals/; Matt Ford, "America's Largest Mental Hospital Is a Jail," *Atlantic*, June 8, 2015, https://www.theatlantic.com/politics/archive/2015/06/americas-largest-mental-hospital-is-a-jail/395012/.

28. Shannon Lee Dawdy, "Clockpunk Anthropology and the Ruins of Modernity," *Current Anthropology* 51, no. 6 (December 1, 2010): 771.

29. Dawdy, "Clockpunk Anthropology and the Ruins of Modernity," 771.

30. Anthony Giddens, *The Consequences of Modernity* (Cambridge: Polity Press, 1991), 37. Pierre Bourdieu, *Esquisse pour une auto-analyse* (Paris: Éditions Raisons d'agir, 2004), and *Science de la science et réflexivité: Cours du Collège de France 2000–2001* (Paris: Éditions Raisons d'agir, 2007).

31. See Mervat Nasser, "The Rise and Fall of Anti-Psychiatry," *Psychiatric Bulletin* 19, no. 12 (December 1995): 743–746.

32. Frantz Fanon, *Peau Noire, Masques Blancs* (Paris: Éditions du Seuil, 1952); Frantz Fanon, *L'An V de la révolution algérienne* (Paris: Maspero, 1959); Frantz Fanon, *Les damnés de la terre* (Paris: Éditions La Découverte, 1961).

33. Raja Ben Slama, "La psychanalyse en Égypte, Psychoanalysis in Egypt—A Problematic Case of Non-Accession," *Topique*, no. 110 (October 1, 2010): 91. For a different take on psychoanalysis and Islam in Egypt, see Omnia S. El Shakry, *The Arabic Freud: Psychoanalysis and Islam in Modern Egypt* (Princeton, NJ: Princeton University Press, 2017).

34. Sadik al-Azm, *Self-Criticism after the Defeat*, trans. George Stergios (London: Saqi, 2011).

35. Sadik al-Azm, *Critique of Religious Thought*, trans. George Stergios and Mansour Ajami (Berlin: Gerlach Press, 2015), 1.

36. Al-Azm, *Critique of Religious Thought*, 10.

37. Hisham Sharabi, *Neopatriarchy: A Theory of Distorted Change in Arab Society* (Oxford: Oxford University Press, 1988), 104–124.

38. Sadik al-Azm, "Orientalism and Orientalism in Reverse," in A. L. Macfie, ed., *Orientalism: A Reader* (New York: New York University Press, 2000), 217–238. The article was originally published in 1980.

39. Albert Hourani, "The Road to Morocco," *New York Review of Books*, March 8, 1979, https://www.nybooks.com/articles/1979/03/08/the-road-to-morocco/. For Fred Halliday—another early critic of Said's work—see Roger Owen, "Edward Said and the Two Critiques of Orientalism," *Middle East Institute*, April 20, 2012, https://www.mei.edu/publications/edward-said-and-two-critiques-orientalism. For a Marxist critique of Said's *Orientalism*, see Gilbert Achcar, *Marxism, Orientalism, Cosmopolitanism* (Chicago: Haymarket Books, 2013), especially 68–96.

40. Mona Abaza, "A Tribute to Sadek Jalal Al 'Azm," Open Democracy, December 23, 2016, https://www.opendemocracy.net/en/tribute-to-sadek-jalal-al-azm/; Achcar, *Marxism, Orientalism, Cosmopolitanism*, 40–56.

41. On the brain drain of physicians, see A. B. Zahlan, "The Arab Brain Drain," *Middle East Studies Association Bulletin* 6, no. 3 (1972): 1–16. On the reproduction of the elite through self-preservation, see Pierre Bourdieu, *Homo academicus* (Paris: Éditions de Minuit, 1984).

42. Mohammed Yahia, "Dealing with Mental Illness in the Middle East," *Nature Middle East*, July 24, 2012, https://www.natureasia.com/en/nmiddleeast/article/10.1038/nmiddleeast.2012.103; Lesley Pocock, "Mental Health Issues in the Middle East—An Overview," *Middle East Journal of Psychiatry and Alzheimer's* 8, no. 1 (June 2017): 10–15.

43. Joelle M. Abi-Rached, "Psychiatry in the Middle East: The Rebirth of Lunatic Asylums?," *British Journal of Psychiatry International*, May 2020, https://doi.org/10.1192/bji.2020.22.

44. State of Israel, Sha'ar Menashe Mental Health Center, accessed April 7, 2020, http://www.shaar-menashe.org/. Strikingly, Palestine, a third of whose population suffers from issues related to mental health, is almost entirely missing from WHO's statistics on world health. Palestine is mentioned only in terms of the public health-related contributions made by UNRWA to Palestinian refugees residing in Jordanian territories. See World Health Organization, *World Health Statistics 2013* (Geneva: World Health Organization, 2013), 141. On the state of mental health care in Palestine, see Abdel Hamid Afana, Samir Qouta, and Eyad El Sarraj, "Mental Health Needs in Palestine," Humanitarian Practice Network, November 2004, https://odihpn.org/magazine/mental-health-needs-in-palestine/.

45. Official numbers at Dayr al-Ṣalīb are not published consistently, and the hospital's website has not been updated since 2004. See Hôpital Psychiatrique de la Croix, "Situation géographique," accessed April 7, 2020, http://www.hopitalpsychiatriquedelacroix.org.lb/french/situation/index.htm. For ʿAbbasiyya, see General Secretariat of Mental Health and Addiction Treatment, "Mustashfa al-ʿAbbāsiyya lil-Suḥa al-Nafsiyya," accessed April 7, 2020, http://www.mentalhealthegypt.com/index.php/ar/2015-10-11-01-10-32/abbasia/abbasia, and Mohamad Ali, "Tastaqbel 100 alf Marīḍ Sanawiyyan ... Jibhat al-Difāʿ ʿAn Mustashfa al-ʿAbbāsiyya Tuṭāleb bi-Inqādhuha min-al-Naql," *Buwwābat al-Ahram*, January 14, 2019, http://gate.ahram.org.eg/News/2097342.aspx. For Al-Khanqa, see General Secretariat of Mental Health and Addiction Treatment, "Mustashfa al-Khanka lil-Suḥa al-Nafsiyya," accessed April 7, 2020, http://www.mentalhealthegypt.com/index.php/ar/2015-10-11-01-10-32/khanka/khanka. For Al-Rashad, see Hamed el-Sayyed, "Saāa Fī Mustashfa al-Rashād lil-Amrād al-ʿAqliyya," September 7, 2019, https://www.youtube.com/watch?v=Y0ZBy87LSek; Sabah Sadik and Abdul-Monaf Al-Jadiry, "Mental Health Services in Iraq: Past, Present and Future," *International Psychiatry* 3, no. 4 (October 1, 2006): 11–13.

46. For Iraq, see Jennifer Percy, "How Does the Human Soul Survive Atrocity?," *New York Times Magazine*, October 31, 2019, https://www.nytimes.com/interactive/2019/10/31/magazine/iraq-mental-health.html.

47. Andrew Scull, "A Convenient Place to Get Rid of Inconvenient People: The Victorian Lunatic Asylum," in *Buildings and Society: Essays on the Social Development of the Built Environment*, ed. Anthony D. King (London: Routledge and Kegan Paul, 1980), 37–60.

48. Julia Hell and Andreas Schönle, eds., *Ruins of Modernity* (Durham, NC: Duke University Press, 2008).

49. Ann Laura Stoler, ed., *Imperial Debris: On Ruins and Ruination* (Durham, NC: Duke University Press, 2013).

50. Achille Mbembe, "Nécropolitique," *Raisons politiques* 1, no. 21 (March 14, 2006): 29–60.

51. See Andrew Curry, "Here Are the Ancient Sites ISIS Has Damaged and Destroyed," *National Geographic*, September 1, 2015, http://news.nationalgeographic.com/2015/09/150901-isis-destruction-looting-ancient-sites-iraq-syria-archaeology/; Ahmed Rasheed and Isabel Coles, "Iraq Says Islamic State Militants Raze Ancient Hatra City," *Reuters*, March 7, 2015, http://www.reuters.com/article/us-mideast-crisis-iraq-hatra-idUSKBN0M30GR20150307.

52. Eric J. Hobsbawm, *The Age of Extremes: A History of the World, 1914–1991* (New York: Vintage Books, 1996).

53. Yael Navaro-Yashin, "Affective Spaces, Melancholic Objects: Ruination and the Production of Anthropological Knowledge," *Journal of the Royal Anthropological Institute* 15, no. 1 (2009): 14.

54. See survey results in "Notes."

55. Zygmunt Bauman, *Wasted Lives: Modernity and Its Outcasts* (Oxford: Polity, 2004).

56. See Gastón Gordillo, *Rubble: The Afterlife of Destruction* (Durham, NC: Duke University Press, 2014); Dora Apel, *Beautiful Terrible Ruins: Detroit and the Anxiety of Decline* (New Brunswick, NJ: Rutgers University Press, 2015).

57. See, for instance, Gerard Russell, *Heirs to Forgotten Kingdoms: Journeys into the Disappearing Religions of the Middle East* (New York: Basic Books, 2014); Paul Veyne, *Palmyre: L'irremplaçable trésor* (Paris: Albin Michel, 2015).

58. William Cunningham Bissell, "Engaging Colonial Nostalgia," *Cultural Anthropology* 20, no. 2 (2005): 240.

59. *Human Flow*, the 2018 documentary by the Chinese dissident artist, activist, and critic Ai Weiwei (Berlin: NFP Marketing & Distribution), captures the massive scale of what has been referred to as "the greatest human displacement" since the Second World War, see the official website of the documentary, accessed April 6, 2020, https://www.humanflow.com/synopsis/.

60. See, for instance, Will Kymlicka, *Multicultural Citizenship: A Liberal Theory of Minority Rights* (Oxford: Oxford University Press, 1995).

61. See, for instance, Pierre Dardot and Christian Laval, *Commun: Essai sur la révolution du XXIe siècle* (Paris: Découverte, 2014).

62. Robert D. Kaplan, "The Ruins of Empire in the Middle East," *Foreign Policy*, May 25, 2015, https://foreignpolicy.com/2015/05/25/ruins-of-empire-in-the-middle-east-syria-iraq-islamic-state-iran/; Brynjar Lia, "The Arab Mukhabarat State and Its 'Stability': A Case of Misplaced Nostalgia," *New Middle East Blog* (blog), April 26, 2016, https://newmeast.wordpress.com/2016/04/26/the-arab-mukhabarat-state-and-its-stability-a-case-of-misplaced-nostalgia/.

63. Sune Haugbolle, *War and Memory in Lebanon* (New York: Cambridge University Press, 2010), especially 96–131.

64. Haugbolle, *War and Memory in Lebanon*, especially 96–131.

65. The most vocal nongovernmental organization is the Association for the Protection of the Lebanese Heritage, created in 2010. Other initiatives include Save Beirut Heritage and the Civil Coalition against the Highway Project "Hekmeh-Turk" Axis.

66. Russell, *Heirs to Forgotten Kingdoms*. In the Arab press, for instance, the online magazine *Raseef* has published an entire issue on the various ancient Jewish communities in the Arab world and their abandoned synagogues. See "Al-Yahūdī al-ʿArabī al-Akhīr," *Raṣīf22*, February 19, 2016.

67. See Jon Lee Anderson, "ISIS and the Destruction of History," *New Yorker*, March 18, 2015, http://www.newyorker.com/news/daily-comment/isis-and-the-destruction-of-history.

68. Pierre Nora, *Présent, nation, mémoire* (Paris: Gallimard, 2011), 374–376, and "Between Memory and History: Les Lieux de Mémoire," trans. Marc Roudebush, *Representations* 26 (Spring 1989): 1–24. This historiographical approach has its own shortcomings. For a subtle critique, see Claire Gantet, "Entre appropriation et neutralization: La commemoration de la paix de Westphalie (1648–1660)," in *De la guerre juste à la paix juste: Aspects confessionnels de la construction de la paix dans l'espace franco-allemand (XVIe–XXe siècles)*, ed. Jean-Paul Cahn, Françoise Knopper, and Anne-Marie Saint-Gille (Villeneuve d'Ascq, France: Presses Universitaires du Septentrion, 2008), especially 104–105.

69. On the metamorphosis of public memorials in Lebanon, see Lucia Volk, *Memorials and Martyrs in Modern Lebanon* (Bloomington: Indiana University Press, 2010).

70. Philemon Wehbe wrote the song, titled "ʿAl-ʿAṣfūriyyeh" (To ʿAṣfūriyyeh) in 1978.

71. Ziad Rahbani, *Fīlm Amīrikī Tawīl* (Beirut: Mukhtārāt, 1994). See also Wissam Matta, "'Fīlm Amīrkī Ṭawīl' Bayn al-Ams wal-Yawm: Al-ʿAsfūriyyeh al-Lubnāniyyeh Bāqiat wa-Tatamaddad," *Raṣīf22*, September 22, 2016.

72. Louis Althusser, *L'avenir dure longtemps; suivi de, Les faits* (Paris: Stock/IMEC, 1992), especially 18–25.

73. Marc Augé, *Non-Lieux: Introduction à une anthropologie de la surmodernité* (Paris: Seuil, 1992).

74. Theophilus Waldmeier letter to "Friends and other Christians to whom this may come," October 20, 1898, LH/07/04, box 9, LH, SOAS.

75. Louis Althusser, *The Future Lasts a Long Time and the Facts*, ed. Olivier Corpet, trans. Yann Moulier Boutang (London: Chatto and Windus, 1993), xi.

76. For more on the concept of the duty to remember, see Avishai Margalit, *The Ethics of Memory* (Cambridge, MA: Harvard University Press, 2002); Myriam Bienenstock, ed., *Devoir de mémoire: Les lois mémorielles et l'histoire* (Paris: Éclat, 2014); Sébastien Ledoux, *Le devoir de mémoire: Une formule et son histoire* (Paris: CNRS Éditions, 2016).

77. Paul Ricoeur, "Memory and Forgetting," in *Questioning Ethics: Contemporary Debates in Philosophy*, ed. Richard Kearney and Mark Dooley (New York: Routledge, 1999), especially 9–10.

78. Jean-Claude Monod, "Qu'est-ce qu'une 'mémoire juste'?," in *Devoir de mémoire: Les lois mémorielles et l'histoire*, ed. Myriam Bienenstock (Paris: Éclat, 2014), 39–52.

79. Ricoeur, "Memory and Forgetting," 10. See also, Hannah Arendt, *The Human Condition*, 2nd ed. (Chicago: The University of Chicago Press, 2018), especially 175–247.

80. Ricoeur, "Memory and Forgetting," 11.

81. See Haugbolle, *War and Memory in Lebanon*.

82. Jalal Toufic, *Undeserving Lebanon* (Beirut: Forthcoming Books, 2007), 9. For more on the cultural productions of memory and amnesia, see Haugbolle, *War and Memory in Lebanon*, especially 64–95.

83. Hans Gebhardt, Dorothee Sack, and Ralph Bodenstein, eds., *History, Space and Social Conflict in Beirut: The Quarter of Zokak El-Blat* (Beirut: Orient-Institut, 2005); Serge Yazigi, Rita Chedid, and Marieke Krijnen, "Zokak el-Blat: A Neighborhood of Contrasts," September 22, 2014, https://www.area-arch.it/en/zokak-el-blat-a-neighborhood-of-contrasts/.

84. Margalit, *The Ethics of Memory*.

85. See Rochelle Davis, *Palestinian Village Histories: Geographies of the Displaced* (Stanford, CA: Stanford University Press, 2011).

86. Jalal Toufic, "Ruins," in *Thinking: The Ruin*, ed. Matthew Gumpert and Jalal Toufic (Istanbul: Istanbul Studies Center, 2010), 37.

87. Kendall R. Phillips and G. Mitchell Reyes, introduction to *Global Memoryscapes: Contesting Remembrance in a Transnational Age*, ed. Kendall R. Phillips and G. Mitchell Reyes (Tuscaloosa: University of Alabama Press, 2011), 1–26.

Index

Note: Page numbers in italic type indicate illustrations

Post, George E., 25, 31, 44, 52, 219n59
Post-traumatic stress disorder (PTSD), 13. *See also* Shell shock
Potet, Maurice, 76
Poujoulat, Jean-Joseph-François, 221n102
Poverty, 103–104. *See also* Assistance publique
Prefrontal leucotomy, 132
Prisons and prisoners, 6, 86, 93, 110, 117, 124, 140–144, 180, 183–184, 269n27. *See also* Forensic unit
Proselytism
  civilizing missions linked to, 64
  not an end in itself, 9
  psychiatry in Middle East attributed to motives of, 8, 9, 19, 48, 50, 161–163
  See also Missionaries
Protestant Missionary Press, 175
Protestants
  and ʻAṣfūriyyeh, 14, 58, 75
  nominal Christians criticized by, 5
  opposition to, 8, 39, 53–54, 71, 78–80, 88, 162–163
  rationalist approach of, 56–57, 76
  sect of, 174–177
  SPC founded by, 38, 52
  and waqf associated with ʻAṣfūriyyeh, 160
  See also Missionaries
Provincial Municipal Law (Ottoman Empire, 1877), 82
Prussian (Johanniter) hospital, Beirut, 52, 243n202
Psychiatry
  birth of, in Levant, 50
  colonial practices of, 17–18
  expansion of, in mid-twentieth century, 83
  failures of, 185–188
  legitimacy granted to, 82
  in medical school curricula, 73, 75, 76, 85–86, 88–89
  in the Middle East, 18–21
  progressive methods in, 3–4
  See also Alienists; Asylums; Clinical psychiatry; Deinstitutionalization; Forensic psychiatry; Moral treatment; Neuropsychiatry
Psychoanalysis, 133, 186
Psychological mindedness, 148
Psychology
  journals with articles on, 39–47
  mental sciences as precursor of, 57
Psychoneurosis, 120
Psychopathic personality, 108–110, 148
Psychosomatic, 100, 130, 266n1
Psychotherapy, 133
Psychotic disorders, 120–121
Puzantian, Vahé, 110, 115

Qabbani, Mufti, 174
Qasr al-ʻAini Medical School, Egypt, 51
Quakerism, 1, 3, 4, 27, 58, 61, 62, 64, 129, 150, 164, 166, 168, 175–178, 180
Quran, 29, 172

Racy, John, 107–108, 121, 253n143
Rahbani, Ziad, "Fīlm Amīrkī Ṭawīl," 191
Red Cross. *See* American Red Cross; Lebanese Red Cross
Regulation for Lunatic Asylums (Ottoman Empire, 1876), 42, 81–82
Religious excess, 102–103
Religious fanaticism, 32
Ricoeur, Paul, 191–192
Robertson, Robert, 83
Roché, Louis, 49, 88, 90–91
Rockefeller Foundation, 71, 72, 164
Rogan, Eugene, 11, 18, 138, 161
Royal College of Physicians, Britain, 61
Royal Edinburgh Asylum, 59
Royal Glasgow Asylum, 59
Royal Medico-Psychological Association, 61, 81, 88